Kidney Disease

Editors

KIM ZUBER
JANE S. DAVIS

W9-ALZ-841

PHYSICIAN ASSISTANT CLINICS

www.physicianassistant.theclinics.com

Consulting Editor
JAMES A. VAN RHEE

January 2016 • Volume 1 • Number 1

ELSEVIER

1600 John F. Kennedy Boulevard • Suite 1800 • Philadelphia, Pennsylvania, 19103-2899

http://www.theclinics.com

PHYSICIAN ASSISTANT CLINICS Volume 1, Number 1
January 2016 ISSN 2405-7991, ISBN-13: 978-0-323-43128-6

Editor: Jessica McCool
Developmental Editor: Casey Jackson

© 2016 Elsevier Inc. All rights reserved.

This periodical and the individual contributions contained in it are protected under copyright by Elsevier, and the following terms and conditions apply to their use:

Photocopying
Single photocopies of single articles may be made for personal use as allowed by national copyright laws. Permission of the Publisher and payment of a fee is required for all other photocopying, including multiple or systematic copying, copying for advertising or promotional purposes, resale, and all forms of document delivery. Special rates are available for educational institutions that wish to make photocopies for non-profit educational classroom use. For information on how to seek permission visit www.elsevier.com/permissions or call: (+44) 1865 843830 (UK)/(+1) 215 239 3804 (USA).

Derivative Works
Subscribers may reproduce tables of contents or prepare lists of articles including abstracts for internal circulation within their institutions. Permission of the Publisher is required for resale or distribution outside the institution. Permission of the Publisher is required for all other derivative works, including compilations and translations (please consult www.elsevier.com/permissions).

Electronic Storage or Usage
Permission of the Publisher is required to store or use electronically any material contained in this periodical, including any article or part of an article (please consult www.elsevier.com/permissions). Except as outlined above, no part of this publication may be reproduced, stored in a retrieval system or transmitted in any form or by any means, electronic, mechanical, photocopying, recording or otherwise, without prior written permission of the Publisher.

Notice
No responsibility is assumed by the Publisher for any injury and/or damage to persons or property as a matter of products liability, negligence or otherwise, or from any use or operation of any methods, products, instructions or ideas contained in the material herein. Because of rapid advances in the medical sciences, in particular, independent verification of diagnoses and drug dosages should be made.

Although all advertising material is expected to conform to ethical (medical) standards, inclusion in this publication does not constitute a guarantee or endorsement of the quality or value of such product or of the claims made of it by its manufacturer.

Physician Assistant Clinics (ISSN: 2405–7991) is published quarterly by Elsevier Inc., 360 Park Avenue South, New York, NY 10010-1710. Months of issue are January, April, July, and October. Periodicals postage paid at New York, NY and additional mailing offices. Subscription prices are $150.00 per year (US individuals), $195.00 (US institutions), $100.00 (US students), $150.00 (Canadian individuals), $245.00 (Canadian institutions), $100.00 (Canadian students), $150.00 (international individuals), $245.00 (international institutions), and $100.00 (international students). Foreign air speed delivery is included in all *Clinics* subscription prices. All prices are subject to change without notice. POSTMASTER: Send address changes to *Physician Assistant Clinics*, Elsevier Periodicals Customer Service, 11830 Westline Industrial Drive, St. Louis, MO 63146. Customer Service Health Sciences Division, Subscription Customer Service, 3251 Riverport Lane, Maryland Heights, MO 63043. **Customer Service: 1-800-654-2452 (U.S. and Canada); 314-447-8871 (outside U.S. and Canada). Fax: 314-447-8029. E-mail: journalscustomerservice-usa@elsevier.com (for print support); journalsonlinesupport-usa@elsevier.com (for online support).**

Reprints. For copies of 100 or more, of articles in this publication, please contact the Commercial Reprints Department, Elsevier Inc., 360 Park Avenue South, New York, NY 10010-1710. Tel. 212-633-3874; Fax: 212-633-3820; E-mail: reprints@elsevier.com.

Physician Assistant Clinics is covered in *MEDLINE/PubMed (Index Medicus) and EMBASE/Excerpta Medica, Current Contents/Clinical Medicine, and ISI/BIOMED.*

Printed in the United States of America.

PROGRAM OBJECTIVE
The goal of the *Physician Assistant Clinics* is to keep practicing physician assistants up to date with current clinical practice by providing timely articles reviewing the state of the art in patient care.

TARGET AUDIENCE
Physician Assistants and other healthcare professionals.

LEARNING OBJECTIVES
Upon completion of this activity, participants will be able to:
1. Review methods in managing chronic kidney disease and acute kidney injury.
2. Discuss the social aspects of kidney disease, such as lifestyle, diet, and health disparities among kidney patients.
3. Recognize advances in kidney transplant in the 21st century.

ACCREDITATION
The Elsevier Office of Continuing Medical Education (EOCME) is accredited by the Accreditation Council for Continuing Medical Education (ACCME) to provide continuing medical education for physicians.

The EOCME designates this enduring material for a maximum of 15 *AMA PRA Category 1 Credit*(s)™. Physicians should claim only the credit commensurate with the extent of their participation in the activity.

All other health care professionals requesting continuing education credit for this enduring material will be issued a certificate of participation.

DISCLOSURE OF CONFLICTS OF INTEREST
The EOCME assesses conflict of interest with its instructors, faculty, planners, and other individuals who are in a position to control the content of CME activities. All relevant conflicts of interest that are identified are thoroughly vetted by EOCME for fair balance, scientific objectivity, and patient care recommendations. EOCME is committed to providing its learners with CME activities that promote improvements or quality in healthcare and not a specific proprietary business or a commercial interest.

The planning committee, staff, authors and editors listed below have identified no financial relationships or relationships to products or devices they or their spouse/life partner have with commercial interest related to the content of this CME activity:
Molly E. Band, MHS, PA-C; Catherine G. Brown, CRNP, MSN; April Crunk, PA-C; Cynthia D'Alessandri-Silva, MD; Joseph Daniel; Erica N. Davis, MHS, PA-C; Jane S. Davis, CRNP, DNP; Harvey A. Feldman, MD, FACP; Anjali Fortna; Cheryl Gilmartin, PharmD; Alexis Anne Harris, MD; Niveen Hilal; David Hughes; Casey Jackson; Denise K. Link, MPAS, PA-C; Jessica McCool; Becky Ness, MPAS, PA-C; Jenna Norton, MPH; Amy Barton Pai, PharmD, BCPS; Fawad Qureshi, MD; Megan Suermann; Arlene Keller Surós, MSHS, RD, PA-C; Laura Troidle, PA; Mandy Trolinger, MS, RD, PA-C; Catherine Clark Wells, DNP, ACNP-BC, CNN-NP, FNKF; Kim Zuber, PA-C.

The planning committee, staff, authors and editors listed below have identified financial relationships or relationships to products or devices they or their spouse/life partner have with commercial interest related to the content of this CME activity:
James A. Van Rhee, MS, PA-C, DFAAPA receives royalties/patents from Kaplan, Inc.

UNAPPROVED/OFF-LABEL USE DISCLOSURE
The EOCME requires CME faculty to disclose to the participants:
1. When products or procedures being discussed are off-label, unlabelled, experimental, and/or investigational (not US Food and Drug Administration [FDA] approved); and
2. Any limitations on the information presented, such as data that are preliminary or that represent ongoing research, interim analyses, and/or unsupported opinions. Faculty may discuss information about pharmaceutical agents that is outside of FDA-approved labelling. This information is intended solely for CME and is not intended to promote off-label use of these medications. If you have any questions, contact the medical affairs department of the manufacturer for the most recent prescribing information.

TO ENROLL
The CME program is available to all *Physician Assistant Clinics* subscribers at no additional fee. To subscribe to the *Physician Assistant Clinics*, call customer service at 1-800-654-2452 or sign up online at www.physicianassistant.theclinics.com.

METHOD OF PARTICIPATION

In order to claim credit, participants must complete the following:

1. Complete enrolment as indicated above.
2. Read the activity.
3. Complete the CME Test and Evaluation. Participants must achieve a score of 70% on the test. All CME Tests and Evaluations must be completed online.

CME INQUIRIES/SPECIAL NEEDS

For all CME inquiries or special needs, please contact elsevierCME@elsevier.com.

Contributors

CONSULTING EDITOR

JAMES S. VAN RHEE, MS, PA-C, DFAAPA
Associate Professor, Program Director, Physician Associate Program, Yale Physician Associate Program, New Haven, Connecticut

EDITORS

KIM ZUBER, PA-C
Past Chair, National Kidney Foundation's Council of Advanced Practitioners; American Academy of Nephrology PAs, Oceanside, California

JANE S. DAVIS, CRNP, DNP
Communication Chair, National Kidney Foundation's Council of Advanced Practitioners; Division of Nephrology, University of Alabama Medical Center at Birmingham, Birmingham, Alabama

AUTHORS

MOLLY E. BAND, MHS, PA-C
Pediatric Nephrology, Connecticut Children's Medical Center, Hartford, Connecticut

CATHERINE G. BROWN, CRNP, MSN
Director of Advanced Practice Providers; Lead Nurse Practitioner, Hospitalist Service, University of Alabama at Birmingham, Birmingham, Alabama

APRIL CRUNK, PA-C
Department of Interventional Radiology, University of Alabama at Birmingham, Birmingham, Alabama

CYNTHIA D'ALESSANDRI-SILVA, MD, FAAP
Pediatric Nephrology, Connecticut Children's Medical Center, Hartford, Connecticut

ERICA N. DAVIS, MHS, PA-C
Metropolitan Nephrology Associates, Alexandria, Virginia

JANE S. DAVIS, CRNP, DNP
Communication Chair, National Kidney Foundation's Council of Advanced Practitioners; Division of Nephrology, University of Alabama Medical Center at Birmingham, Birmingham, Alabama

HARVEY A. FELDMAN, MD, FACP
Physician Assistant Program, Nova Southeastern University, Ft. Lauderdale, Florida

CHERYL GILMARTIN, PharmD
Clinical Assistant Professor, Department of Medicine, University of Illinois Hospital and Health Sciences System, Chicago, Illinois

ALEXIS ANNE HARRIS, MD
Director of Nephropathology, Ameripath/Quest Diagnostic Laboratories, Renal Pathology, Oklahoma City, Oklahoma

NIVEEN HILAL
Doctor of Pharmacy Candidate, University of Illinois at Chicago College of Pharmacy, Chicago, Illinois

DAVID HUGHES
Doctor of Pharmacy Candidate, Albany College of Pharmacy and Health Sciences, Albany, New York

DENISE K. LINK, MPAS, PA-C
Associate Clinical Provider, The University of Texas Southwestern Medical Center, Nephrology: Chronic Kidney Disease Clinic, Dallas, Texas

BECKY NESS, MPAS, PA-C
Nephrology, SWMN Mayo Clinic Health System, Mankato, Minnesota

JENNA NORTON, MPH
Kidney and Urologic Science Translation, National Kidney Disease Education Program, Department of Kidney, Urologic and Hematologic Diseases, National Institute of Diabetes and Digestive and Kidney Diseases, National Institutes of Health, Bethesda, Maryland

AMY BARTON PAI, PharmD, BCPS, FASN, FCCP
Professor, Department of Pharmacy Practice, Albany College of Pharmacy and Health Sciences, Albany, New York

FAWAD QURESHI, MD
Interventional Nephrologist/Transplant Nephrologist/Critical Care Medicine/General Nephrologist, Department of Nephrology, SWMN Mayo Clinic Health System, Mankato, Minnesota

ARLENE KELLER SURÓS, MSHS, RD, PA-C
The Hospitalist Group, Virginia Hospital Center, Arlington, Virginia

LAURA TROIDLE, PA
Metabolism Associates, New Haven, Connecticut

MANDY TROLINGER, MS, RD, PA-C
Denver Nephrology, Lone Tree, Colorado

CATHERINE CLARK WELLS, DNP, ACNP-BC, CNN-NP, FNKF
Associate professor, Division of Nephrology, University of Mississippi, Jackson, Mississippi

KIM ZUBER, PA-C
Past Chair, National Kidney Foundation's Council of Advanced Practitioners; American Academy of Nephrology PAs, Oceanside, California

Contents

> The incidence of kidney disease, acute and chronic, has increased expo-
> nentially, and yet the diagnosis is often missed by the non-nephrology
> practitioner. Twenty million Americans are living with kidney disease,
> and this number is expected to increase. Highlights of the common causes
> of kidney injury, along with details of incidence and differential diagnoses
> are reviewed for the non-nephrology practitioner.

> More than 26 million people have chronic kidney disease (CKD), with less
> than 10% aware of their diagnosis and another 73 million are at risk of
> CKD. Hypertensive diabetic patients are easily recognized as potentially
> having kidney disease, but what about atypical patients? CKD can be
> caused by other entities: focal segmental glomerulosclerosis, nephrolithia-
> sis, lupus nephritis, glomerulonephritis, autosomal dominant polycystic
> kidney disease, immunoglobulin A nephropathy, and scleroderma, among
> others. This article is a review of those other kidney diagnoses including
> images and a review of staging of patients with kidney disease using Kid-
> ney Disease Improving Global Outcomes 2012 criteria.

> Chronic kidney disease (CKD) is progressive with multiple implications for
> the patient, family, and health care providers. Effectively treating CKD and
> reducing cardiovascular mortality is a challenge requiring a team effort in
> which the patient plays a major role. Screening all at-risk patients becomes
> paramount. The primary care clinician must modify the disease progres-
> sion and limit cardiovascular mortality. This article reviews methods to
> slow CKD progression and discusses modifiable risk factors. It reviews
> recent guidelines regarding hypertension goals and treatments, evaluation
> and management of albuminuria, and reduction of risk factors for cardio-
> vascular disease.

In the clinical setting, patients with chronic kidney disease and the elderly with age-related kidney decline in addition to comorbid conditions are largely unrecognized and therefore vulnerable to dosing errors. Concerted efforts have been made to reduce errors in these patient populations without yielding significant results. Awareness of the poor clinical outcomes and adherence to consensus dosing guidelines are needed to minimize medication errors.

Chronic kidney disease (CKD) is a worldwide public health problem. Diet plays an important role in the management CKD. Following renal diet guidelines is an extremely cost-effective means of promoting renal health and decreasing morbidity. This article investigates the development of the current dietary guidelines for CKD. It explores the difficulties and controversies associated with the current recommendations and discusses multiple aspects of the renal diet. The goal of this article is to define the most recent dietary guidelines and recommendations and highlight the importance of diet and nutrition in treating this complex patient population.

Physician assistants should recognize risk factors for kidney disease when preparing a patient for surgery. Acute kidney injury is a common sequel to the surgical experience. A thorough history and physical examination are essential preoperatively, along with close follow-up after the procedure. For patients with known kidney disease, it is essential to adjust and monitor medication dosing.

Cardiorenal disease refers to a host of insults that arise from a decline in either cardiac or renal function. The entwined relationship of the kidney with the heart is complex. Therefore, there are 5 different types of cardiorenal disease. The disease processes ignite a cascade of pathophysiologic events that upset the natural balance between the heart and the kidney. The identification of the initiating factor and subsequent result may lead to an expedient and appropriate therapy. Biomarkers may be particularly useful.

The prevalence, costs, and morbidity of kidney stones have been increasing significantly. Although improved operative techniques have facilitated the treatment of obstructing stones, less attention has been given to preventing future recurrences. Physician assistants, especially those in primary care, must play a central role in preventing recurrent nephrolithiasis. This paper focuses on the medical evaluation and nonsurgical management of nephrolithiasis.

in CKD risk factors, social determinants of health, and implicit biases among clinicians, that likely contribute to racial/ethnic disparities in CKD, with special emphasis on social factors that are often underappreciated and may be more amenable to intervention. Additionally, this article suggests ways practicing clinicians may be able to counteract CKD disparities in the clinical setting.

Mandy Trolinger

Kidney transplant patients are seen and managed by primary care providers in every specialty. However, there are special considerations for the transplant recipient including cancer incidence, immunization schedules, pregnancy, glycemia, and hyperlipidemia issues. Most importantly, there are medication interactions that can cause failure of the graft. In 2014, a new kidney allocation system was introduced in the United States to more fairly distribute deceased donor kidneys. This article highlights the most common issues encountered in the primary care office regarding the kidney transplant patient and explains transplant as practiced in the twenty-first century.

PHYSICIAN ASSISTANT CLINICS

THE CLINICS ARE AVAILABLE ONLINE!
Access your subscription at:
www.theclinics.com

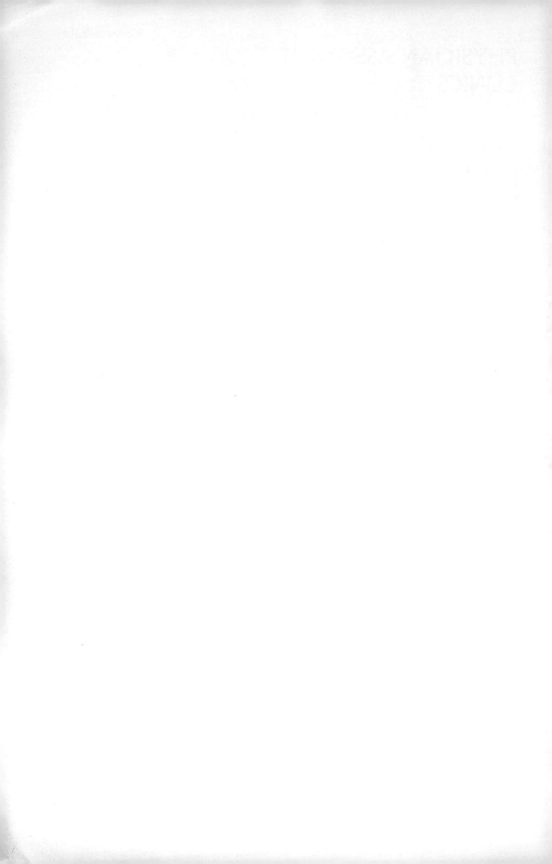

Foreword

Not Just Another Physician Assistant Journal

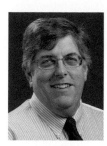

James A. Van Rhee, MS, PA-C, DFAAPA
Consulting Editor

 Video content accompanies this article at www.physicianassistant.theclinics.com

Welcome to the first issue of *Physician Assistant Clinics*.

Four times a year, you will receive a comprehensive review of numerous topics in medicine, surgery, pediatrics, or others. Written largely by clinical physician assistant experts, *Physician Assistant Clinics* will provide you the information you need for clinical practice, as a review for board preparation, and CME for continued certification.

Physician Assistant Clinics is about getting practicing physician assistants the comprehensive review and latest information they need for clinical practice. Issues will focus on a specific topic and provide the reader with detailed information on a number of subjects related to the issue topic. Plus, special topics related to the latest trends in physician assistant practice and education will be presented in each issue.

The first *Physician Assistant Clinics* topic is Kidney Disease. Whether you are practicing in primary care or in a specialty area of medicine or surgery, patients with kidney disease will be part of the clinical practice. After reviewing the table of contents for this issue, I think you will agree there is something for everyone in this issue.

For example, Erica Davis provides an excellent review of acute kidney injury. Cheryl Gilmartin and others discuss the effects of medications on the patient with chronic kidney disease. Jena Norton describes the role of social factors in the health disparities seen in patients with chronic kidney disease, and an article that hits close to home is an overview of nephrolithiasis by Harvey Feldman.

Thank you to our guest editors, Jane S. Davis, CRNP, DNP of the University of Alabama at Birmingham, and Kim Zuber, PA-C of Alexandria, Virginia. They have pulled together some of the most relevant and current topics in kidney disease. The articles are fascinating and illuminating and make you realize that there is much more to kidney disease than you ever thought. Their clear and concise presentations will be greatly appreciated by all the readers.

Physician Assist Clin 1 (2016) xiii–xiv
http://dx.doi.org/10.1016/j.cpha.2015.10.003
2405-7991/16/$ – see front matter © 2016 Published by Elsevier Inc.

physicianassistant.theclinics.com

I sincerely believe that you will find the first issue of *Physician Assistant Clinics* as informative and enjoyable as I have. See you again with the second issue, where the topic will be Dermatology.

SUPPLEMENTARY DATA

Supplementary data related to this article can be found online at http://dx.doi.org/10.1016/j.cpha.2015.10.003.

James A. Van Rhee, MS, PA-C, DFAAPA
Yale School of Medicine
Yale Physician Associate Program
100 Church Street South, Suite A250
New Haven, CT 06519, USA

E-mail address:
james.vanrhee@yale.edu

Preface

From Alphabet Soup to Manuscript

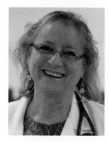 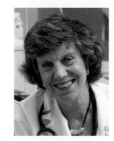

Kim Zuber, PA-C   Jane S. Davis, CRNP, DNP
Editors

Nephrology and kidney disease have emerged from the shadows. At the turn of the century, national and international organizations jointly defined kidney disease by stages and function. Gone was the myriad of names—renal insufficiency, dropsy, nephritis, nephrosis, uremia and Bright's disease—and in its place was a unified nomenclature and specific parameters for identifying and thus treating patients with chronic kidney disease (CKD).

This was accompanied by an explosion in research leading to a realization that kidney disease was much more than dialysis, and the incidence was higher than anyone expected. The primary practitioner has moved to the forefront in identifying and managing CKD. We now recognize that the CKD patient is seen in all types of practices, and the one-size-fits-all theory definitely does not fit.

As kidney disease was defined and monitored, allowing for more robust research, the 21st century has also identified the "high-risk" patient. We know CKD is found more often in the minority populations, but we have also learned it is a disease of the older American, a disease with a strong genetic component and one that is silent in early stages. In addition, it follows on the coattails of diabetes and hypertension, both of which are epidemic in the United States today. We have identified CKD as a risk factor for cardiovascular disease, stroke, dementia, and liver disease. CKD can be found with other chronic diseases: HIV, osteoarthritis, depression, orthopedic issues, lupus, and rheumatologic diseases, to name a few. Often, it accompanies the disease process but frequently is an unwanted side effect of treatments.

The last 20 years have led to novel therapies to decrease progression. Some of these have been successful; some less successful. What is known to the entire kidney community is that by the time the CKD patient has progressed to stage 4 and shows up in the nephrology office, much of the damage has been done. It is nonreversible, and the expense, in personal, monetary, and societal cost, is massive. The only way to slow the

Physician Assist Clin 1 (2016) xv–xvi
http://dx.doi.org/10.1016/j.cpha.2015.10.002
2405-7991/16/$ – see front matter © 2016 Published by Elsevier Inc.
physicianassistant.theclinics.com

relentless pace of kidney disease is to recognize the disease early enough for the progression to be slowed, if not halted.

It is at this juncture, when the kidney community admits they cannot do this alone, that the need for the PA is tantamount. Whether it is the primary care PA, the orthopedic PA, the OB/GYN PA, the urgent care PA, or the surgical PA; it does not matter. We are all in this together, and only by all working as a team can we slow the scourge of kidney disease. As described in the "butterfly theory" that one small change can progress around the world and change the wind, so too can one small change by just one PA make a difference to the kidney patient.

If you think you do not see kidney patients, you are wrong. We all lose kidney function as we age, and as PAs, we see patients at all times, ages, and aspects of their life spans. The goal of this issue of *Physician Assistant Clinics* is to open your eyes to the kidney patient hiding in plain sight: the elephant in the room.

We, the editors, appreciate the contributions of the diverse group of authors who came together to share their expertise and knowledge with you, the readers of this, the inaugural issue of *Physician Assistant Clinics.* We hope you enjoy reading it as much as we enjoyed developing it.

Kim Zuber, PA-C
American Academy of Nephrology PAs (AANPA)
535 Gillingham Cir
Oceanside, CA 92058, USA

Jane S. Davis, CRNP, DNP
University of Alabama at Birmingham
Center at Birmingham
Department of Nephrology
1720, 2nd Ave south
Birmingham, AL 35294, USA

E-mail addresses:
zuberkim@yahoo.com (K. Zuber)
jsdavis@uab.edu (J.S. Davis)

Will the Real Kidney Patient Please Stand up?

 CrossMark

Kim Zuber, PA-C[a,b,*], Jane S. Davis, CRNP, DNP[b,c]

KEYWORDS

- Chronic kidney disease • Kidney patient • Differential diagnosis

KEY POINTS

- All adults lose kidney function as they age, and thus the kidney patient can be hiding in plain sight.
- Often kidney disease is not considered in the differential although it may be a component and should not be overlooked.
- A kidney patient will be seen in every specialty, every setting, and every age group. It is vital that one knows how to evaluate and manage these patients.

I think I'll go back to ignoring the creatinine until it gets so high it scares me. Kidney disease is confusing, and I can't figure out what I'm supposed to do.
—*Andy Narva, MD, Director, National Institutes of Health (NIH), National Kidney Disease Education Program, (NKDEP)*

The National Kidney Foundation (NKF) recently reported that Americans are "kidney clueless," with more than half of those surveyed unsure what the kidneys do, the signs or symptoms of kidney disease, or even who is at risk of developing kidney disease.[1] This would be less concerning if their practitioners were kidney disease experts and could educate patients regarding risk factors and symptoms. However, in a 2014 study, NKF reported a severe lack of knowledge among practitioners as to the diagnosis and treatment of chronic kidney disease (CKD).[2] In this inaugural issue of *PA Clinics*, the authors hope to highlight kidney disease in all its permutations, the patient population, the presence of kidney disease in every specialty and increase the comfort zone of the PA who is not in nephrology. One should start with the basics: who is the kidney patient?

The standard risk factors for CKD include diabetes, hypertension and race.

But few practitioners, however, look outside the box and realize that age alone will increase one's risk of CKD. In addition, patients face risk factors daily. A recent

[a] American Academy of Nephrology PAs, 535 Gillingham Cir, Oceanside, CA 92058, USA; [b] National Kidney Foundation's Council of Advanced Practitioners; [c] Division of Nephrology, University of Alabama Medical Center at Birmingham, Birmingham, AL, USA
* Corresponding author.
E-mail address: zuberkim@yahoo.com

Physician Assist Clin 1 (2016) 1–12
http://dx.doi.org/10.1016/j.cpha.2015.10.001
2405-7991/16/$ – see front matter © 2016 Elsevier Inc. All rights reserved.

A 20 year old female presents with white-coat hypertension and an inability to lose weight, primarily centrally.

Kidney diagnosis?

Autosomal-dominant polycystic kidney disease

A 60 year old healthy woman presents for her annual Pap smear and pelvic.

Kidney diagnosis?

Age-related chronic kidney disease

A 45 year old African-American man presents with new-onset hypertension.

Kidney diagnosis?

Apoliproprotein L1 gene variant

A 50 year-old Japanese man presents with recurrent hematuria although his present urine is bland.

Kidney diagnosis?

IGA nephropathy

A thin 17 year-old wrestler attempts to lose 5 pounds to qualify at a lower weight class. He is running sprints in a rubber suit. He presents with multiple joint pains.

Kidney diagnosis?

Rhabdomyolysis

A 55 year-old diabetic presents to the office with an A1C of 9.8, overt neuropathy, retinopathy, and microalbuminuria.

Kidney diagnosis?

End Organ Diabetic Nephropathy

A 35 year-old man with long-standing human immunodeficiency virus (HIV) well-controlled with triple therapy presents for his quarterly management laboratory tests.

Kidney diagnosis?

Human immunodeficiency-associated nephropathy

A 28 year-old African American federal employee presents for a physical examination prior to posting overseas. Routine screening laboratory tests show a serum creatinine (SCr) of 5.9.

Kidney diagnosis?

Glomerulonephritis

A 45 year-old construction worker presents with complaints of knee pain. He has been using over-the-counter nonsteroidal anti-inflammatory steroids (NSAIDS) for pain management.

Kidney diagnosis?

Acute tubular necrosis secondary to nonsteroidal anti-inflammatory drugs

---

A teenager is seen in the emergency room with complaints of nausea and vomiting. Laboratory tests are done and show a serum creatinine (SCr) of 4.5. She admits to smoking synthetic marijuana earlier in the day.

Kidney diagnosis?

Spice-induced acute kidney injury

A 16 year-old football player comes into the office for a sports physical prior to the football season. He admits to taking creatine supplements to bulk up, and his blood pressure is 135/90.

Kidney diagnosis?

Creatine-induced hypertension

An 8-year old boy presents to the office. His mother is concerned, because he still wets the bed. Under further questioning, it is discovered that he has never had a dry night.
Kidney diagnosis?
Pediatric vesicoureteral reflux disease
A 45 year mother presents with an influenza-like illness. She is running a temperature of 102°F, has 2 school-aged children and a sick husband at home. She has not been able to keep any food or liquids down but is taking over-the-counter cold medications.
Kidney diagnosis?
Acute kidney injury due to dehydration
A 28 year-old woman presents to the urgent care center with severe flank pain. She admits to drinking 16 diet sodas per day.
Kidney diagnosis?
Phosphate-induced nephrolithiasis
A 68 year-old man with a history of congestive heart failure (CHF) is admitted to the hospital for monitoring. His ejection fraction is 15% with crackles heard throughout his lung fields.
Kidney diagnosis?
Fluid overload

publication from Johns Hopkins highlighted that close to 60% of all Americans will develop CKD Stage 3 or greater within their lifetimes.[3]

Smoking is a known risk for CKD, and yet many practitioners do not realize this or share this information with patients.[4] Perhaps a push on how smoking affects the function of kidneys and a glimpse into life on dialysis will scare a teenager a bit. Perhaps not.

Obesity is a risk factor for diabetes and thus a risk factor for diabetic nephropathy. Yet, obesity alone is a risk factor for progression of CKD. A recent article in the *Clinical Journal of the American Society of Nephrology (CJASN)* highlighted the recovery of some kidney function with a small weight loss, even at the extremes decrease in kidney function[5] (**Fig. 1**).

More than 20 million Americans have kidney disease, which is the eighth most common cause of death.[6,7] It is a more common diagnosis than heart disease, but somehow it is not taken as seriously.[8] An American is more likely to die of kidney disease than breast or prostate cancer. Two hundred thousand American children and adolescents have kidney disease. As obesity and diabetes in the pediatric population increase, this number will only grow and expand. In 2014, 150,000 children were either on dialysis or living with a kidney transplant.[9]

There were a half a million Americans on dialysis in the United States in 2014 and another 100,000 who declined dialysis and were living with kidney failure.[9] (**Fig. 2**) There are 185,000 Americans with a kidney transplant and more than 100,000 on the kidney transplant wait list as of January 2015.[6] The kidney wait list dwarfs all other transplant lists. In some areas of the country where the wait list can be 8 to 10 years long, a patient is more likely to die waiting than to receive a transplant.[10] Twelve people die of kidney disease complications every day waiting for a transplant.[11] (**Fig. 3**) Kidney disease reduces quality of life and reduces lifespan. As a kidney patient stated: "You can go on vacation and forget patients for awhile, but I can never go on vacation from kidney disease."[12]

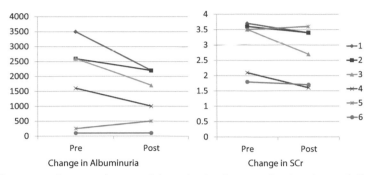

Fig. 1. Short-term changes after a weight reduction intervention in advanced diabetic nephropathy. (*Data from* Friedman AN, Chambers M, Kamendulis M, et al. Short term changes after a weight reduction intervention In advanced diabetic nephropathy. Clin J Am Soc Nephrol 2013;8(11):1892–8.)

The cost of kidney failure to the Medicare system is tremendous. In the November 9, 1962, issue of *Life Magazine*, Shana Alexander highlighted the new treatment for kidney disease: "kidney dialysis."[13] She also highlighted the cost, the lack of machines, and the inability to offer the treatment to all patients who needed it. Her article "They Decide who Lives, Who Dies: Medical Miracle Puts a Moral Burden on a Small Committee" was the first time the public was made aware of selection committees. Known colloquially as the "God Squad," the committee was made up of 7 members of the public included a minister and representatives from the community with a physician as an expert consultant. These committees weighed the importance of each patient to both society and their families, choosing only a limited few who could be offered dialysis. As Medicare was in Congress for authorization at this time, a separate section called "The End Stage Renal Disease (ESRD) Program" was inserted into Medicare regulations. This means that no matter one's age, a person diagnosed with kidney failure requiring dialysis will be covered by Medicare.[14] This program has grown large and costly (as medical programs tend to do) and now accounts for 7% of the entire Medicare budget. Thus, for the less than 1% of the Medicare population, $35 billion or 7% of the entire Medicare budget pays for the ESRD patients. This does not include the one-third of the Medicare budget used to pay for the older Medicare patient with a diagnosis of CKD or acute kidney injury (AKI) (CPT code 585 and 584).[8]

Kidney disease is everywhere. The statistics regarding AKI and CKD are truly astounding. The fact that the less than 1% of the Medicare population costs the American taxpayer more than the entire budget of the National Institutes of Health only makes the identification of the kidney patient all the more imperative.[15] Unless one stems the influx of kidney patients, treating them early and decreasing the sequelae of chronic issues, the cost to society, and each particular patient, will be insurmountable.

One in three Americans is at risk for developing kidney disease. Those with usual risk factors are more likely to develop CKD but there are a few surprising facts:

- Men with CKD are more likely to progress to kidney failure than women.[10]
- Many blacks of African American descent can carry the APOL-1 gene which will protect them from sleeping sickness (African trypanosomiasis) but will increase their chance of progression of hypertension-induced kidney disease.[16,17]
- Hispanics have a 1.5% increased risk of kidney disease.[10]

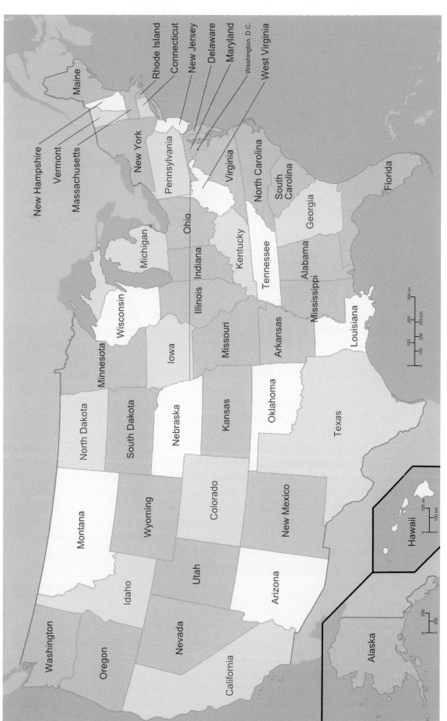

Fig. 2. Interactive map on the ASN Web site to link that allows the online reader to click on any state and view state specific kidney disease data. (Available at: http://www.asn-online.org/policy/fact-sheets.aspx). Accessed April 30, 2015.

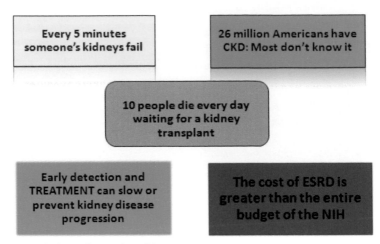

Fig. 3. Chronic kidney disease factoids.

Research into kidney disease is lacking and lagging. For a long time, descriptors of kidney disease were not standardized, and thus research on progression was difficult to define both in the US and worldwide. In 2001, the NKF under the Kidney Disease Outcomes Quality Initiative (KDOQI) defined kidney disease by stages and with standardized formulas[18] (**Table 1**). The Glomerular Filtration Rate (GFR) was accepted as the measurement to be used for all research and this allowed significant amounts of data to be collected and analyzed. In 2012, KDIGO (Kidney Disease Improving Global Outcomes), an international kidney coalition including the United States, defined kidney disease stages by both GFR and albuminuria[19] (**Fig. 4**). Albuminuria has been shown to be pathognomonic for kidney disease and a highly prognostic factor in progression.[20–24]

Another issue with research is defining endpoints in kidney disease: a doubling of the serum creatinine or the halving of the GFR was considered the gold standard in defining kidney endpoints. However, these can take many years to reach, and research studies are often of a shorter span. Thus, the US Food and Drug Administration (FDA) and NKF sponsored an international consensus workshop in December

Table 1 Stages of CKD 2002		
Stage	Description	GFR (mL/min/1.73 m²)
1	Kidney damage with normal or ↑ GFR	≥90
2	Kidney damage with mild ↓ GFR	60–89
3	Moderate ↓ GFR	30–59
4	Severe ↓ GFR	15–29
5	Kidney failure	<15 (or dialysis)

Chronic kidney disease is defined as either kidney damage or GFR less than 60 mL/min/1.73 m² for ≥3 months. Kidney damage is defined as pathologic abnormalities or markers of damage, including abnormalities in blood or urine tests or imaging studies.

Adapted from National Kidney Foundation. K/DOQI Clinical practice guidelines for chronic kidney disease: evaluation, classification and stratification. Am J Kidney Dis 2002; 39(Suppl 1):S1–266.

		Prognosis of CKD by GFR and Albuminuria Categories: KDIGO 2012		Persistent albuminuria categories Description and range		
				A1 Normal to mildly increased <30 mg/g <3 mg/mmol	A2 Moderately increased 30–300 mg/g 3–30 mg/mmol	A3 Severely increased >300 mg/g >30 mg/mmol
GFR categories (mL/min/ 1.73 m²) Description and range	G1	Normal or high	≥90			
	G2	Mildly decreased	60–89			
	G3a	Mildly to moderately decreased	45–59			
	G3b	Moderately to severely decreased	30–44			
	G4	Severely decreased	15–29			
	G5	Kidney failure	<15			

Fig. 4. Prognosis of CKD by GFR and albuminuria category. (*From* KDIGO 2012 clinical practice guideline for the evaluation and management of chronic kidney disease. Kidney Int Suppl 2013;3: p. 1–150; with permission. Available at: http://www.kdigo.org/clinical_practice_guidelines/pdf/CKD/KDIGO_2012_CKD_GL.pdf.)

2014 with the international kidney community to consider a 30% to 40% GFR decline as an endpoint for clinical trials in CKD.[25] The kidney community believes this would increase research outcomes and provide more analyzed data to treat the CKD patient with outcome driven, peer-reviewed statistics and information shown to help patients.

Although kidney disease is common, and research is lacking, the PA in every specialty is treating these patients right now.[26] The American Academy of Nephrology PAs (AANPA), the PA and nurse practitioners from the NKF (NKF/CAP), and the pharmacists who help on a day-to-day basis with patients want to share their collective knowledge and insights into this challenging population. Thus, this issue of *PA Clinics* will highlight what is vital for every PA to know regarding kidney disease.

Because many PAs can identify the standard diabetic, hypertensive CKD patient, Becky Ness, PAC, and her colleagues from Mayo Clinic will present the more unusual CKD diagnoses in "Introduction of the Kidney Patient." Knowing a picture is worth a thousand words, Alexis Snead, MD, renal pathologist from the University of Oklahoma and Ameripath, has collected slides detailing the changes seen with each diagnosis. Becky has used a case-based presentation format in order to encourage the PA to open up the differential and consider a kidney diagnosis rather than jumping into treatment. As is often said: failure to diagnose can be due to a failure to consider a diagnosis.

Kidney patients frequently undergo surgical procedures. This is often not just for kidney-specific conditions or dialysis access procedures but also for any cause found in the general population. The kidney patient is often diabetic, which leads to multiple surgical risks and procedures; is older and thus has years of outdoor exposure increasing dermatologic procedures; and can be obese with the orthopedic risks that this entails and has multiple medical comorbidities. Thus, the surgical PA is often faced perioperatively with a multitude of risk factors from the kidney patient. Catherine Brown, CRNP, and April Crunk, PAC, of the University of Alabama at Birmingham, bring their considerable experience together, along with protocols developed and refined using peer-reviewed outcome-driven results to help the surgical PA in crossing the red line.

Cardiology and nephrology are intertwined and complementary. As a nephrology PA noted when she was moved by her university from the nephrology suite to run the heart failure clinic: "I was afraid it would be a huge learning curve but when I walked in the front door, it was all my same kidney patients! It was like 'Old Home Week'." Just as she realized, kidney patients are heart patients and vice versa. In "The Pump and the Filter," Laura Troidle, PA, from Hypertension and Metabolism Associates and Yale University, presents the newest research and management to balance competing diagnoses in these complicated patients.

Renal medication dosing is fraught with errors and often the scariest part of caring for the kidney patient. The average kidney patient takes 12 to 15 different medications, and the chance of either dosing errors or medication interactions is real. Cheryl Gilmartin Pharm D, and Amy Barton Pai, Pharm D, at University of Illinois and Albany College of Pharmacy & Health Sciences respectively, bring their many years of experience in treating kidney patient in all stages of CKD along with their extensive knowledge of the interactions of medication classes to "Risky Business: Lessons in Medication Misadventures in CKD." Using a Socratic method of teaching, they highlight the most common dosing errors made with the kidney patient by the non-nephrology practitioner.

With a large percentage of intensive care unit (ICU) patients having some level of kidney disease, appropriate management of these fragile patients is vital. Catherine Wells, DNP, takes a break from training the residents and fellows at the University of Mississippi, a hotbed of kidney disease, to share her expertise. "The ABCs of the ICU," is based on her presentations to medical practitioners regarding when, how, why, and what kind of renal replacement therapies (continuous renal replacement therapy [CRRT] and intermittent hemodialysis [IHD]) are needed. For those treating the hospital-based patient, this is a valuable educational addition.

AKI is one of the most frequent diagnoses of the hospitalized patient. If one is not diagnosed with AKI on admission, often a procedure or treatment will cause an AKI episode. For the over 80 year old hospitalized patient, data show 80% will have an AKI diagnosis before discharge (**Fig. 5**). Erica Davis, PAC, of Metropolitan Nephrology, has been on both sides of this issue both as a hospitalist PA and as a nephrology PA. She is able to combine both views and share research-driven diagnosis and management of the AKI patient with the non-nephrology PA in "Acute Kidney Injury: The Ugly Truth".

"Pediatrics: the Forgotten Stepchild of Nephrology" is a reminder that not every kidney patient is the older, hypertensive diabetic. There are over 200,000 children and adolescents living with kidney disease. Mandy Trolinger, PAC, and author of the transplant article in this issue, was diagnosed with kidney disease when she was a teenager. These children often have missed diagnoses or are marginalized at school and the medical clinic. Molly Band, PAC, from Connecticut Children's Hospital has been caring for them for years and highlights her view from the other side.

As the most common site to see the kidney patient is the outpatient arena, Denise Link, PAC, helps guide the evaluation and treatment of CKD in "Management of the CKD Patient". As a long-time instructor at the University of Texas, Dallas PA program, Link is well positioned to share standards of care while also highlighting the direction research is headed in kidney disease. When one meets a CKD patient, this is often

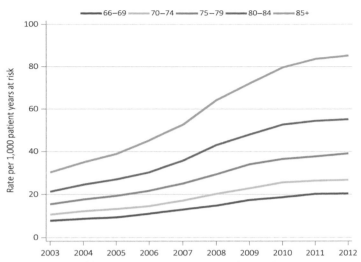

Fig. 5. Unadjusted rates of first hospitalization with AKI for Medicare patients aged 66 + by age and year, 2003 to 2012. AKI, acute kidney injury. (*From* Saran R, Li Y, Robinson B, et al. US Renal Data System 2014 annual data report: epidemiology of kidney disease in the United States. Am J Kidney Dis. 2015;66(1)(suppl 1):S1–S306. Available at: http://www. usrds.org/2014/view/v1_05.aspx. Accessed December 05, 2014.)

the beginning of a lifetime relationship. As she often notes, she has known her CKD patients longer than her husband.

One of the risk factors for kidney disease is nephrolithiasis or kidney stones. In "The Rolling Stones," Harvey Feldman, MD, discusses the diagnosis and prognosis of stones and stone management. As an experienced professor of nephrology in the Florida NOVA Southeastern PA program, Feldman has the ability to make kidney disease, and even stones, less painful to learn. As the incidence of patients with stones is increasing each year, this is a timely and important subject.

"Kidney Transplant for the 21st Century" is written by a PA with a special connection to the subject; Mandy Trolinger, PAC, is a 2 time transplant patient. In fact, Tronlinger is a PA because of the interaction she had with PAs during her experience as a kidney patient. She is all that more empathetic with her patient population by being one of them, but she is also more effective at teaching others what transplant is really like and what one can do to help these patients. With the new protocols and listing rules that took effect in December 2014, she highlights what is new and what effects have been seen because of these changes.

In "Health Disparities in CKD: The Role of Social Factors", Jenna Norton, MPH, of the NIH, reports on a vitally important fact of kidney disease: there are more minorities and urban poor with kidney disease than are found in the general population. Is this a nurture or nature issue? Is there a modifiable risk factor that one can adjust? Change? Using the research breakthroughs that she has participated in at the NIH, Norton leads readers through the minefield that can be found when one tries to tease out disparities in evaluation and treatment in medicine.

Finally, but certainly not least, Arlene Suros, PAC and RD, shares "Food for Thought." The diet one learned in school is very 'last century, and she shows what can and cannot be done to slow progression in kidney patients through nutrition. She discusses the importance of diet and what is ground breaking for the 21st century. She highlights the direction research is going and what can be expected in the future.

Whether kidney disease is the lead in the differential or not, it should be a consideration in diagnosing and treating patients. Practitioners also need to be vigilant to slow progression of CKD. This inaugural issue highlights the incidence, risk factors, and management of the patient with mild, moderate, and severe kidney disease from the child to the older adult. These patients present not challenges but opportunities to employ knowledge and critical thinking skills.

NATIONAL KIDNEY FOUNDATION FACTOIDS[10]

- 1 in 3 American adults is currently at risk for developing kidney disease.
- 26 million American adults have kidney disease, and most do not know it.
- High blood pressure and diabetes are the 2 leading causes of kidney disease.
- Major risk factors for kidney disease include diabetes, high blood pressure, family history of kidney failure, age greater than 60 years old. Additional risk factors include kidney stones, smoking, obesity, and cardiovascular disease.
- Those at risk should have simple blood and urine tests to check if their kidneys are working properly.
- Kidney disease is the ninth leading cause of death in the United States.
  - Every year, kidney disease kills more people than breast or prostate cancer.
  - In 2013, more than 47,000 Americans died from kidney disease.
- Men with kidney disease are more likely than women to progress to kidney failure.
- Black Americans are 3 times more likely to experience kidney failure.
- Hispanics are 1½ times more likely to experience kidney failure.
- Once the kidneys fail, dialysis or a kidney transplant is required.
- Approximately 450,000 Americans are on dialysis, and approximately 185,000 live with a functioning kidney transplant.
- Of more than 123,000 Americans currently on the waiting list for a lifesaving organ transplant, over 101,000 need a kidney. Fewer than 17,000 people receive one each year.
- Every day, 12 people die waiting for a kidney transplant.

REFERENCES

1. National Kidney Foundation. Americans are kidney clueless. Available at: https://www.kidney.org/news/americans-are-kidney-clueless. Accessed May 15, 2015.
2. Szczech L, Stewart RC, Su HL, et al. Primary care detection of chronic kidney disease in adults with type-2 diabetes: the ADD-CKD Study (awareness, detection and drug therapy in type 2 diabetes and chronic kidney disease). PLoS One 2014;9(11):e110535.
3. Grams ME, Chow EKH, Segev DL. Lifetime incidence of CKD Stages 3-5 in the United States. Am J Kidney Dis 2013;62(2):245–52.
4. Garcia-Esquinas E, Loeffler LF, Weaver VM, et al. Kidney function and tobacco smoke exposure in US adolescents. Pediatrics 2013;131(5):e1415–23.
5. Friedman AN, Chambers M, Kamendulis M, et al. Short term changes after a weight reduction intervention in advanced diabetic nephropathy. Clin J Am Soc Nephrol 2013;8(11):1892–8.
6. United States Renal Data System, 2014 annual data report: an overview of the epidemiology of kidney disease in the United States. Bethesda (MD): National Institutes of Health, National Institute of Diabetes and Digestive and Kidney Diseases; 2014.

7. U.S. Renal data system, USRDS 2013 annual data report: Atlas of chronic kidney disease and end-stage renal disease in the United States. Bethesda (MD): National Institutes of Health, National Institute of Diabetes and Digestive and Kidney Diseases; 2013.

8. Cho S. ASN President urges kidney disease innovation. Nephrol News Issues. Available at: http://www.newswise.com/articles/asn-president-calls-for-kidney-disease-innovation-in-congressional-testimony. Accessed April 9, 2014.

9. ASN. State-specific statistics on the burden of kidney disease. Available at: http://www.asn-online.org/policy/fact-sheets.aspx. Accessed May 15, 2015.

10. NKF. CKD facts. Available at: https://www.kidney.org/news/newsroom/factsheets/FastFacts#Ref. Accessed May 01, 2015.

11. United Network of Organ Sharing (UNOS). Available at: http://optn.transplant.hrsa.gov/data/. Accessed October 28, 2014.

12. Trollinger M. Pregnancy and the CKD patient. Dallas (TX): NKF Spring Clinical Meetings; 2015.

13. Available at: http://www.lifemagazineconnection.com/LIFE-Magazines-1960s/LIFE-Magazines-1962/1962-November-9-LIFE-Magazine-CUBAN-MISSILE-CRISIS; http://ihatedialysis.com/forum/index.php?topic=23860.0. Accessed May 01, 2015.

14. Medicare end stage renal disease program. Available at: www.cms.gov/Medicare/End-Stage-Renal-Disease/ESRDGeneralInformation/index.html?redirect=/ESRDGeneralInformation/. Accessed May 25, 2015.

15. Olan G. Prospects looking better for NIH funding in 2014. ASN Kidney News 2014;7.

16. Genovese G, Friedman DJ, Ross MD, et al. Association of trypanolytic ApoL1 variants with kidney disease in African Americans. Science 2010;329(5993):841–5.

17. Freedman BI, Skorecki K. Gene-gene and gene-environment interactions in apolipoprotein L1 gene-associated nephropathy. Clin J Am Soc Nephrol 2014;9(11):2006–13.

18. National Kidney Foundation. K/DOQI Clinical practice guidelines for chronic kidney disease: evaluation, classification and stratification. Am J Kidney Dis 2002;39(Suppl 1):S1–266.

19. Kidney Disease: Improving Global Outcomes (KDIGO) CKD Work Group. KDIGO 2012 clinical practice guideline for the evaluation and management of chronic kidney disease. Kidney Int Suppl 2013;3:1–150.

20. Lea J, Greene T, Hebert L, et al. The relationship between magnitude of proteinuria reduction and risk of end-stage renal disease: results of the African American study of kidney disease and hypertension. Arch Intern Med 2005;165(8):947–53.

21. Turin TC, James M, Ravani P, et al. Proteinuria and rate of change in kidney function in a community-based population. J Am Soc Nephrol 2013;24(10):1661–7.

22. Eriksen BO, Ingebretsen OC. The progression of chronic kidney disease: a 10-year population-based study of the effects of gender and age. Kidney Int 2006;69(2):375–82.

23. Hallan SI, Ritz E, Lydersen S, et al. Combining GFR and albuminuria to classify CKD improves prediction of ESRD. J Am Soc Nephrol 2009;20(5):1069–77.

24. Hemmelgarn BR, Manns BJ, Lloyd A, et al, Alberta Kidney Disease Network. Relation between kidney function, proteinuria, and adverse outcomes. JAMA 2010;303(5):423–9.

25. The NKF/FDA Scientific Workshop. GFR decline as an endpoint for clinical trials in CKD. Available at: https://www.kidney.org/professionals/research/research_info. Accessed May 25, 2015.

26. Coresh J, Selvin E, Stevens LA, et al. Prevalence of chronic kidney disease in the United States. JAMA 2007;298(17):2038–47.

Introduction to Kidney Patients

Becky Ness, MPAS, PA-C[a],*, Fawad Qureshi, MD[b], Alexis Anne Harris, MD[c]

KEYWORDS

- CKD • Proteinuria • Hematuria • Acute kidney failure

KEY POINTS

- Many common medical conditions are associated with chronic kidney disease (CKD). Unfortunately, these are too often overlooked regarding their impact on kidney health until a crisis occurs or CKD has progressed to stage III or beyond.
- Early identification of patients with other conditions that impact kidney health is crucial in allowing the maintenance of current kidney health and slowing the progression between CKD stages.
- Prompt referral to nephrology on identification of these other conditions and recognition of CKD progression is a key element to managing patients with CKD.

More than 26 million people have chronic kidney disease (CKD) and another 73 million are at risk of CKD; yet less than 10% are aware of their diagnosis.[1] Identification of those patients at risk is crucial but often overlooked. Hypertensive diabetic patients are easily recognized as potentially having kidney disease, but what about atypical patients? CKD can be caused by other entities: focal segmental glomerulosclerosis (FSGS), lupus nephritis, glomerulonephritis, autosomal dominant polycystic kidney disease (ADPKD), immunoglobulin A (IgA) nephropathy, nephrolithiasis, and scleroderma, among others. This article is a review of those other kidney diagnoses including images and a review of staging of kidney patients using Kidney Disease Improving Global Outcomes (KDIGO) 2012 criteria.

CKD is primarily staged using the glomerular filtration rate (GFR), which takes into account age, race, gender, and serum creatinine. Kidney function is normal in stage I and minimally reduced in stage II; from stage III to V there is progression from

No disclosures.
[a] Nephrology, SWMN Mayo Clinic Health System, 1015 Marsh Street, Mankato, MN 56001, USA;
[b] Department of Nephrology, SWMN Mayo Clinic Health System, 1015 Marsh Street, Mankato, MN 56001, USA; [c] Ameripath/Quest Diagnostic Laboratories, Renal Pathology, 225 Northeast 97th Street, Suite 600, Oklahoma City, OK 73114, USA
* Corresponding author.
E-mail address: ness.becky@mayo.edu

Physician Assist Clin 1 (2016) 13–41
http://dx.doi.org/10.1016/j.cpha.2015.09.001
2405-7991/16/$ – see front matter © 2016 Elsevier Inc. All rights reserved.

moderate to severe disease culminating in end-stage renal disease (ESRD) (stage V) and often requiring dialysis. Most laboratories report GFR as greater than 60 mL/min for those in stage I or II, not listing a specific value until the GFR is less than 60 mL/min. This reporting, coupled with a busy primary care practice causing time constraints on visits, is a driving force behind this review which highlights the importance of increasing awareness of other kidney diagnoses with directions of when to refer (**Fig. 1**).

Patients will present with a myriad of complaints, many of which could implicate the kidney and signal the presence of, or a risk factor for, the development of CKD. Because of the escalating costs associated with treatment of ESRD, the identification of those at risk for CKD and early treatment is imperative. The following are case studies highlighting patients, much like those that walk into primary care provider's (PCP) offices daily, who are at risk for or have already developed CKD.

CASE STUDY 1
History of Present Illness

A 28-year-old Caucasian man presents Monday morning to his PCP's office complaining of severe left flank pain that lasted for 2 days over the weekend. During this time, he had a single episode of red-colored urine. He denies any significant trauma or

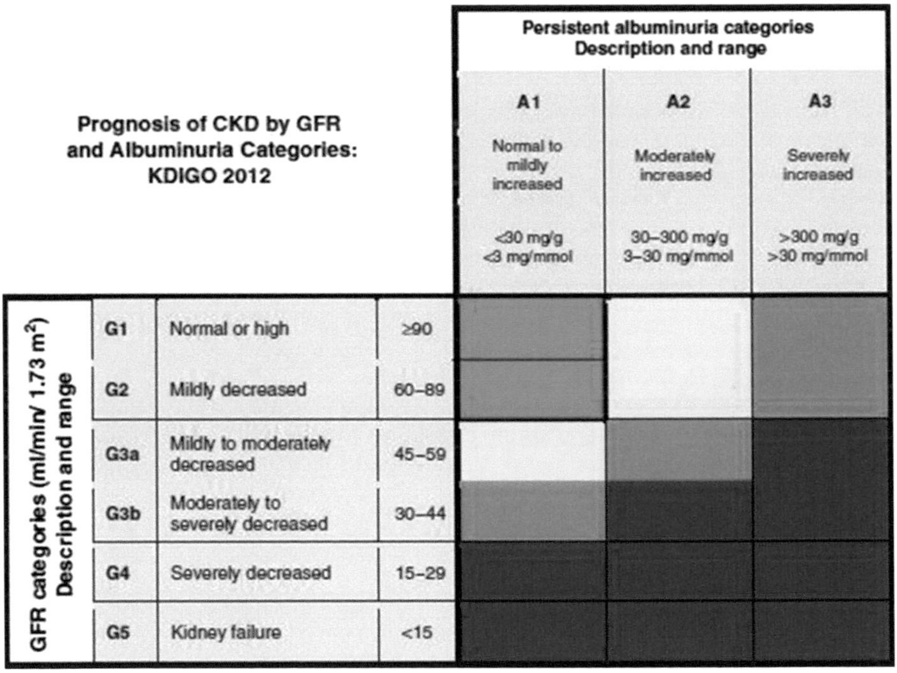

Fig. 1. Prognosis of CKD by GFR and albuminuria category. Green: low risk (if no other markers of kidney disease, no CKD); Yellow: moderately increased risk; Orange: high risk; Red, very high risk. (*From* KDIGO 2012 clinical practice guideline for the evaluation and management of chronic kidney disease. Kidney Int Suppl 2013;3:pp. 1–150; with permission. Available at: http://www.kdigo.org/clinical_practice_guidelines/pdf/CKD/KDIGO_2012_CKD_GL.pdf.)

change in physical activity. He played lacrosse Saturday morning, per his weekend routine. At the time of presentation, the pain had resolved and there had been no additional episodes of red urine. He states that he had a fever measuring 38°C (100.4°F) on Saturday evening. This fever resolved with the use of over-the-counter (OTC) pain medications (the patient is vague on what type). He denies further use of OTC pain medications or return of the fever. He denies changes in urination, painful urination, or bloody semen.

Social History

Single: lives with a roommate who brought him into the clinic
Alcohol: social: 2 to 5 beverages weekly, mostly beer
Tobacco: one-half pack daily for the last 10 years
Drugs: nothing illicit
Employed full time: construction

Past Medical History

There is no known diagnosis.

Family History

His parents have no known kidney disease. His siblings include 2 brothers and a sister, none of whom have known kidney disease. A paternal uncle had a kidney transplant at 55 years of age; however, the patient does not recall the reason. His paternal grandfather was diagnosed with bladder cancer at 80 years old and was a smoker.

Physical Examination

Vitals
The vitals are as follows: blood pressure (BP) 150/90, heart rate (HR) 68 (regular), Respirations (R) 18 (nonlabored), temperature 36°C (96.8°F), weight 79.5 kg (174.9 lb).

General
The patient is in no distress and communicates without difficulty. The patient is polite, cooperative, appropriately dressed, and of normal hygiene.

Heent
Head is of expected size and shape without irregularity or evidence of trauma. Eyes are anicteric, with intact extra ocular movements and pupils that are equal, round and reactive to light and accommodation. Ears demonstrate no abnormal external appearance and the tympanic membranes are healthy in appearance without perforation or evidence of infection. The oropharynx is without lesion of mucosa. The pharynx rises symmetrically without exudate.

Neck
There are no nodes and no thyromegaly. No bruit is auscultated.

Heart
The heart has a regular rate and rhythm. No murmurs, gallops, or rubs noted.

Lungs
The lungs are clear to auscultation bilaterally. There is no expiratory wheeze. There are no accessory muscles of respiration noted.

Abdomen
The abdomen is nontender to palpation. There is no hepatosplenomegaly or mass. There are normal bowel sounds in all 4 quadrants.

Genitalia/rectum
The patient has normal external male genitalia. The patient is previously circumcised. A prostate examination is deferred. The anus appears normal.

Extremities
There is no neurovascular compromise. There is no cyanosis, clubbing, or edema. There is no abnormal limb length.

Differential Diagnosis
1. Trauma: played lacrosse the day symptoms began
2. Nephrolithiasis: gross hematuria with left flank pain
3. Polycystic kidney disease: hematuria, pain (seen with cyst rupture)
4. Bladder cancer: hematuria in a smoker

Laboratory Evaluation

CBC		
	Current Value	Normal Range
WBC	5.8	3.5–10.5 × 10(9)/L
Hgb	15.8	12.0–15.5 g/dL
Hct	48	34.9%–44.5%
RBC	4.2	3.90–5.03 × 10(12)/L
MCV	86	81.6–98.3 fL
RDW	14	11.9%–15.5%
Platelet	275	150–450 × 10(9)/L

Abbreviations: CBC, complete blood count; Hct, hematocrit; Hgb, hemoglobin; MCV, mean corpus volume; RBC, red blood cell; RDW, red (blood cell) diameter width; WBC, white blood cell.

Basic metabolic panel		
	Current Value	Normal Range
Sodium	140	135–145 mmol/L
Potassium	3.8	3.5–5.1 mmol/L
Chloride	100	98–107 mmol/L
CO_2	25	22–29 mmol/L
AGAP	12	7–15 mmol/L
Glucose	99	70–140 mg/dL
Creatinine	0.8	0.6–1.1 md/dL
GFR (MDRD)	78	≥60 mL/min
GFR African American (MDRD)	—	≥60 mL/min
BUN	15	6–24 mg/dL
Calcium	9	8.8–10.3 mg/dL

Abbreviations: AGAP, anion gap; BUN, serum urea nitrogen; CO_2, carbon dioxide; MDRD, modification of diet in renal disease.

Urinalysis with micro		
	Current Value	Normal Range
UA source	Clean catch	—
UA color	Yellow	—
UA clarity	Clear	—
UA specific gravity	1.005	1.005–1.030
UA pH	5	4.6–8.0
UA protein	Negative	Negative mg/dL
UA glucose	Negative	Negative mg/dL
UA ketones	Negative	Negative mg/dL
UA bilirubin	Negative	Negative
UA urobilinogen	Negative	Negative
UA blood	Negative	Negative
UA nitrite	Negative	Negative
UA Leuk Est	Negative	Negative
UA WBC	None seen	—
UA RBC	None seen	—
UR % dysmorphic RBC	None seen	—
UR squamous Epi cells	None seen	—
UR bacteria	None seen	—
UR crystals	None seen	—

Abbreviations: Epi, epithelial cells; Leuk set, leukocyte esterase; RBC, red blood cell; UA, urinalysis; UR, urine; WBC, white blood cell.

Radiology Evaluation

Renal ultrasound
Renal ultrasound demonstrates no evidence of hydronephrosis or nephrolithiasis. Multiple cysts are noted bilaterally along with enlargement of the kidneys, with the right kidney measuring 15 cm and the left measuring 16 cm.

Discussion

The patient returns to the clinic to discuss the results of the laboratory and ultrasound examinations and mentions that his uncle was diagnosed with ADPKD, which was the reason for his transplant. He also reveals that his father had episodes of bloody urine periodically without pain or sequelae but had not been assessed for ADPKD despite his brother's (the uncle) diagnosis and subsequent need for transplant.

In this patient, the pain and frank hematuria were secondary to cyst rupture. The patient was advised of the diagnosis of ADPKD (**Fig. 2**). The diagnosis was reached based on presentation and ultrasound findings (Ravine criteria used, **Table 1**). He was educated regarding the increased risk of progression to CKD and ultimately ESRD requiring transplant and/or renal replacement therapy. Recommendations were made to follow closely with his PCP to monitor for the development of hypertension (at his return visit his BP measured 118/65), the need for routine evaluation of a metabolic panel to assess for the progression of CKD (CKD present because of anatomic diagnosis), and the importance of monitoring cholesterol levels (treating with a statin when indicated) as well as the risk for coronary vascular disease. The importance of hydration was emphasized (60 to 90 oz of water daily), and a handout

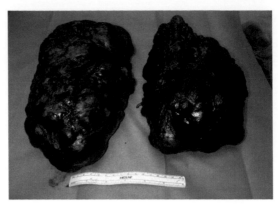

Fig. 2. Polycystic kidneys removed from a patient with APKD. (*Courtesy of* Alex Gilbert, MD, Medstar Georgetown University Hospital; with permission.)

regarding lifestyle modifications necessary to preserve kidney function was provided (**Box 1**). Smoking cessation was encouraged and he was provided with resources.

ADPKD, the most common inherited cause of kidney disease, affects 4 to 6 million people worldwide and occurs equally in men and women across all ethnic groups.[2,3] Despite the fact that abnormal kidney cyst development is thought to start in utero, most patients do not have noticeable symptoms for many years, with half of patients remaining asymptomatic and undiagnosed during their lifetime.[4] The average age for

Table 1		
Ravine ultrasound criteria for diagnosis of ADPKD		
Age (y)	**Positive Family History**	**Negative Family History**
<30	At least 2 in 1 or both kidneys	At least 5
30–59	At least 2 in each kidney	At least 5
>60	At least 4 in each kidney	At least 8

Box 1
CKD education

1. Keep your BP less than 130/80 or preferably less than 125/75.

2. Goal cholesterol: Use statin medications when indicated.
   a. Low-density lipoprotein less than 80
   b. Triglyceride less than 150
   c. High-density lipoprotein greater than 45

3. Eat less animal protein (pork, beef, chicken, and fish) (about 70 g/d that is size of a deck of cards) and stay well-hydrated.

4. Follow a low-calorie diet and increase physical activity to achieve/maintain a healthy weight.

5. Follow a low-salt diet (<2000 mg/d).

6. Do not smoke.

7. Do not take nonsteroidal antiinflammatory drugs (naproxen [Aleve], ibuprofen [Advil], piroxicam [Feldene], acetaminophen/aspirin/caffeine [Excedrin], and so forth).
   a. *It is ok* to take acetaminophen if you do not have any liver problems.

8. Follow up with your medical providers.

onset of symptoms is 42 to 56 years of age depending on the type of ADPKD.[5] Although family history is known by some patients, often the variable symptoms within a family means that ADPKD may not be known by all members of that family. Suspicion must be high in a patient who presents with hematuria and hypertension, the two most common symptoms of ADPKD.

CASE STUDY 2
History of Present Illness

A 38-year-old Caucasian man presents to his PCP's office on Monday with a history of red urine and sore throat over the weekend; both symptoms have since resolved. He has also noted swelling of his feet and ankles over the last month, and it is his concern with the swelling that brought him to the clinic. There is no complaint of pain with this edema, and he has not recently traveled any distance or had a change in his activity level. He does mention that each time he gets sick, such as the sore throat over the weekend, he notes red urine.

Social History

Married: lives with his wife and 2 children
Alcohol: none
Tobacco: none
Drugs: nothing illicit
Employed full time: teacher

Past Medical History

He has stage 1 hypertension, and the current treatment is lifestyle modifications.

Family History

His parents are alive and without chronic medical conditions. He has 3 brothers, all healthy. He has a daughter and son, both healthy.

Physical Examination

Vitals
The vitals are as follows: BP 152/94, HR 76 (regular), R 16 (nonlabored), weight 86 kg (189.2 lb).

General
The patient is in no distress and capable of full communication without difficulty. The patient is polite and cooperative, appropriately dressed, and of normal hygiene.

Heent
Head is of expected size and shape without irregularity or evidence of trauma. Eyes are anicteric, with intact extra ocular movements and pupils that are equal, round and reactive to light and accommodation. Ears demonstrate no abnormal external appearance and the tympanic membranes are healthy in appearance without perforation or evidence of infection. The oropharynx is without lesion of mucosa. The pharynx rises symmetrically without exudate.

Neck
There are no nodes or thyromegaly, and no bruit is auscultated.

Heart
The heart has a regular rate and rhythm. There are no murmurs, gallops, or rubs noted.

Lungs

The lungs are clear to auscultation bilaterally. There is no expiratory wheeze. There are no accessory muscles of respiration noted.

Abdomen

The abdomen is nontender to palpation. There is no hepatosplenomegaly or mass. There are normal bowel sounds in all 4 quadrants. He is overweight.

Extremities

There is no neurovascular compromise. There is no cyanosis or clubbing. There is 2 + pitting edema bilaterally of the lower extremities, which is greatest over the pretibial region. There is no abnormal limb length.

Differential Diagnosis

1. Poststreptococcal glomerulonephritis
2. End-organ hypertensive nephropathy
3. IgA nephropathy

Laboratory Evaluation

CBC		
	Current Value	Normal Range
WBC	6.5	3.5–10.5 × 10(9)/L
Hgb	13.5	12.0–15.5 g/dL
Hct	40.5	34.9%–44.5%
RBC	4.6	3.90–5.03 × 10(12)/L
MCV	86.2	81.6–98.3 fL
RDW	13	11.9%–15.5%
Platelet	355	150–450 × 10(9)/L

Abbreviations: CBC, complete blood count; Hct, hematocrit; Hgb, hemoglobin; MCV, mean corpus volume; RBC, red blood cell; WBC, white blood cell.

Basic metabolic panel		
	Current Value	Normal Range
Sodium	138	135–145 mmol/L
Potassium	4.3	3.5–5.1 mmol/L
Chloride	102	98–107 mmol/L
CO_2	24	22–29 mmol/L
AGAP	12	7–15 mmol/L
Glucose	123	70–140 mg/dL
Creatinine	**1.4**	0.6–1.1 mg/dL
GFR (MDRD)	**58**	≥60 mL/min
GFR African American (MDRD)	—	≥60 mL/min
BUN	22	6–24 mg/dL
Calcium	9.2	8.8–10.3 mg/dL

Abbreviations: BUN, serum urea nitrogen; CO_2, carbon dioxide; MDRD, modification of diet in renal disease.

Urinalysis with micro		
	Current Value	Normal Range
UA source	Clean catch	—
UA color	Yellow	—
UA clarity	Clear	—
UA specific gravity	1.005	1.005–1.030
UA pH	5	4.6–8.0
UA protein	2+	Negative mg/dL
UA glucose	Negative	Negative mg/dL
UA ketones	Negative	Negative mg/dL
UA bilirubin	Negative	Negative
UA urobilinogen	Negative	Negative
UA blood	**Trace**	Negative
UA nitrite	Negative	Negative
UA Leuk Est	Negative	Negative
UA WBC	None seen	—
UA RBC	**10–20**	—
UR % dysmorphic RBC	None seen	—
UR squamous Epi cells	None seen	—
UR bacteria	None seen	—
UR crystals	None seen	—
RBC casts	2	—

Abbreviations: RBC, red blood cell; WBC, white blood cell.

Radiology Evaluation

Renal ultrasound

Renal ultrasound demonstrated no evidence of hydronephrosis or nephrolithiasis, a negative renal ultrasound.

Discussion

Because of the presence of hematuria, a renal ultrasound was ordered with results as stated. Given the presence of uncontrolled hypertension and pedal edema, treatment was initiated with an angiotensin-converting enzyme inhibitor (ACEi) and diuretic. The patient was referred to nephrology for further evaluation of hematuria and proteinuria.

Nephrology evaluation

Additional evaluation included the following:

- Urine and serum protein electrophoresis (UPEP and SPEP, respectively) were obtained to provide further analysis of the protein.
- There was 3.5 g proteinuria noted on UPEP. No abnormal proteins or M-spike were noted on either UPEP or SPEP.

Immunologic evaluation including the following:

- Hepatitis B and C serology: negative
- Anti–glomerular basement membrane (GBM): negative

- Antineutrophil cytoplasmic autoantibody (ANCA): negative
- Complements (C3 and C4): within normal range

Renal biopsy (performed because of amount of proteinuria, reoccurrence of symptoms, and lack of diagnosis from laboratory testing) revealed IgA nephropathy (**Figs. 3** and **4**).

Clinical manifestations of IgA nephropathy include microscopic hematuria and usually mild proteinuria, sometimes with one or more bouts of gross hematuria associated with acute mucosal infections and an indolent, slowly progressive course.[6] The course of progression can be more rapid in the setting of persistent proteinuria greater than 1 g. IgA nephropathy is characterized morphologically by IgA deposition in the glomerular mesangium. IgA nephropathy is recognized as the most common primary glomerulonephritis in the world and initially was thought to be a benign condition; however, it is now the second or third most common primary glomerulonephritis to result in ESRD in many areas of the world.[7]

Current treatment options for IgA nephropathy are limited and include nonimmunosuppressive and immunosuppressive therapies. Nonimmunosuppressive therapies that have been shown to slow the progression of IgA nephropathy include ACEi or angiotensin II receptor blockers (ARBs), with slowing of CKD progression independent of the effect of these agents on blood pressure. KDIGO clinical practice guidelines for glomerulonephritis reflect the importance of using ACEi or ARBs. Immunosuppressive agents include corticosteroids, which are first-line therapy in patients with significant proteinuria (>1 g/d) after 6 months of conservative therapy and preserved kidney function.[8] Oral cyclophosphamide in addition to corticosteroids can be used as well, especially in the setting of persistent proteinuria, and is a common course of therapy in many practices.[9]

The case patient followed up with his PCP about 1 month later; his BP was improving (130/80) on lisinopril 40 mg and furosemide 20 mg daily. Repeat urine protein, as requested by the nephrologist, demonstrated a reduction in proteinuria, 1.75 g from 3.5 g. In collaboration with the consulting nephrologist, the patient was then started on therapy with prednisone for 6 months and cyclophosphamide for the next year because of the persistence of proteinuria measuring greater than 1 g and the nature of disease progression when protein measurements exceed 1 g. At his 1-year return visit to nephrology, his urine protein demonstrated a reduction to less than 1 g.

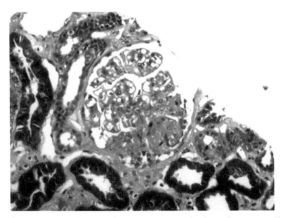

Fig. 3. Glomerulus from case with prominent segmental sclerosis responsible for proteinuria in patient (Masson trichrome stain, original magnification × 20).

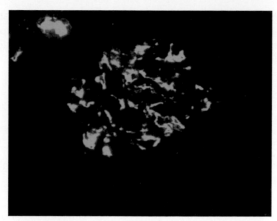

Fig. 4. Staining for IgA within glomerulus on direct immunofluorescence (Mesangial granular staining, original magnification × 20).

CASE STUDY 3
History of Present Illness

A 48-year-old obese black woman presents to the clinic with a complaint of progressive leg swelling over the last 6 months. She denies travel within the last 6 months and has not noted fevers or other symptoms of illness. On further questioning, she recalls noting her urine appearing frothy over the last 1 to 2 years without change in color or the presence of painful urination or blood in her urine.

Social History

Married: 2 children
Tobacco: never
Alcohol: none
Drugs: none
Employment: full time, lawyer

Past Medical History

There is a negative medical history.

Family History

There is a negative family history.

Physical Examination

Vitals
The vitals are as follows: temperature 36°C (96.8°F), BP 170/98, HR 82 (regular), R 18 (nonlabored), weight 98 kg (215.6 lb), height 142.24 cm (56 inches), body mass index (BMI) 48.4.

General
The patient is in no distress and is capable of full communication without difficulty. The patient is polite and cooperative, appropriately dressed, and of normal hygiene.

Heent
Head is of expected size and shape without irregularity or evidence of trauma. Eyes are anicteric, with intact extra ocular movements and pupils that are equal, round

and reactive to light and accommodation. Ears demonstrate no abnormal external appearance and the tympanic membranes are healthy in appearance without perforation or evidence of infection. The oropharynx is without lesion of mucosa. The pharynx rises symmetrically without exudate.

Neck
There are no nodes and no thyromegaly. No bruit is auscultated.

Heart
The hear has a regular rate and rhythm. There are no murmurs, gallops, or rubs noted.

Lungs
The lungs are clear to auscultation bilaterally. There is no expiratory wheeze. No accessory muscles of respiration are noted.

Abdomen
The abdomen is nontender to palpation. There is no hepatosplenomegaly or mass. There are normal bowel sounds in all 4 quadrants. The patient is morbidly obese.

Extremities
There is no neurovascular compromise. There is no cyanosis or clubbing. There is 3 + pitting edema bilaterally of the lower extremities. There is no abnormal limb length.

Differential Diagnosis

1. Minimal change disease
2. Membranous nephropathy
3. FSGS
4. Hypertensive nephrosclerosis

Laboratory Evaluation

Comprehensive metabolic panel		
	Current Value	Normal Range
Sodium	137	135–145 mmol/L
Potassium	4.3	3.5–5.1 mmol/L
Chloride	102	98–107 mmol/L
CO_2	27	22–29 mmol/L
AGAP	8	7–15 mmol/L
Glucose	135	70–140 mg/dL
Creatinine	1.6	0.6–1.1 mg/dL
GFR (MDRD)	—	≥60 mL/min
GFR African American (MDRD)	45.16	≥60 mL/min
BUN	20	6–24 mg/dL
Calcium	9	8.8–10.3 mg/dL
Protein	7	6.3–7.9 g/dL
Albumin	4	3.5–5.2 g/dL
AST	12	8–43 U/L
ALT	9	7–45 U/L
Bili total	0.8	≤1.2 mg/dL

Abbreviations: ALT, alanine transaminase; AST, aspartate transaminase; Bili, total bilirubin; BUN, serum urea nitrogen; CO_2, carbon dioxide; MDRD, modification of diet in renal disease.

CBC		
	Current Value	Normal Range
WBC	4.2	3.5–10.5 × 10(9)/L
Hgb	12.4	12.0–15.5 g/dL
Hct	37.2	34.9%–44.5%
RBC	4.2	3.90–5.03 × 10(12)/L
MCV	85	81.6–98.3 fL
RDW	12.3	11.9%–15.5%
Platelet	287	150–450 × 10(9)/L

Abbreviations: CBC, complete blood count; Hct, hematocrit; Hgb, hemoglobin; MCV, mean corpus volume; RBC, red blood cell; WBC, white blood cell.

UA with micro		
	Current Value	Normal Range
UA source	Clean catch	—
UA color	Yellow	—
UA clarity	**Frothy**	—
UA specific gravity	1.008	1.005–1.030
UA pH	5	4.6–8.0
UA protein	**4+**	Negative mg/dL
UA glucose	Negative	Negative mg/dL
UA ketones	Negative	Negative mg/dL
UA bilirubin	Negative	Negative
UA urobilinogen	Negative	Negative
UA blood	Negative	Negative
UA nitrite	Negative	Negative
UA Leuk Est	Negative	Negative
UA WBC	None	—
UA RBC	None	—
UR % dysmorphic RBC	None	—
UR squamous Epi cells	None	—
UR bacteria	None	—
UR crystals	None	—

Abbreviations: RBC, red blood cell; WBC, white blood cell.

Random urine protein: 12 g.

Radiology Evaluation

Renal ultrasound
Renal ultrasound demonstrated no evidence of hydronephrosis or nephrolithiasis; the kidneys were normal size, and the renal ultrasound was negative.

Discussion
1. The patient was referred to nephrology for further evaluation because of the significant proteinuria noted on spot urine in the presence of pedal edema.

2. While waiting for the nephrology appointment, the following medications were begun in the setting of elevated BP readings, noted CKD 3, and proteinuria:
   a. Lisinopril 20 mg daily
   b. Furosemide 20 mg daily
3. At the patient's 1-month follow-up with the PCP, her BP improved to 150/80, at which time her lisinopril was increased to 40 mg daily, her furosemide was increased to 20 mg twice daily, and diltiazem 120 mg daily was started.
4. At the 2-month follow-up with the PCP, her BP was 130/90 with persistent edema; therefore, furosemide was increased to 40 mg twice daily and diltiazem was further increased to 240 mg daily; the lisinopril dose remained at 40 mg daily.

Nephrology Evaluation

Repeat random urine protein.

- 8 g proteinuria, reduced from 12 g initially

Immunologic evaluation including the following:

- Hepatitis B and C serology: negative
- Anti-GBM: negative
- ANCA: negative
- Complements (C3 and C4): within normal range

Renal biopsy (performed because of the amount of proteinuria and lack of diagnosis) revealed FSGS (**Fig. 5**).

In FSGS, there is scarring present in some of the glomeruli. Most often no specific cause can be identified; however, human immunodeficiency virus (HIV) infection, obesity, sickle cell disease, birth defects of the kidney, drug use (such as heroin), and rarely genetic causes can cause FSGS. Left untreated, FSGS can result in kidney failure.[10] FSGS has become one of the leading causes of nephrotic syndrome in adults, especially in African Americans.[11] In patients with FSGS who have proteinuria, the initial therapy consists of optimal BP control using ACEi or ARBs and conservative therapy, such as weight loss, dietary modifications, and so forth. For those patients who remain nephrotic despite a conservative course, therapy with prednisone and other immunosuppressive agents is indicated.[11]

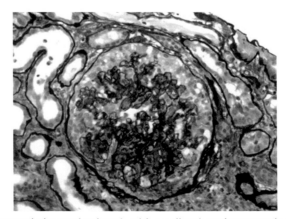

Fig. 5. Focal segmental glomerulosclerosis with a collapsing phenotype in patient. Note the prominent wrinkling and collapsing sclerosis of capillary walls. Epithelial cells are enlarged and increased in number (Jones Silver stain, original magnification × 20).

The patient was followed by nephrology and her PCP, and 6 months from diagnosis proteinuria reduced to 6 g. Treatment options at that time included weight loss or initiation of steroids and cyclophosphamide. The patient elected weight loss, and at her 1-year appointment her BMI had decreased to 38 and proteinuria measured 4 g. She continued with weight loss as she did not want to take steroids or cytotoxic medications, and at her 2-year appointment her BMI was 33 and her proteinuria reduced to 2.8 g.

CASE STUDY 4
History of Present Illness

A 26-year-old black woman presents to the clinic with a history of a facial rash and leg swelling that she has noticed over the last year. The rash and swelling are not constant, but she thinks they are both occurring more often and are more noticeable. She also mentions 1 to 2 episodes of blood in her urine not related to menses. She has otherwise felt well without significant fatigue or fevers or other symptoms of illness.

Social History

Married: one child
Tobacco: never
Alcohol: none
Drugs: none
Employment: full time

Past Medical History

1. She had preeclampsia with her pregnancy and progressively elevated BPs; however, these resolved on delivery. During her pregnancy, there were no seizures or eclampsia.
2. Left lower leg deep vein thrombosis following a car trip from New York to Chicago about 2 years prior. She presented to her PCP with leg swelling at that time. It was treated with baby aspirin without recurrence.

Family History

There is a negative family history; her parents are alive and well, and she has 3 siblings without health issues.

Physical Examination

Vitals
The vitals are as follows: BP 155/95, HR 78 (regular), R 18 (nonlabored), dioxygen 98%, BMI 21.

General
The patient is in no distress and capable of full communication without difficulty. The patient is polite and cooperative, appropriately dressed, and of normal hygiene.

Heent
Head is of expected size and shape without irregularity or evidence of trauma. Eyes are anicteric, with intact extra ocular movements and pupils that are equal, round and reactive to light and accommodation. Ears demonstrate no abnormal external appearance and the tympanic membranes are healthy in appearance without perforation or evidence of infection. The oropharynx is without lesion of mucosa. The pharynx rises symmetrically without exudate. There is a slightly reddened rash noted along the cheeks bilaterally, across the bridge of her nose but sparing the nasolabial folds. The rash is well demarcated and macular in appearance.

Neck
There are no nodes or thyromegaly. No bruit is auscultated.

Heart
The heart has a regular rate and rhythm. There are no murmurs, gallops, or rubs noted.

Lungs
The lungs are clear to auscultation bilaterally. There is no expiratory wheeze. No accessory muscles of respiration are noted.

Abdomen
The abdomen is slender and nontender to palpation. There is no hepatosplenomegaly or mass. There are normal bowel sounds in all 4 quadrants.

Extremities
There is no neurovascular compromise. There is no cyanosis, clubbing, or edema. There is no abnormal limb length.

Differential Diagnosis

1. Lupus erythematosus with nephritis
2. Pellagra
3. Dermatomyositis

Laboratory Evaluation

CBC		
	Current Value	**Normal Range**
WBC	4.5	$3.5–10.5 \times 10(9)$/L
Hgb	12.8	12.0–15.5 g/dL
Hct	38.4	34.9%–44.5%
RBC	4.3	$3.90–5.03 \times 10(12)$/L
MCV	85	81.6–98.3 fL
RDW	13.2	11.9%–15.5%
Platelet	225	$150–450 \times 10(9)$/L

Abbreviations: CBC, complete blood count; Hct, hematocrit; Hgb, hemoglobin; MCV, mean corpus volume; RBC, red blood cell; WBC, white blood cell.

BMP		
	Current Value	**Normal Range**
Sodium	137	135–145 mmol/L
Potassium	3.8	3.5–5.1 mmol/L
Chloride	99	98–107 mmol/L
CO_2	26	22–29 mmol/L
AGAP	12	7–15 mmol/L
Glucose	98	70–140 mg/dL
Creatinine	**1.5**	0.6–1.1 mg/dL
GFR (MDRD)	—	$\geq$60 mL/min
GFR African American (MDRD)	**48.03**	$\geq$60 mL/min
BUN	22	6–24 mg/dL
Calcium	9.8	8.8–10.3 mg/dL

Abbreviations: BMP, basic metabolic panel; BUN, serum urea nitrogen; CO_2, carbon dioxide; MDRD, modification of diet in renal disease.

Erythrocyte sedimentation rate (ESR) – 89
Antinuclear antibody (ANA) – 4.2

UA with micro		
	Current Value	**Normal Range**
UA source	Clean catch	—
UA color	Yellow	—
UA clarity	Clear	—
UA specific gravity	1.03	1.005–1.030
UA pH	5	4.6–8.0
UA protein	**3+**	Negative mg/dL
UA glucose	Negative	Negative mg/dL
UA ketones	Negative	Negative mg/dL
UA bilirubin	Negative	Negative
UA urobilinogen	Negative	Negative
UA blood	Negative	Negative
UA nitrite	Negative	Negative
UA Leuk Est	Negative	Negative
UA WBC	None	None
UA RBC	**5–10**	Negative
UR % dysmorphic RBC	None	—
UR squamous Epi cells	None	None
UR bacteria	None	None
UR crystals	None	None
UA casts	**+ RBC**	None

Abbreviations: RBC, red blood cell; WBC, white blood cell.

Discussion

1. Treatment of hypertension was initiated with lisinopril 20 mg daily and furosemide 20 mg daily following a detailed discussion regarding the need to continue taking her oral contraceptives given the contraindications to the use of ACEi agents in pregnancy after the first trimester.
2. She was referred to nephrology because of abnormal laboratory results; lupus antibodies were pending at the time of referral.

Nephrology Evaluation

Additional laboratory studies included the following:

- dsDNA: 85 IU/mL
- Compliment levels (C3 and C4): 70 mg/dL and 10 mg/dL, respectively
- Hepatitis B and C antibodies: negative
- HIV: negative
- Random urine protein: 4g

Renal ultrasound was ordered and returned without any abnormality noted.

Hypertension agent changed because of development of angioedema from lisinopril. Diltiazem was initiated, but the patient developed heart block; therefore, nifedipine was introduced and BP improved to 130/80.

At the 3-month nephrology follow-up visit, the patient gained 5 lb and BP is nicely controlled at 112/78; unfortunately, proteinuria increased to 5 g on repeat random urine protein analysis. Biopsy is performed and reveals membranous lupus nephritis (**Figs. 6** and **7**).

Treatment was initiated with oral prednisone and cyclophosphamide.

Discussion occurred regarding future pregnancies; given history of preeclampsia with her first pregnancy, her kidney function needs to be closely monitored. If her creatinine would increase to greater than 1.5, her risk for repeat preeclampsia is greater.

The exact cause of systemic lupus erythematosus (SLE) is not clear, but there have been several genetic and environmental factors implicated. SLE can have varying ranges of kidney involvement from mild to severe and occurs in 50% to 70% of patients with lupus.[12] SLE is increasing in incidence and prevalence, with a higher percentage of African Americans and those of African Caribbean descent being affected. Women are affected more often than men, especially those of childbearing age.[13] A predictor of the development of lupus nephritis is the presence of anti–double-stranded DNA antibodies (dsDNA).[13] Research demonstrates that the presence of dsDNA antibodies and tissue deposition of immune complexes (some trapped passively in the glomeruli, others attached directly to the glomerular structure) results in glomerulonephritis.[14] Several different clinical manifestations of lupus nephritis have been reported, with proteinuria and nephrotic syndrome as dominant features. Nephrotic syndrome can occur with or without kidney function impairment. Microscopic hematuria is almost always noted but rarely isolated; macroscopic hematuria is rare.[14]

Lupus nephritis is currently classified using the International Society of Nephrology/Renal Pathology Society/2003 system (**Table 2**), which incorporates a revision of modifications around activity and chronicity. The treatment of lupus nephritis depends on the class identified. The aim of induction therapy is to achieve rapid clinical remission, which is associated with an improved long-term prognosis. The aim of maintenance therapy is to maintain remission of renal manifestations without increasing morbidity for patients. Oral corticosteroids, along with oral (and at times intravenous) cyclophosphamide, are fairly standard as the combination improves kidney outcomes over corticosteroids alone and allows for lower recurrence rates.[14] There have been

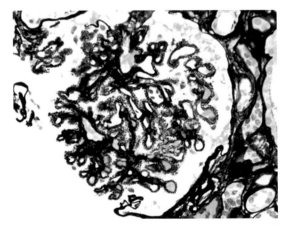

Fig. 6. Lupus membranous glomerulonephritis (class V lupus nephritis). Note the extreme capillary loop thickening and spiking (Jones Silver stain, original magnification × 40).

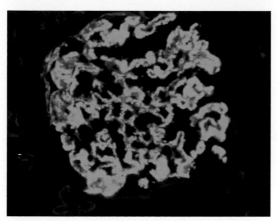

Fig. 7. Granular capillary wall C1q staining on direct immunofluorescence (IgG direct immunofluorescence × 40). The presence of C1q supports lupus nephritis.

studies looking at the use of antimalarial agents (such as hydroxychloroquine) as well as how to evaluate response criteria, such as urine sediment; however, there is no consensus between nephrologists and rheumatologists regarding use and monitoring.[10]

Table 2 Activity and chronicity index	
Activity Index	**Chronicity Index**
Glomerular abnormalities	
1. Cellular proliferation	1. Glomerular sclerosis
2. Fibrinoid necrosis, karyorrhexis	2. Fibrous crescents
3. Cellular crescents	
4. Hyaline thrombi, wire loops	
5. Leukocyte infiltration	
Tubulointerstitial abnormalities	
1. Mononuclear cell infiltrates	1. Interstitial fibrosis
	2. Tubular atrophy

CASE STUDY 5
History of Present Illness

A 28-year-old Caucasian man presents to the clinic for a follow-up after an emergency department (ED) visit. The patient was seen over the weekend with a complaint of severe left flank pain for 3 days with notable bloody urine. At the time of clinical follow-up, the symptoms have resolved; he denies additional complaints, such as painful urination, fever, chills, or discharge from the penis.

Social History

Single: no children
Tobacco: never
Alcohol: none
Drugs: none
Employment: dairy farmer
Soda: 6 cans of cola daily

Past Medical History

He has a negative medical history.

Medications

The medications include the following: vitamin C supplement 1000 mg daily, fish oil 1000 mg daily, and coenzyme Q 10 1 tablet daily.

Family History

His mother has a positive history of kidney stones, and his father has coronary artery disease.

Physical Examination

Vitals

The vitals are as follows: BP 120/80, HR 72 (regular), R 16 (nonlabored), weight 90.9 kg (199.98 lb).

General

The patient is in no distress and capable of full communication without difficulty. The patient is polite and cooperative, appropriately dressed, and of normal hygiene.

Heent

Head is of expected size and shape without irregularity or evidence of trauma. Eyes are anicteric, with intact extra ocular movements and pupils that are equal, round and reactive to light and accommodation. Ears demonstrate no abnormal external appearance and the tympanic membranes are healthy in appearance without perforation or evidence of infection. The oropharynx is without lesion of mucosa. The pharynx rises symmetrically without exudate.

Neck

There are no nodes or no thyromegaly. No bruit is auscultated.

Heart

The heart has a regular rate and rhythm. There are no murmurs, gallops, or rubs noted.

Lungs

The lungs are clear to auscultation bilaterally. There is no expiratory wheeze. No accessory muscles of respiration are noted.

Abdomen

The abdomen is nontender to palpation. There is no hepatosplenomegaly or mass. There are normal bowel sounds in all 4 quadrants.

Genitalia/rectum

The patient has normal external male genitalia. The patient is previously circumcised. A prostate examination was not done. The anus appears normal.

Extremities

There is no neurovascular compromise. There is no cyanosis, clubbing, or edema. There is no abnormal limb length.

Differential Diagnosis

1. Trauma: injury on the farm
2. Nephrolithiasis

Laboratory Evaluation

BMP		
	Current Value	Normal Range
Sodium	136	135–145 mmol/L
Potassium	3.8	3.5–5.1 mmol/L
Chloride	99	98–107 mmol/L
CO_2	23	22–29 mmol/L
AGAP	14	7–15 mmol/L
Glucose	82	70–140 mg/dL
Creatinine	1.0	0.6–1.1 mg/dL
GFR (MDRD)	>60	≥60 mL/min
GFR African American (MDRD)	—	≥60 mL/min
BUN	22	6–24 mg/dL
Calcium	8.9	8.8–10.3 mg/dL

Abbreviations: BMP, basic metabolic panel; BUN, serum urea nitrogen; CO_2, carbon dioxide; MDRD, modification of diet in renal disease.

CBC		
	Current Value	Normal Range
WBC	4.3	3.5–10.5 × 10(9)/L
Hgb	14.8	12.0–15.5 g/dL
Hct	44	34.9%–44.5%
RBC	4.7	3.90–5.03 × 10(12)/L
MCV	95	81.6–98.3 fL
RDW	13	11.9%–15.5%
Platelet	350	150–450 × 10(9)/L

Abbreviations: CBC, complete blood count; Hct, hematocrit; Hgb, hemoglobin; MCV, mean corpus volume; RBC, red blood cell; WBC, white blood cell.

UA		
	Current Value	Normal Range
UA source	Clean catch	—
UA color	Yellow	—
UA clarity	Clear	—
UA specific gravity	1.007	1.005–1.030
UA pH	4.9	4.6–8.0
UA protein	Negative	Negative mg/dL
UA glucose	Negative	Negative mg/dL
UA ketones	Negative	Negative mg/dL
UA bilirubin	Negative	Negative
UA urobilinogen	Negative	Negative

(continued on next page)

(continued)		
	Current Value	Normal Range
UA blood	Negative	Negative
UA nitrite	Negative	Negative
UA Leuk Est	Negative	Negative
UA WBC	Negative	—
UA RBC	Negative	—
UR % dysmorphic RBC	Negative	—
UR squamous Epi cells	Negative	—
UR bacteria	Negative	—
UR crystals	Negative	—

Abbreviations: RBC, red blood cell; WBC, white blood cell.

Radiology Evaluation

Kidney, ureter, and bladder
A 2-mm opacity was noted in each kidney consistent with kidney stones (done in the ED).

Discussion

A referral was made to nephrology based on the family history of nephrolithiasis and presentation in the ED.

Nephrolithiasis (kidney stones) is a common condition. There are a variety of types of kidney stones, and the cause depends on the type of stone identified. Some stones are familial; others can form if the urine contains too much of a specific substance, which results in the formation of crystals. The formation of kidney stones usually occurs over time, from weeks to months. The most common stone is a calcium stone, in which calcium often combines with other substances to form the stones, such as phosphate, carbonate, or oxalate. Uric acid stones are more common in men than women and can occur in the presence (or absence) of gout as well as with chemotherapy. Of the familial stones, cystine stones are the most common and form in those who have cystinuria. Struvite stones occur more often in women than men and are usually found in the presence of a urinary tract infection. Struvite stones can grow very large resulting in obstruction of the renal pelvis, ureter, or bladder.[15] Many times stones are composed of layers of different minerals with yet a different mineral core.

Risk factors for stone formation include not drinking enough water (the greatest risk factor) as well as diet composition and medications (OTC as well as prescribed). Treatment of nephrolithiasis depends on stone formation and the severity of symptoms. Increased hydration is recommended for all patients with stones: 3000 to 4000 mL daily in some practices, but 48 to 60 oz (1 oz = 30 mL) is a standard recommendation. Dietary modifications are recommended, again based on the stone type, and include oxalate reduction, reduction of sodium, and reduction of animal protein (to reduce sodium levels), to name a few. Medications prescribed include allopurinol for uric acid stones to reduces uric acid levels, thiazide diuretics as they help to reduce urinary excretion of calcium, and sodium citrate to increase citrate levels (although lemonade is much cheaper and often recommended first).[15,16] At times sodium bicarbonate is also prescribed if there is an acid-base correction needed (Figs. 8–10).

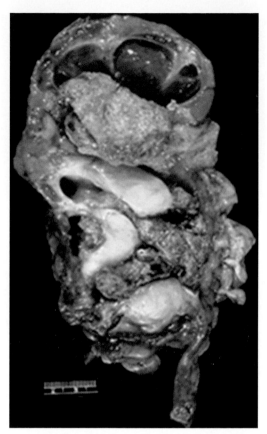

Fig. 8. Resected kidney containing large Staghorn calculus. (*Courtesy of* J. Charles Jennette, MD; with permission.)

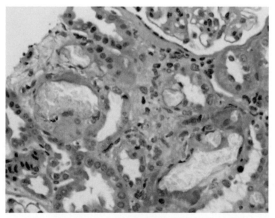

Fig. 9. Intratubular oxalate casts in renal biopsy (hematoxylin-eosin, original magnification × 40).

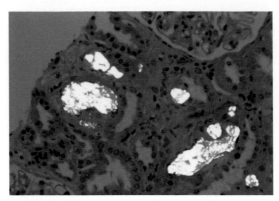

Fig. 10. Oxalate casts polarized (original magnification × 40).

Nephrology Evaluation

- Laboratory studies
  - Serum uric acid: 9.5 mg (3.5–7.2 mg)
  - 24-hour urine (**Table 3**)
- Radiology studies
  - Computed tomography (CT) abdomen stone protocol: 6 stones noted in each kidney

INITIAL RECOMMENDATIONS

1. Strain the urine to capture stone for analysis.
2. Increase hydration toward a goal of greater than 2 L of urine output daily.
3. Stop drinking dark sodas to help reduce oxalate level. Dark sodas contain significant levels of oxalate and are a major contributing factor to stone formation.
4. Decrease meat and sodium consumption in diet to help reduce the sodium level in urine.
5. Drink lemonade to improve citrate level in urine, which will help reduce stone formation.

Table 3 24-hour urine test results				
	Normal Range	Initial Results	Follow-up (3 mo)	Follow-up (6 mo)
Oxalate	20–40 mg/d	120 mg	60 mg	40 mg
Sodium	50–150 mmol/d	350 mmol	270 mmol	220 mmol
Calcium	M <250 mg/d F <200 mg/d	320 mg	250 mg	230 mg
Uric acid	M <0.800 g/d F <0.750 g/d	1.2 g	0.7 g	0.4 g
Protein	—	110 mg	110 mg	110 mg
Creatinine	—	1363.5 mg	1295 mg	1295 mg
Citrate	M >450 mg/d F >550 mg/d	280 mg	300 mg	300 mg
Total urine volume	—	1200 mL	1800 mL	2100 mL

Abbreviations: F, female; M, male.

6. Return to nephrology in 3 months with a repeat 24-hour urine study and laboratory work.
    ○ Laboratory results at the 3-month follow-up
        ▪ 24-hour urine (see **Table 3**)
        ▪ Serum uric acid 8.5 mg
        ▪ Stone analysis: uric acid core with calcium oxalate and calcium phosphate outer layers

TREATMENTS INITIATED

1. Potassium citrate 2 tablets twice daily: increase citrate levels
2. Allopurinol 300 mg daily: reduce uric acid levels
3. Hydrochlorothiazide 12.5 mg daily: reduce stone formation
4. Continue to increase hydration with water and lemonade
5. Focus on dietary calcium sources and avoid calcium supplements
6. A 6-month follow-up in nephrology
    ○ Repeat the 24-hour urine (see **Table 3**).
    ○ CT stone protocol: Reduction in size of stones was noted and 1 less stone identified.
    ○ The patient was advised to stop vitamin C supplement and follow up in 1 year.

CASE STUDY 6
History of Present Illness

A 56-year-old Native American woman with a history of scleroderma presents to the ED secondary to elevated BP readings. She has several specialists involved in her outpatient care working collaboratively with her PCP as she has noted an escalation in Raynaud-type symptoms over the last year. In the ED, her BP is 222/120 and laboratory work showed an increase in her creatinine to 4.0 mg/dL (baseline is 1.2–1.5 mg/dL). The patient reports she has not urinated for the last 36 hours. She is admitted for malignant hypertension management, and the attending hospitalist on duty happens to be her PCP.

Social History

Married: 3 children
Tobacco: never
Alcohol: none
Drugs: none
Employment: administrative assistant

Past Medical History

1. Gastroesophageal reflux disease: currently being evaluated for gastrointestinal involvement of scleroderma
2. Scleroderma

Family History

Her mother and sister have scleroderma and Raynaud disease, and her father has hypertension. Her children are healthy and without chronic medical disease.

Physical Examination

Vitals
The vitals are as follows: BP 180/100 (on a nitroprusside drip), HR 72 (regular), R 16 (nonlabored), weight 59 kg (129.8 lb).

General

The patient is in no distress and capable of full communication without difficulty. The patient is polite and cooperative, appropriately dressed, and of normal hygiene.

Heent

Head is of expected size and shape without irregularity or evidence of trauma. Eyes are anicteric, with intact extra ocular movements and pupils that are equal, round and reactive to light and accommodation. Ears demonstrate no abnormal external appearance and the tympanic membranes are healthy in appearance without perforation or evidence of infection. The oropharynx is without lesion of mucosa. The pharynx rises symmetrically without exudate. Tightening of the perioral skin is noted.

Neck

There are no nodes or no thyromegaly. No bruit is auscultated.

Heart

The heart has a regular rate and rhythm. There are no murmurs, gallops, or rubs noted.

Lungs

The lungs are clear to auscultation bilaterally. There is no expiratory wheeze. There are no accessory muscles of respiration noted.

Abdomen

The abdomen is nontender to palpation. There is no hepatosplenomegaly or mass. There are normal bowel sounds in all 4 quadrants.

Extremities

There is no neurovascular compromise. There is no cyanosis, clubbing, or edema. There is no abnormal limb length. Strictures are noted at the tips of the digits.

Differential Diagnosis

1. Hypertensive crisis
2. Acute renal failure of unknown cause
3. Scleroderma renal crisis

Laboratory Evaluation

BMP		
	Current Value	Normal Range
Sodium	136	135–145 mmol/L
Potassium	3.8	3.5–5.1 mmol/L
Chloride	99	98–107 mmol/L
CO_2	18	22–29 mmol/L
AGAP	14	7–15 mmol/L
Glucose	82	70–140 mg/dL
Creatinine	4.0	0.6–1.1 md/dL
GFR (MDRD)	12	≥60 mL/min
GFR African American (MDRD)	—	≥60 mL/min
BUN	80	6–24 mg/dL
Calcium	8.9	8.8–10.3 mg/dL

Abbreviations: BMP, basic metabolic panel; BUN, serum urea nitrogen; CO_2, carbon dioxide; MDRD, modification of diet in renal disease.

CBC		
	Current Value	**Normal Range**
WBC	**2.8**	3.5–10.5 × 10(9)/L
Hgb	**10.1**	12.0–15.5 g/dL
Hct	30	34.9%–44.5%
RBC	4.7	3.90–5.03 × 10(12)/L
MCV	95	81.6–98.3 fL
RDW	13	11.9%–15.5%
Platelet	**120**	150–450 × 10(9)/L

Abbreviations: CBC, complete blood count; Hct, hematocrit; Hgb, hemoglobin; MCV, mean corpus volume; RBC, red blood cell; WBC, white blood cell.

UA		
	Current Value	**Normal Range**
UA source	Clean catch	—
UA color	Yellow	—
UA clarity	Clear	—
UA specific gravity	1.007	1.005–1.030
UA pH	4.9	4.6–8.0
UA protein	**2+ (500 mg measured)**	Negative md/dL
UA glucose	Negative	Negative md/dL
UA ketones	Negative	Negative mg/dL
UA bilirubin	Negative	Negative
UA urobilinogen	Negative	Negative
UA blood	**Trace**	Negative
UA nitrite	Negative	Negative
UA Leuk Est	Negative	Negative
UA WBC	Negative	—
UA RBC	**3–5**	—
UR % dysmorphic RBC	Negative	—
UR squamous Epi cells	Negative	—
UR bacteria	Negative	—
UR crystals	Negative	—

Abbreviations: RBC, red blood cell; WBC, white blood cell.

Radiology Evaluation

The renal ultrasound was negative.

DISCUSSION

Given the history of scleroderma with increasing Raynaud symptoms and the hypertensive presentation, renal biopsy was performed, confirming the diagnosis of scleroderma renal crisis (**Fig. 11**).

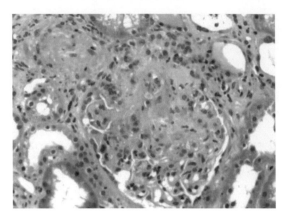

Fig. 11. Glomerulus from patient with scleroderma-renal crisis with typical thrombotic microangiopathic features. Notice how the glomerulus has a very swollen appearance that also involves the afferent arteriole (hematoxylin-eosin, original magnification × 20).

Treatment

1. High-dose ACEi reduced BP to 170/100, at which point nitroprusside was weaned off.
2. Diuretic therapy was initiated because of renal failure with oliguria; no improvement was noted, and the patient began hemodialysis in the hospital. Three months later, renal function improved, creatinine (Cr) 1.5. Hemodialysis was stopped, and ACEi therapy remains in place.

Scleroderma is a chronic connective tissue disease that is classified as local (skin alone) or systemic with impact on multiple organs, including the kidney. Scleroderma renal crisis occurs in those with systemic scleroderma, affecting about 5% to 10% of these patients. Presentation can include abrupt onset of hypertension, acute renal failure, fevers, malaise, headaches, encephalopathy, pulmonary edema, and hypertensive retinopathy.[17] Patients who have diffuse cutaneous forms or a rapidly progressing form of systemic scleroderma are at greatest risk for developing scleroderma renal crisis.[17] Aggressive and early initiation of ACEi therapy has been shown to improve prognosis, as ACEi have drastically improved the outcome for patients who develop scleroderma renal crisis. Unfortunately 40% of these patients may still require dialysis, and the 5-year mortality is about 30% to 40%.[17]

SUMMARY

Many other disease processes potentiate the development of CKD or accelerate its progression. The intent of this article is to increase awareness of some of these disease processes as well as improve the PCP's ability to identify changes in symptoms and laboratory results, prompting a referral to your local nephrology care team. The awareness of this potential and the implementation of a means to evaluate and diagnose the more unusual causes of CKD are important. You can never predict when one of the zebras will come along.

REFERENCES

1. Tuot DS, Plantinga LC, Hsu CY, et al. Chronic kidney disease awareness among individuals with clinical markers of kidney dysfunction. Clin J Am Soc Nephrol 2011;6(8):1838–44.

2. Nishiura JNR, Eloi S. Evaluation of nephrolithiasis in autosomal dominant polycystic kidney disease patients. Clin J Am Soc Nephrol 2009;4(4):838–44.
3. Srivastava APN. Autosomal dominant polycystic kidney disease. Am Fam Physician 2014;90(5):303–7.
4. Yoo DJ, Agodoa L, Yuan CM, et al. Risk of intracranial hemorrhage associated with autosomal dominant polycystic kidney disease in patients with end stage renal disease. BMC Nephrol 2014;15:39.
5. Igarashi PSS. Genetics and pathogenesis of polycystic kidney disease. J Am Soc Nephrol 2002;13(9):2384–98.
6. D'Amico G. Natural history of idiopathic IgA nephropathy: role of clinical and histological prognostic factors. Am J Kidney Dis 2000;36(2):227–37.
7. Lukasz P, Bartosik M, Lajoie G, et al. Predicting progression in IgA nephropathy. Am J Kidney Dis 2001;38(4):728–35.
8. Hogan J, Mohan P, Appel G. Diagnostic tests and treatment options in glomerular disease: 2014 update. Am J Kidney Dis 2014;63(4):656–66.
9. Roccatello D, Ferro M, Cesano G, et al. Steroid and cyclophosphamide in IgA nephropathy. Nephrol Dial Transplant 2000;15(6):833–5.
10. NephCure Foundation. Available at: www.Nephcure.org.
11. Korbet S. Treatment of primary FSGS in adults. J Am Soc Nephrol 2012;23(11): 1769–76.
12. Bose B, Silverman E, Bargman J. Ten common mistakes in the management of lupus nephritis. Am J Kidney Dis 2014;63(4):667–76.
13. Lisnevskaia L, Murphy G, Isenberg D. Systemic lupus erythematosus. Lancet 2014;384:1878–88.
14. Molino C, Fabbian F, Longhini C. Clinical approach to lupus nephritis: recent advances. Eur J Intern Med 2009;20:447–53.
15. Available at: http://www.nlm.nih.gov/medlineplus/ency/article/000458.htm.
16. Reilly R, Peixoto A, Desir G. The evidence-based use of thiazide diuretics in hypertension and nephrolithiasis. Clin J Am Soc Nephrol 2010;5(10):1893–903.
17. Denton CP, Lapadula G, Mouthon L, et al. Renal complications and scleroderma renal crisis. Rheumatology 2009;48(suppl 3):iii32–5.

Management of the Chronic Kidney Disease Patient

Denise K. Link, MPAS, PA-C

KEYWORDS

- Chronic kidney disease • Primary care • Angiotensin-converting enzyme inhibitor
- Angiotensin receptor blocker • Antihypertensive • Albuminuria

KEY POINTS

- Chronic kidney disease (CKD) is a deadly and progressive disease.
- Effectively treating CKD and reducing cardiovascular mortality is a challenging task that cannot be done by a sole provider. It requires a team effort in which the patient plays a large role.
- Screening all at-risk patients is paramount.
- As the number of nephrology providers decrease along with increase rates of incident CKD, the primary care clinician can be confident in modifying the disease progression and limiting cardiovascular mortality through: (1) aggressive hypertension treatment with multiple medications and intentional lifestyle changes to achieve recommended blood pressure targets; (2) using angiotensin converting enzyme inhibitor or angiotensin receptor blocker as the initial medication of choice in patients with albuminuria; (3) reduction in proteinuria through renin-angiotensin-aldosterone system blockade, along with adherence to reduction in dietary sodium intake; and (4) reduction of both traditional and nontraditional risk factors for cardiovascular disease.

The incidence of end-stage renal disease (ESRD) is increasing rapidly and resulting in more patients requiring renal replacement therapy (RRT), defined as kidney transplant, hemodialysis, and peritoneal dialysis. For patients who decline interventions, medical management is indicated.[1] Nearly 1 in 6 Americans will develop stage 3 to 5 kidney disease in their lifetime; by comparison, lifetime risk for diabetes, myocardial infarction, or invasive cancer is about 4 in 10.[2,3]

Although only 1% of the Medicare population has ESRD, this diagnosis accounted for 8.1% of the Medicare budget and $49.3 billion in total costs in 2011.[1] Diabetes is the leading cause of ESRD in patients in the United States, followed by hypertension (**Fig. 1**).[1]

The author has disclosed no potential conflicts of interest, financial or otherwise.
The University of Texas Southwestern Medical Center, Nephrology: Chronic Kidney Disease Clinic, 5939 Harry Hines Blvd Suite 700, Dallas, Tx 75390, USA
E-mail address: Denise.Link@utsw.edu

2405-7991/16/$ – see front matter © 2016 Elsevier Inc. All rights reserved.

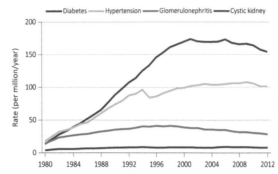

Fig. 1. CKD and diabetes, 1980 to 2012. Incident counts ESRD, by primary diagnosis. USRDS ESRD 2014. (*From* Saran R, Li Y, Robinson B, et al. US Renal Data System 2014 annual data report: epidemiology of kidney disease in the United States. Am J Kidney Dis. 2015;66(1)(suppl 1):S1–S306.)

Knowing this, clinicians should evaluate each at-risk patient for the potential development of chronic kidney disease (CKD), the precursor to ESRD. Although kidney transplant is the preferred treatment of patients with ESRD, with more than 100,000 people on the transplant list, dialysis or medical management is the answer for most patients. Dialysis treatments have made tremendous advances in prolonging the lives of patients with ESRD but take a physical, financial, and emotional toll on most patients, their families, and loved ones. For these reasons, evaluating kidney function is critical, especially in patients with CKD risk factors.

STEP 1: IDENTIFY PATIENTS AT RISK

Risk factors for developing CKD include[4]

- Age greater than 60 years
- Diabetes
- Hypertension
- Cardiovascular disease (CVD)
- Family history of CKD
- History of autoimmune disease
- History of recurrent urinary tract infections
- Nephrolithiasis
- Kidney cancer
- Systemic infections
- Abnormal serum creatinine (SCr), low glomerular filtration rate (GFR), or previous acute kidney injury (AKI)
- Transplant of any organ (due to the use of antirejection drugs, which are nephrotoxic).[2]

STEP 2: DIAGNOSIS

Using the accepted international definition developed by Kidney Disease Improving Global Outcomes (KDIGO) 2012 guidelines, CKD is present if 1 or more of the following criteria occur for more than 3 months:[2]

- A persistent and usually progressive reduction in GFR to less than 60 mL/min/ 1.73 m^2

- Albuminuria greater than or equal to 30 mg in 24 hours or urine albumin to creatinine ratio (UACR) greater than or equal to 30gm/g
- Urine sediment abnormalities (ie, hematuria or red cell casts)
- Electrolyte and other tubular disorders
- Histologic abnormalities
- Structural abnormalities (ie, polycystic kidneys) detected by imaging
- History of kidney transplantation.[2]

Kidney function is determined by calculating the GFR, which requires the patient's age, race, sex, and SCr level. Most laboratories report the GFR with the metabolic panel: normal is 90 mL/min or greater. The GFR approximates the percentage of remaining kidney function. That is, if the GFR is 40 mL/min, there is about 40% of kidney function remaining and, conversely, about 60% of kidney function has been irreversibly damaged. The kidneys age over time. The rate of decline in kidney function accelerates with advancing age, even without the presence of kidney disease; however, the aging kidney alone will rarely result in ESRD.[5] Normal age-related loss is 8 ml/min for each decade after the age of 40.[6] Thus, an 85-year-old African American woman with a GFR of 55 would be considered to have normal age-related loss of kidney function (8 mL/min × 4 decades, subtracted from 90).

The GFR and SCr are used to detect CKD and monitor remaining kidney function.[7] Many factors determine SCr independent of kidney function: muscle mass, dietary animal protein intake, use of certain medications (eg, trimethoprim, cimetidine), and the presence of liver disease. In patients with extremes in muscle mass and/or dietary animal protein intake, SCr will not accurately reflect kidney function. Thus, 2 patients with identical SCr values of 1.3 mg/dL may have significantly different kidney function. A male bodybuilder may have his GFR underestimated by SCr, whereas an 80-year-old thin white woman will be overestimated by the same formula. Although these formulas do not take into consideration the outliers, they are more precise than the SCr alone (**Table 1**).

CKD is a progressive disease but prompt intervention can often slow the march. CKD progression is based on factors that can be influenced by various treatments. Although most patients worry about requiring dialysis, in actuality less than 2% of patients with CKD will require RRT. This is likely due to the increased risk of death from cardiovascular causes before reaching ESRD.[8] In this day of electronic medical records, trends of any laboratory value can be graphically displayed. Monitor the trends, not just an individual GFR and/or SCr value to determine if CKD is stable or progressing. A SCr or GFR can be influenced by the amount and type of fluid consumed, medications, the diet (salt, protein), and outside factors (heat, exercise). Thus, a single reading is not enough to classify and/or stage a patient. A trend is more correct.

CKD staging is determined by GFR with prognosis determined by amount of albuminuria (**Fig. 2**).[2] Determining the stage of CKD anticipates when the patient will

Table 1 Glomerular filtration rate versus serum creatinine					
	SCr	Race	Age	GFR	CKD Stage
Male gender	1.5	Black	17	78	2
Male gender	1.5	Other	70	46	3a
Female gender	1.5	Black	17	48	3a
Female gender	1.5	White	70	35	3b

GFR calculator available at: https://www.kidney.org/professionals/KDOQI/gfr_calculator.

Prognosis of CKD by GFR and Albuminuria Categories: KDIGO 2012			Persistent albuminuria categories Description and range		
			A1	A2	A3
			Normal to mildly increased	Moderately increased	Severely increased
			<30 mg/g <3 mg/mmol	30–300 mg/g 3–30 mg/mmol	>300 mg/g >30 mg/mmol
GFR categories (ml/min/ 1.73 m²) Description and range	G1	Normal or high	≥90		
	G2	Mildly decreased	60–89		
	G3a	Mildly to moderately decreased	45–59		
	G3b	Moderately to severely decreased	30–44		
	G4	Severely decreased	15–29		
	G5	Kidney failure	<15		

Fig. 2. Prognosis of CKD by GFR and albuminuria category. Green: low risk (if no other markers of kidney disease, no CKD); Yellow: moderately increased risk; Orange: high risk; Red, very high risk. (*From* KDIGO 2012 clinical practice guideline for the evaluation and management of chronic kidney disease. Kidney Int Suppl 2013;3: p. 1–150; with permission. Available at: http://www.kdigo.org/clinical_practice_guidelines/pdf/CKD/KDIGO_2012_CKD_GL.pdf.)

develop signs of kidney dysfunction. The kidneys perform many functions: removing toxins from the blood, acid-base regulation, blood pressure (BP) control, fluid balance, maintaining normal hemoglobin through production of erythropoietin, regulation of vitamin D, and balance of minerals and electrolytes, including sodium, potassium, calcium, phosphorus, magnesium, and so forth. As CKD advances from stage 1 to 5, or even 5d (dialysis dependent), comorbid conditions will develop due to the loss of the kidneys' ability to perform these various functions. In early stage 1 or 2, hypertension usually develops. As early as stage 2, bone and mineral abnormalities may begin to surface; however, these abnormalities may not be reflected as abnormal laboratory values until stage 3.[9] In late stage 3 and early stage 4, evidence of anemia of CKD might begin to show. By stage 4, patients will need aggressive management of these comorbid conditions. Patients with CKD benefit from interdisciplinary care focusing on treatment of blood pressure, albuminuria, anemia, hyperphosphatemia, secondary hyperparathyroidism, hyperkalemia, and metabolic acidosis.[10,11]

KDIGO recommends referral to nephrologist for patients with CKD in the following circumstances[2]:

- AKI or abrupt, sustained fall in GFR
- GFR less than 30 ml/min
- Consistent albuminuria greater than 300 mg/g
- CKD progression defined as a sustained decline in estimated GFR (eGFR) of more than 5 mL/min/1.73 m2/y

- CKD and hypertension refractory to treatment with 4 or more antihypertensive agents
- Hereditary kidney disease
- Progression to kidney failure expected within 1 year.

It is essential that every patient with CKD start discussing and preparing for RRT when GFR is less than 30 ml/min; therefore, timely referral should be a major priority of the primary clinician. Late referral to kidney specialist is associated with worse health status at time of dialysis initiation and higher mortality after starting dialysis.[11]

STEP 3: PREDICTING PROGRESSION OF CHRONIC KIDNEY DISEASE—ALBUMINURIA

There are many proteins found in the urine, including serum globulins, albumin, and proteins secreted by the nephron. The terms proteinuria and albuminuria are often used interchangeably; however, they are not quite the same. Patients with early diabetic nephropathy can have normal GFR with microalbuminuria (UACR 30–300 mg/g) indicating kidney damage is occurring but has not yet impaired kidney function.[12] Microalbuminuria is UACR of 30 to 300 mg/g and macroalbuminuria is greater than 300 mg/g. Proteinuria is an indicator that kidney disease is present although transient or small amounts of protein can be also be found in healthy individuals. Albuminuria is specific to kidney disease. The amount of albuminuria is used for both diagnostic and prognostic indicators in managing CKD.[13–15] Albuminuria is pathognomonic for CKD and can occur before a decrease in GFR.

Albuminuria can be evaluated by 3 methods:

- Urine dipstick is a relatively crude quantification of urinary proteinuria and does not accurately determine the presence of microalbuminuria.[5,16] This test can detect multiple urinary proteins but the results can be affected by urine concentration or dilution.[16] Most kidney diseases lead to albuminuria except for rare exceptions; multiple myeloma and/or monoclonal gammopathy of undetermined significance (MGUS) produce nonalbumin urinary proteins that cannot be detected on urine dipstick. For this reason, a dipstick is often followed by a confirmatory and quantified urinalysis at the laboratory. If the urine dipstick is positive for proteinuria or to stage a patient with CKD, the albuminuria must be quantified.
- A 24-hour urine collection can quantify the total amount of total urinary proteins both in normal and pathognomonic parameters. Healthy adults normally excrete 80 to 150 mg of protein in the urine daily. A 24-hour urine collection can provide data on many kidney parameters and comorbidities, including total urinary sodium excretion and staging of CKD for those outliers described above. The accuracy of 24-hour urine test depends on adherence to proper collecting techniques including keeping specimens away from heat or sun exposure. Undercollection results in an underestimation of the true level of proteinuria, albuminuria, creatinine clearance, and sodium consumption. Due to inherent collection inaccuracies, 24-hour urine for total protein is not the preferred method for routine screening for albuminuria.
- A random or spot urine sample for UACR is the preferred method of screening for albuminuria and a spot total protein to creatinine ratio (UPCR) is the preferred study for proteinuria.[2,11,17] The UACR is especially useful for detecting microalbuminuria, which may be the only early clue to the development of CKD in a diabetic.[12] The National Kidney Disease Education Program (NKDEP) has many references for primary care providers focused on CKD diagnosis and management, including a quick reference for albuminuria: http://nkdep.nih.gov/resources/quick-reference-uacr-gfr.shtml.[18] UACR and UPCR are used to approximate the amount of albumin

and total urinary protein excreted in 24 hours. These ratios correct for the amount of dietary creatinine intake and standardize the collection; subsequently, a normal UACR is less than 30 mg/g and UPCR is less than 150 mg/g.

Following a screening algorithm allows both management of the albuminuric patient with CKD and reminds the practitioner of the importance of the UACR (**Fig. 3**). Once albuminuria is detected, repeat testing within 3 months ensures albuminuria is chronic and not transient. Benign proteinuria comes from various sources, including vigorous exercise, infections, fever, uncontrolled serum glucose, or stress.

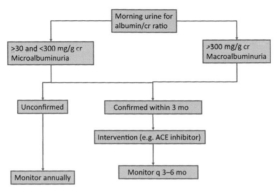

Fig. 3. Evaluation of proteinuria: based on presence of albuminuria. cr, creatinine; g cr, gram of creatinine.

STEP 4: TREATMENT STRATEGIES

Initially, the cause of CKD must be determined and treatment must be focused on the primary kidney disease.[19] Referral to nephrology may be necessary to determine the diagnosis. Although most patients have hypertension or diabetes as the cause of their CKD, there are other causes: glomerular, interstitial, genetic, or vascular disorders that should not be missed because they may be reversible. Immunosuppression may be the initial treatment of primary glomerular disorders, whereas diabetic CKD requires aggressive serum glucose control.

In addition to treating primary kidney disease, the following interventions have been shown to slow the progression of CKD and decrease cardiovascular mortality.

Treatment of Hypertension

Again and again, the evidence has shown that controlling blood pressure slows the rate of progression in CKD.[2,13–15,20] Although management is important, the goal blood pressure has evolved and multiple guidelines currently available do not match each other. Based on the 2002 Kidney Disease Outcomes Quality Initiative (KDOQI) guidelines, a target BP is less than 130/80 mm Hg.[17] Newer 2012 KDIGO and Eighth Joint National Committee (JNC 8) guidelines suggest relaxing early BP targets for most patients. KDIGO suggests a target less than 130/80 mm Hg in patients with albuminuria and less than 140/90 mm Hg in patients without albuminuria.[21] On Dec 10, 2015, KDIGO announced they will evaluate BP goals for CKD patients via a sub-analysis of the SPRINT data http://www.kdigo.org/News%20Release/SPRINT%20Trial%20News%20Release%202015.pdf. JNC 8 does not differentiate between patients with or without albuminuria but recommends a goal of less than 140/90 mm Hg for all patients with CKD.[22]

Selection of a first-line antihypertensive medication depends on the UACR to guide choice of therapy and goal of medication. Often a UACR is omitted but it is vital to staging and treatment in CKD.[1]

Based on the KDOQI and KDIGO guidelines, renin-angiotensin-aldosterone system (RAAS) blocking agent, angiotensin-converting enzyme inhibitor (ACEi), or angiotensin receptor blocker (ARB) drug classes are indicated as first-line therapy in patients who have CKD and albuminuria and those with kidney disease secondary to diabetes.[2,21] JNC 8 recommends ACEi or ARB drugs as initial or add-on therapy in patients with CKD.[22] Therapy should be tailored based on comorbidities with the main goal of achieving BP targets.

RAAS blocking agents are recommended over other drug classes due to their renal protective qualities which are independent of their antihypertensive effects.[23] In addition to reducing systemic hypertension, RAAS blocking agents also reduce glomerular hypertension and ameliorate glomerular sieving properties, thus reducing albuminuria.[24]

Patients need to take an active role in achieving BP targets. The first step is lifestyle modifications: reducing daily sodium intake, achieving modest weight loss, smoking cessation, limiting alcohol, and exercising. Eating a high sodium diet may decrease efficacy of antihypertension medications and the antiproteinuric effects of ACEi or ARB drugs.[25] It is imperative to teach patients with CKD the proper technique and importance of daily BP monitoring. Studies have noted that home BPs are more accurate than intermittent office readings.[26] Be sure that patients are aware of their BP targets.

In most cases of hypertension in a patient with CKD, a single agent will not be sufficient and most patients will require a multidrug regimen to achieve maximal kidney and cardiovascular protection.[9,26] To encourage medication adherence, prescribe once-daily dosing or combination drugs if possible.

Reduction of Albuminuria

Not only is albuminuria a marker and criteria for CKD, it also is a prognostic indicator.[13,15,20,27,28] The more albuminuria, the faster the rate of progression to kidney failure.[13,27,28] A patient with a normal GFR with albuminuria has a greater risk of progressing to kidney failure than a person with a GFR less than 60 mL/min without albuminuria.[29] Because albuminuria predicts progression, treatment is aimed at reducing albuminuria to slow the progression to kidney failure.

ACEi and ARB drugs have been shown to reduce albuminuria, leading to reduced rate of decline in GFR.[24,30–35] Additionally, ACEi and ARBs have been shown to reduce risk of CKD progression, CVD, and death, even when administered to patients with advanced CKD.[30,31] Reduction of albuminuria to less than 300 to 500 mg/d has been shown to slow progression of CKD.[36]

Observational data suggest weight loss, sodium restriction, and tobacco cessation may lower albuminuria.[11]

Albuminuria also is an independent risk factor for CVD and mortality in patients with and without CKD.[28,37,38]

Minimizing Risk of Cardiovascular Disease

The leading cause of death for patients with CKD is not kidney failure but is CVD. A reduced GFR of less than 49 ml/min has been shown to be associated with an increased risk of death, cardiovascular event, and hospitalization, independent of known risk factors such as medical history of CVD or albuminuria.[39] Treatment strategies must focus on rigorous management of comorbidities to reduce the risk of CVD.[39]

CKD has a high burden of traditional CVD risk factors; hypertension, diabetes, obesity, and dyslipidemia. In addition, the patient with CKD has a range of nontraditional risk factors, including inflammation, oxidative stress, anemia, proteinuria, imbalance of calcium, phosphate metabolism, and hyperhomocysteinemia.[40] The pathophysiology of these nontraditional risk factors is complex and treatment is ever-evolving. CVD risk remains high in patients with kidney disease and death due to a cardiac cause represents the major risk for patients with CKD, more than the risk of ever needing dialysis.[41] The United States Renal Data System (USRDS) is a national data system that collects, analyzes, and distributes information about CKD and ESRD in the United States.[1] USRDS has found that among CV causes for patients with CKD, only 20% are due to atherosclerotic coronary heart disease (CAD), whereas most deaths result from arrhythmia, sudden cardiac death, or heart failure.[42]

In the general population, there is a well-known association between increasing plasma lipids and coronary risk. This is less true for the patient with CKD. In 2003, KDOQI published guidelines recommending lipid goals and encouraging statin therapy for all patients with CKD.[43] The KDOQI guidelines were based on post hoc analysis of large trials conducted in the general population, not in those with CKD. These post hoc analyses demonstrated that statin therapy significantly reduces cholesterol synthesis and CVD morbidity and mortality either directly, by reducing the lipid profile, or via pleiotropic effects; supposedly reducing both the progression of CKD and proteinuria.[41]

In 2011, the Study of Heart and Renal Protection (SHARP) trial published results involving more than 9000 subjects with CKD questioning whether lowering low-density-lipoprotein cholesterol (LDL-C) with statins reduced the risk of myocardial infarction, ischemic stroke, and/or the need for coronary revascularization in subjects with moderate-to-severe CKD.[44] SHARP aimed to assess the efficacy and safety of the combination of simvastatin plus ezetimibe in the CKD population. Subjects were randomized to treatment with simvastatin 20 mg plus ezetimibe 10 mg or placebo. For the first time ever, approximately 50% of the 9000 subjects enrolled were on dialysis or CKD stage 5 with an GFR of less than 15 mL/min. Among non-dialysis subjects, 80% had albuminuria, a known predictor of increased CVD. Additionally, 46% of the 9000 subjects enrolled were diabetics. The SHARP trial results demonstrated a 17% proportional reduction in first major atherosclerotic events in the simvastatin plus ezetimibe arm. However, there was no significant difference in coronary mortality of the treatment arm versus the placebo arm. There was no evidence of a renal protective effects (defined as dialysis starts, transplantation, or a doubling of baseline SCr) between the treatment and placebo arms.[41] Reduction in LDL-C does not retard CKD progression.[44] There appears to be a different pathogenesis of atherosclerosis in patients with CKD compared with the general population. Thus, the role of statins in reducing CVD death among patients with CKD remains in question.[41]

Based on the SHARP trial results, the newer KDIGO guidelines differ drastically from the older KDOQI guidelines.[42] They suggest the following:

- Newly diagnosed patients with CKD should have a baseline lipid panel (do not follow lipid levels on patients with CKD).
- For patients 50 years or older with eGFR less than 60 ml/min, treat with a statin or statin/ezetimibe combination.
- For patients 50 years or older and eGFR greater than or equal to 60 ml/min, treat with a statin.
- For patients 18 to 49 years old with CKD and known CAD, treat with a statin.
- For patients 18 to 49 years old with CKD and diabetes, treat with a statin.

- For patients 18 to 49 years old with CKD and a prior ischemic stroke, treat with a statin.
- For patients 18 to 49 years old with CKD and an estimated 10-year incidence of coronary death or nonfatal, treat with a statin.

Glycemic Control

Hyperglycemia is a fundamental cause for diabetic kidney disease. Newer KDIGO guidelines advise caution with intensive treatment to achieve normal glycemia due to increased risk of severe hypoglycemia.[11,45] There is little evidence that intensive treatment (hemoglobin A1C < 6.5) has an effect on maintaining GFR and delaying progression of CKD. A target hemoglobin A1C of 7.0% is recommended to prevent or delay progression of CKD but caution is recommended in patients prone to hypoglycemia. Additionally, a hemoglobin A1C target of greater than 7.0% is recommended in patients with comorbidities, limited life expectancy, or risk for hypoglycemia.[45] There are no randomized controlled trials that have evaluated the effect of glycemic control on CKD progression in patients with advanced CKD.

There has been much discussion regarding metformin in a CKD population. In patients with decreased kidney function, the plasma and blood half-life of metformin is prolonged and the renal clearance is decreased in proportion to the decrease in creatinine clearance.[46] Additionally, metformin is known to be substantially excreted by the kidney, and the risk of metformin accumulation and lactic acidosis increases with the degree of impairment of renal function. Metformin is not nephrotoxic; however, in those with decreased kidney function, the drug accumulation can lead to a rare but serious metabolic complication: lactic acidosis. Metformin's Food and Drug Administration package insert states discontinuation of the medication should occur in patients with a SCr of greater than 1.5 (for males) and greater than 1.4 (for females) mg/dl.[47] Yet, KDIGO recommendations are patient-specific, based on GFR not SCr. Thus, KDIGO recommends discontinuation of metformin at a GFR less than 30 ml/min.[2] KDIGO asks practitioners to review metformin use in patients with eGFR of 30 to 44 ml/min, knowing that this a danger zone.

SUMMARY

CKD is a common and progressive disease. Effectively treating CKD and reducing cardiovascular mortality is a challenging task that cannot be done by a sole provider.[48] It requires a team effort in which the patient plays a major role. For this reason, the National Institute of Health, the auspices of the National Kidney Disease Education Program (NKDEP), has developed an easy-to-read, bulleted guide that summarizes all the guidelines and opinions into an accessible portable document format (PDF).[11] It can be downloaded for free at: http://nkdep.nih.gov/resources/ckd-primary-care-guide-508.pdf.

While on the NKDEP website, download the free (well, tax dollars did pay for them) patient guides and handouts. With practitioners working together, CKD does not have to mean dialysis or death for our patients.

REFERENCES

1. Saran R, Li Y, Robinson B, et al. US Renal Data System 2014 Annual Data Report: epidemiology of kidney disease in the United States. Am J Kidney Dis 2015; 66(Suppl 1):S1–306.

2. Kidney Disease: Improving Global Outcomes (KDIGO) CKD Work Group. KDIGO 2012 clinical practice guideline for the evaluation and management of chronic kidney disease. Kidney Int Suppl 2013;3:1–150.
3. Grams ME, Chow EKH, Segev DL, et al. Lifetime incidence of CKD stages 3-5 in the United States. Am J Kidney Dis 2013;62:245–52.
4. Moyer V, US Preventative Services Task Force. Screening for chronic kidney disease: US Preventive Task Force Recommendation statement. Ann Intern Med 2012;157(8):567–70.
5. Eriksen BO, Ingebretsen OC. The Progression of CKD: A 10-year population-based study of the effects of gender and age. Kidney Int 2006;69(2):375–82.
6. Weinstein J, Anderson J. The aging kidney: physiological changes. Adv Chronic Kidney Dis 2010;17(4):302–7.
7. Stevens LA, Coresh J, Greene T, et al. Assessing kidney function: measured and estimated glomerular filtration rate. N Engl J Med 2006;354:2473–83.
8. Keith DS, Nicholas GA, Gullion CM, et al. Longitudinal follow-up and outcomes among a population with chronic kidney disease in a large managed care organization. Arch Intern Med 2004;164:659–63.
9. Levin A, Bakris GL, Molitch M, et al. Prevalence of abnormal serum vitamin D, PTH, calcium and phosphorus in patients with chronic kidney disease: results of the study to evaluate early kidney disease. Kidney Int 2007;71(1):31–8.
10. Wagner LA, Tata A, Fink J. Patient safety issues in CKD: Core Curriculum 2015. Am J Kidney Dis 2015;66(1):159–69.
11. National Kidney Disease Education Program. Making sense of CKD: A concise guide for managing chronic kidney disease in the primary care setting. 2014. Available at: http://nkdep.nih.gov/resources/ckd-primary-care-guide-508.pdf.
12. Remuzzi G, Macia M, Ruggenenti P. Prevention and treatment of diabetic renal disease in type 2 diabetics: the BENEDICT study. J Am Soc Nephrol 2006;17(4):S90–7.
13. Lea J, Greene T, Hebert L, et al. The relationship between magnitude of proteinuria reduction and the risk of ESRD: Results of the AASK study of kidney disease and hypertension. Arch Intern Med 2005;165(8):947–53.
14. Turin TC, James M, Ravani P, et al. Proteinuria and rate of change in kidney function in a community-based population. J Am Soc Nephrol 2013;24(10):1661–7.
15. Hallan SI, Ritz E, Lydersen S, et al. Combining GFR and albuminuria to classify CKD improves prediction of ESRD. J Am Soc Nephrol 2009;20(5):1069–77.
16. Rowe JW, Andres R, Tobin JD, et al. The effect of age on creatinine clearance in men: a cross-sectional and longitudinal study. J Gerontol 1976;31:155–63.
17. National Kidney Foundation. K/DOQI clinical practice guidelines for chronic kidney disease: evaluation, classification and stratification. Am J Kidney Dis 2002;39(Suppl 1):S1–266.
18. National Kidney Disease Education Program. National Institute of Diabetes and Digestive and Kidney Diseases. Bethesda (MD). Available at: http://nkdep.nih.gov/resources/quick-reference-uacr-gfr.shtml.
19. Levey AS, de Jong PE, Coresh J, et al. The definition, classification, and prognosis of chronic kidney disease: a KDIGO Controversies Conference report. Kidney Int 2011;80:17–28.
20. Peterson JC, Adler S, Burkart JM, et al. Blood pressure control, proteinuria, and the progression of renal disease. Ann Intern Med 1995;123:754–62.
21. Kidney Disease: Improving Global Outcomes (KDIGO) Blood Pressure Work Group. KDIGO Clinical Practice Guideline for the Management of Blood Pressure in Chronic Kidney Disease. Kidney Int Suppl 2012;2:337–414.

22. James PA, Oparil S, Carter BL, et al. 2014 evidence-based guideline for the management of high blood pressure in adults; report from the panel members appointed to the Eighth Joint National Committee (JNC 8). JAMA 2014;311(5):507–20.
23. Tylicki L, Lizakowski S, Rutkowski B. Renin-angiotensin-aldosterone system blockade for nephroprotection: current evidence and future directions. J Nephrol 2012;25(6):900–10.
24. Remuzzi G, Ruggenenti P, Perico N. Chronic renal disease: renoprotective benefits of renin-angiotensin system inhibition. Ann Intern Med 2002;136(8):604–15.
25. Esnault VLM, Ekhlas AMR, Delcroix C, et al. Diuretic and enhanced sodium restriction results in improved antiproteinuric response to RAS blocking agents. J Am Soc Nephrol 2005;16:474–81.
26. Bliziotis IA, Destounis A, Stergiou GS. Home versus ambulatory and office blood pressure in predicting target organ damage in hypertension: a systematic review and meta-analysis. J Hypertens 2012;30(7):1289–99.
27. Remuzzi G, Benigni A, Remuzzi A. Mechanisms of progression and regression of renal lesions of chronic nephropathies and diabetes. J Clin Invest 2006;116(2): 288–96.
28. Hammelgam BR, for the Alberta Kidney Disease Network. Relation between kidney function, proteinuria, and adverse outcomes. JAMA 2010;303(5):423–9.
29. Iseki K, Kinjo K, Iseki C, et al. Relationship between predicted creatinine clearance and proteinuria and the risk of developing ESRD in Okinawa, Japan. Am J Kidney Dis 2004;44:806–14.
30. Brenner BM, Cooper ME, de Zeeuw D, et al. Effects of losartan on renal and cardiovascular outcomes in patients with type 2 diabetes and nephropathy. N Engl J Med 2001;345(12):861–9.
31. Lewis E, Hunsicker LG, Clarke WR, et al. Renoprotective effect of the angiotensin-receptor antagonist irbesartan in patients with nephropathy due to type 2 DM. N Engl J Med 2001;345(12):851–60.
32. Lewis EJ, Hunsicker LG, Bain RP. The effect of angiotensin-converting-enzyme inhibition on diabetic nephropathy. The Collaborative Study Group. N Engl J Med 1993;329:1456–62.
33. Yusuf S, Sleight P, Pogue J, et al. Effects of angiotensin-converting-enzyme-inhibitor, ramipril, on cardiovascular events in high risk patients. N Engl J Med 2000;342:145–53.
34. Benigni A, Zoja C, Remuzzi G. The renal toxicity of sustained glomerular protein traffic. Lab Invest 1995;73:461–8.
35. Abbate M, Zoja C, Remuzzi G. How does proteinuria cause progressive renal damage. J Am Soc Nephrol 2006;17(11):2974–84.
36. Ruggenenti P, Cravedi P, Remunzzi G. Proteinuria: increased angiotensin-receptor blocking is not the first option. Nat Rev Nephrol 2009;5:367–8.
37. Kannel WB, Stampfer MJ, Castelli WP, et al. The prognostic significance of proteinuria: the Framingham study. Am Heart J 1984;108(5):1347–52.
38. Grimm RH Jr, Svendsen KH, Kasiske B, et al. Proteinuria is a risk factor for mortality over 10 years of follow-up. MRFIT Research Group. Multiple Risk Factor Intervention Trial. Kidney Int 1997;63:S10–4.
39. Go AS, Chertow GM, Fan D, et al. Chronic kidney disease and the risk of death cardiovascular events and hospitalization. N Engl J Med 2004;351:1296–305.
40. Rucker D, Tonelli M. Cardiovascular risk and management in chronic kidney disease. Nat Rev Nephrol 2009;5:287–96.
41. Scarpioni R, Ricardi M, Albertazzi V, et al. Treatment of dyslipidemia in chronic kidney disease: Effectiveness and safety of statins. World J Nephrol 2012;1(6):184–94.

42. Kidney Disease: Improving Global Outcomes (KDIGO) Blood Pressure Work Group. KDIGO Clinical Practice Guideline for Lipid Management in Chronic Kidney Disease. Kidney Int Suppl 2013;3:259–79.
43. Kidney Disease Outcomes Quality Initiative (K/DOQI) Group. K/DOQI clinical practice guidelines for management of dyslipidemias in patients with kidney disease. Am J Kidney Dis 2003;41:I–IV. S1–91.
44. Sharp Collaborative Group. Study of Heart and Renal Protection (SHARP): randomized trial to assess the effects of lowering low-density lipoprotein cholesterol among 9,438 patients with chronic kidney disease. Am Heart J 2010;160(5): 785–94.
45. National Kidney Foundation. KDOQI Clinical Practice Guideline for Diabetes and CKD: 2012 update. Am J Kidney Dis 2012;60(5):850–86.
46. Hung SC, Chang YK, Liu JS, et al. Metformin use and mortality in patients with advanced chronic kidney disease: national, retrospective, observational, cohort study. Lancet Diabetes Endocrinol 2015;3(8):605–14.
47. FDA [Package Insert]. Glucophage (metformin). Princeton, NJ: Bristol-Myers Squibb Co; 2009.
48. Wouters O, O'Donoghue D, Ritchie J, et al. Early chronic D disease: diagnosis, management and models of care. Nat Rev Nephrol 2015;11(8):491–502.

Risky Business

Lessons from Medication Misadventures in Chronic Kidney Disease

Cheryl Gilmartin, PharmD[a],*, Amy Barton Pai, PharmD, BCPS[b],
David Hughes[c], Niveen Hilal[d]

KEYWORDS

- Chronic kidney disease (CKD) • Medication errors • Elderly
- Community-acquired acute kidney injury(CA-AKI) • Acute kidney injury (AKI)

KEY POINTS

- Improvement in dosing for patients with chronic kidney disease (CKD) and age-related kidney decline accompanied by comorbid conditions requires recognition of the populations at risk and adherence to kidney dosing guidelines.
- Clinical outcomes associated with medication errors include increased emergency department visits, hospitalizations, and lengths of stays as well as considerable morbidity and mortality.
- As kidney function declines, renal and nonrenal absorption, metabolism, distribution, and elimination of medications are affected, causing drugs and their metabolites to accumulate and cause toxic effects.
- Concurrent medication use increases the risk of drug interactions leading to electrolyte disorders, hyperglycemia and hypoglycemia, mental status changes, and acute kidney injury.
- Educating patients and providers on the multifactorial issues related to drug management in CKD may reduce medication errors.

INTRODUCTION

Chronic kidney disease (CKD) affects up to 13% of the people in the United States and is widely underdiagnosed despite improvements in measuring and reporting the estimated glomerular filtration rate (eGFR).[1,2] Dosing errors occur at a greater rate in CKD

Disclosures: None.
[a] Department of Medicine, University of Illinois Hospital and Health Sciences System, 820 South Wood Street, Room 418W, Chicago, IL 60612, USA; [b] Department of Pharmacy Practice, Albany College of Pharmacy and Health Sciences, 106 New Scotland Avenue, O'Brien 232, Albany, NY 12208, USA; [c] Albany College of Pharmacy and Health Sciences, 106 New Scotland Avenue, O'Brien 232, Albany, NY 12208, USA; [d] University of Illinois at Chicago College of Pharmacy, 833 South Wood Street, Chicago, IL 60612, USA
* Corresponding author.
E-mail address: cgilmart@uic.edu

Physician Assist Clin 1 (2016) 55–76
http://dx.doi.org/10.1016/j.cpha.2015.09.003
2405-7991/16/$ – see front matter © 2016 Elsevier Inc. All rights reserved.

and undiagnosed CKD than in a patient with a normal glomerular filtration rate (GFR).[3–6] Patients who are not readily diagnosed with CKD are primarily the elderly with age-related kidney decline and comorbid conditions. Dosing errors are reported to range from 19% to 69% depending on the health care setting.[2]

Farag and colleagues[4] reported that technological capabilities to report GFR and trigger drug dosing alerts have done little to reduce the number of dosing errors in CKD. Two experts who participated in an international conference attempting to reduce renal dosing deficits editorialized that the group failed to identify prescribers' nonadherence to CKD dosing guidelines as a barrier.[7] Although many studies have focused on the patient populations, the improper use of drugs, and the health care institutions associated with medication errors in CKD, few have focused on the clinical course and adverse patient outcomes that occur due improper dosing.[3–6]

The purpose of this article is to describe iatrogenic errors in drugs commonly dosed or prescribed incorrectly in CKD, including age-related kidney dysfunction. A focus is placed on describing patient outcomes, delineating pertinent pharmacodynamics and pharmacokinetic changes, and discussing strategies to improve drug dosing. The case studies that follow have been reported either in the literature or by clinicians. They include the most common medication dosing errors seen by clinicians and described by studies: antimicrobials, hypoglycemic agents, analgesics, anticoagulants, nonsteroidal anti-inflammatory drugs (NSAIDS), and antihypertensive agents.[8]

CONTENT
Antimicrobials and Antivirals

Case 1: Valacyclovir
A 52-year-old man with a history of hypertension (HTN), congestive heart failure, and CKD stage 5 receiving hemodialysis (HD) 3 times a week was diagnosed with herpes zoster virus (HSV) in the emergency department (ED) and given a prescription for valacyclovir (VAL) 1 g orally (PO) 3 times a day for 7 days.[9] After taking 2 doses, the patient was brought back to the ED by his wife who stated the patient had become increasingly irritable and was experiencing visual and auditory hallucinations. The differential diagnosis was narrowed down to varicella zoster virus versus HSV meningoencephalitis. He was admitted for further workup.

Table 1 describes his hospital course.[9]

Table 1
Case 1: Valacyclovir, clinical course

Hospital Day	Clinical Course
1	• ACY 10 mg/kg IV q12h 600 mg/d
6	• Mental status declines • Electroencephalogram[a]
7	• Seizure witnessed • ACY discontinued • Daily HD started
10	• Marked resolution neurologic symptoms
15	• Mental status returns to baseline • Discharged to home

[a] Electroencephalogram (EEG) was nonconclusive. Causes consistent with EEG results included seizure vs metabolic encephalopathy.

Acyclovir (ACY) initiated upon hospitalization further contributed to the already toxic outpatient doses of VAL. It was discontinued when a seizure occurred. VAL is metabolized by the liver to ACY, which is eliminated by the kidney. A metabolite of ACY, 9-carboxymethylguanine, is found in the urine and has been linked to the neurotoxicity associated with ACY and VAL.[10,11] As was the case, the patient was dialysis dependent, and neither VAL nor the metabolites were excreted by the nonfunctioning kidney. The only removal of the drug was via HD.

The patient does not have to be dialysis dependent to experience toxic does of VAL or ACY. Often patients may be on multiple medications (including over-the-counter medications) besides an antiviral and acute kidney injury (AKI) can occur. AKI has been described with antivirals use concomitantly with nephrotoxic drugs, particularly NSAIDS, and in the elderly with gastrointestinal (GI) issues. In each circumstance, close evaluation and avoidance of nephrotoxic or renally eliminated drugs are warranted. Antivirals require dose adjustment in CKD according to the GFR and the indication (**Tables 2** and **3**).[11–14]

Table 2
Acyclovir dosing

Indication and Target Dose (mg)	CrCl (mL/min/1.73 m^2)	Adjusted Dose (mg) and Frequency
Herpes zoster: 800 q4h	>25	No adjustment
	10–25	800 q8h
	≤10	800 q12h
Genital herpes Suppression/ prophylaxis: 400 q12h	>10	No adjustment
	≤10	200 q12h
Genital herpes therapy: 200 q4h	>10	No adjustment
	≤10	200 q12h

Table 3
Valacyclovir dosing

Indication and Target Dose (mg)	CrCl (mL/min/1.73 m^2)	Adjusted Dose (mg) and Frequency
Herpes zoster: 1000 q8h	>50	No adjustment
	30–49	1000 q12h
	10–29	1000 q24h
	≤10	500 q24h
Genital herpes (initial episode): 1000 q12h	>30	No adjustment
	10–29	1000 q24h
	≤10	500 q24h
Genital herpes (recurrent episode): 500 q12h	>30	No adjustment
	≤30	500 q24h
Genital herpes suppression: 500 q24h	>30	No adjustment
	≤30	500 q48h
Herpes labialis: 2000 q12h	>50	No adjustment
	30–49	1000 q12h
	10–29	500 q12h
	≤10	500 single dose

Case 2: Levofloxacin

A 62-year-old Hispanic woman with a medical history including diabetes mellitus (DM) type 2, atrial fibrillation (AFIB), and CKD stage 5 receiving HD 3 times a week presented to her primary care practitioner with a chief complaint of redness, swelling, and some pain in her little toe.

Medication list:
- Darbepoetin 5mcg intravenous (IV) weekly
- Doxercalciferol 4 µg PO 3×/wk
- Warfarin 7.5 mg daily
- Sevelamer 2.4 g with each meal
- Glipizide 2.5 mg daily

She was given clindamycin (Clinda) 450 mg PO every 6 hours for 14 days and was scheduled to return to clinic in 4 days (**Table 4**).

Table 4
Case 2: Levofloxacin clinical course

Clinical Day	Patient Clinical Course
4	• Admitted to hospital from clinic due to worsening infection of toe
5	• Discharged to home • Continue oral Clinda 450 mg q6h • Add Levo 750 mg PO q48h—patient given written prescription • Insurance issues precluded obtaining Levo 750 mg prescription, attempt to obtain insurance coverage for medication started by clinic staff
8	• Prior authorization for Levo obtained and patient started medication on Day 8 • Clinda 450 mg q6h continued
13	• Levo 750 mg q48h taken × 3 doses and Clinda 450 mg q6h × 13 d • Infected toe worsened • Patient returns to ED • Patient admitted to hospital • Patient continues Levo 750 mg q48h & Clinda 450 mg q6h • Electrocardiogram performed in ER showing QT prolongation • Levo discontinued; replaced with cefepime 2 g IVPB

Abbreviation: IVPB, intravenous piggyback.

Levofloxacin (Levo), one of the fluoroquinolones, is minimally metabolized and excreted primarily unchanged in the urine. Consequently, dose reductions and extended intervals are necessitated in the face of kidney disease. Patients greater than 60 years old, patients with CKD, those with kidney, heart, or liver transplants, and patients concurrently taking corticosteroids incur an increased risk of the untoward effects of the fluoroquinolones. The adverse effects of fluoroquinolones include tendon rupture (black box warning), QT prolongation, torsades de pointes, and fatal liver toxicity.

Drug interactions occurring with Levo and other quinolones may be of particular concern in the elderly or patients with CKD. Although this particular case occurred in the dialysis-dependent patient, complications of fluoroquinolones are much more common in the outpatient CKD population, where oral antibiotics are frequently given for infections. Medications commonly taken by the older population include antacids, oral iron products, and multivitamins, and these medications diminish the absorption of the fluoroquinolones. This regimen requires a minimum 2-hour dosing separation before or after concurrent use with quinolones.[15] Concomitant use of NSAIDS with fluoroquinolones may precipitate central nervous system (CNS) effects, including seizures.

Hyperglycemia and hypoglycemia have been reported in predominantly elderly diabetic patients with and without diminished kidney function when Levo is used concomitantly with hypoglycemic agents.[16] Hypoglycemia has been described with the concurrent use of glyburide, glipizide, or insulin. Concurrent utilization of the aforementioned antidiabetic agents with the other fluoroquinolones, clarithromycin, fluconazole, and sulfamethoxazole/trimethoprim (SMZ/TMP) has also been reported to cause hypoglycemia.[17] This means that the diabetic patient placed on a fluoroquinolone for an infection, commonly prescribed in this patient population, should be instructed to increase blood glucose monitoring.

Case 3: Sulfamethoxazole/trimethoprim

A 65-year-old African American man with a history of DM type 2, HTN, and CKD stage 3 was admitted to a hospital for GI distress. The patient had a baseline serum creatinine (SCr) of 1.6 mg/dL that increased to 2.5 mg/dL during the acute phase of his GI distress. At hospital discharge, the SCr returned to baseline. After hospitalization, the patient presented to his primary care office with complaints of urinary frequency. A urinary tract infection, confirmed by a positive culture for MRSA (methicillin resistant staph aureus), was treated with SMZ/TMP 800 mg/160 mg daily. The patient presented to the ED 3 days later with a SCr of 6.3 mg/dL, diagnostic of AKI. Because of the acute nature of the illness and the setting (teaching hospital), a kidney biopsy was done, which indicated predominantly acute tubular necrosis (ATN) and possible acute interstitial nephritis (AIN). The clinical pharmacist who was rotating with the renal fellows pointed out that the SMZ/TMP dose that the case patient was given was adequate for a stable SCr of 1.6 mg/dL, but the dose and perhaps the drug itself may have been inappropriate with AKI.

Drug-dosing guidelines for kidney failure are based on stable chronic kidney function using either GFR or creatinine clearance (CrCl). The equations are interchangeable except in patients with extremes in muscle mass and diet, pregnant women, amputees, or patients with serious comorbid conditions or AKI.

The patient with one episode of AKI incurs an increased risk for episodic AKI, end-stage renal disease (ESRD), and an increased risk of nonrenal morbidity and mortality.[18,19] Although an elevation in SCr with SMZ/TMP has been described as artificial, it has also been implicated in precipitating AIN.[20,21] A Veterans Administration (VA) population-based study of 573 patients concluded that SMZ/TMP is a more common cause for interstitial nephritis (both acute and chronic), ATN, and hyperkalemia than previously reported. The VA study described an incidence of AKI in 11.2% of study patients who received SMZ/TMP. The investigators concluded that those patients with diabetes alone or in concert with HTN (both of which the case patient had) were at an increased risk of AKI with the use of SMZ/TMP.[22] An antibiotic choice, such as Linezolid, with less nephrotoxic potential would have been a better choice.

Hyperkalemia with SMZ/TMP is well described.[21] The incidence of hyperkalemia can be exacerbated in the elderly, patients with CKD, or with concomitant use of drugs that increase potassium. A 14-year population-based study demonstrated a 7-fold increased incidence of admissions for hyperkalemia in patients greater than 65 years old co-prescribed angiotensin-converting enzyme inhibitors (ACEI) or angiotensin receptor blockers (ARB) with SMZ/TMP when compared with amoxicillin with ACEI/ARB.[23] Many elderly and patients with CKD are prescribed ACEI/ARB to slow the progression of their kidney disease, so the use of SMZ/TMP should be avoided in this patient population.

SMZ/TMP also can cause hypoglycemia in patients concurrently taking sulfonylureas, pioglitazone, rosiglitazone, repaglinide, or metformin.[21] In CKD or elderly patients with diabetes, the combination of hypoglycemic agents and SMZ/TMP should be avoided, or if the antibiotic is absolutely needed, increased glucose monitoring is vital.

Hypoglycemic Agents

Case 1: Glyburide and metformin

Interestingly, despite diabetes being a primary cause of CKD in the United States, only a single, brief report describing a 79-year-old woman found unresponsive with a blood glucose level of 32 mmol/L due to hypoglycemic agents could be found.[1,2,24] Many consider this a nonreportable complication, but this leads to fewer reported US Food and Drug Administration (FDA) adverse events and less oversight of patients. The FDA has a simple, on-line reporting system (http://www.fda.gov/Safety/MedWatch/default.htm) and encourages all practitioners to report unusual events.

The patient from the reported case, with the blood glucose level of 32 mmol/L, was taking glyburide 5 mg and metformin 1000 mg both 2 times a day. Glyburide is hepatically metabolized by the cytochrome (CYT) P-450 CYP3A and cyp2C9, producing active metabolites.[25] The CYT P450 CVP3A and 2C9 may be reduced up to 50% in CKD.[26] For these reasons, severe hypoglycemia can occur in patients with an eGFR < 60 mL/min/1.73 m^2, and glyburide should be avoided in the CKD population.[27] A recent study found that elderly patients prescribed only sulfonylureas were significantly more likely to frequent the ED when compared with other hypoglycemic agents.[28] Besides glyburide, metformin and many other antidiabetic drugs require patient-specific considerations, dose reductions, or avoidance at various CKD stages (**Table 5**).[25,27,29–47]

Table 5 Diabetes medication dosing		
Class of Medication, Drug	**Typical Dose**	**Renal Dosing (CrCl: mL/min, SCr: mg/dL, eGFR mL/min/1.73 m^2)**
Biguanide		
Metformin (Glucophage)[27,29]	500–1000 mg BID	eGFR <60 stop concurrently: Malnourished/serious illness Nephrotoxic/renally eliminated drug eGFR 30–59 continue: If none of above exist Closely monitor Package insert do not use: Men SCr ≥1.5, women ≥1.4
Sulfonylureas		
Glipizide (Glucotrol)[30]	2.5–40 mg per day Doses >15 mg, divided	eGFR <60 → 1.25–20 mg per day
Glimepiride (Amaryl)[31]	1–8 mg per day	eGFR <15 avoid
Glyburide (Micronase, Diabeta)[25,27]	1.25–20 mg per day	eGFR <60 avoid
Meglitinides		
Nateglinide (Starlix)[32]	60–120 mg TID AC	eGFR <15 ↓ dose

(continued on next page)

Table 5 (continued)		
Class of Medication, Drug	**Typical Dose**	**Renal Dosing (CrCl: mL/min, SCr: mg/dL, eGFR mL/min/1.73 m^2)**
Repaglinide (Prandin)[33]	0.5–6 mg per day Take 15 min before meals	CrCl 20–40 → initiate 0.5 mg CrCl <20 not studied
Thiazolidinediones		
Rosiglitazone (Avandia)[34]	4–8 mg per day	No dose adjustment
Pioglitazone (Actos)[35]	15–45 mg per day	No dose adjustment, titrate carefully
α-Glucosidase Inhibitors		
Acarbose (Precose)[36]	25–100 mg TID ≤60 kg → max 50 mg TID >60 kg → max 100 mg TID Take doses with meals	eGFR <25 → Avoid
Miglitol (Glyset)[37]	25–100 mg TID	CrCl <25 → Avoid
Sodium Glucose Cotransporter 2 Inhibitor		
Canagliflozin (Invokana)[38]	100–300 mg per day	eGFR 45–59 → max 100 mg per day eGFR <45 → Avoid
Empagliflozin (Jardiance)[39]	10–25 mg per day	eGFR <45 → Avoid
DPP4 Inhibitors		
Sitagliptin (Januvia)[40]	100 mg per day	eGFR 30–50 → 50 mg eGFR <30 → 25 mg
Saxagliptin (Onglyza)[41]	2.5–5 mg per day	eGFR <50 → 2.5 mg
Linagliptin (Tradjenta)[42]	5 mg per day	No dose adjustment
Alogliptin (Nesina)[43]	25 mg per day	eGFR 30–59 → 12.5 mg per day eGFR <30 → 6.25 mg per day
GLP-1 Analogs (injections)		
Exenatide (Byetta: immediate release, Bydureon: extended-release)[44,45]	Byetta: 5–10 µg SC BID (within 1 h AM & PM meal) Bydureon: 2 µg SC every 7 d	eGFR 30–50 → use caution eGFR <30 → avoid
Liraglutide (Victoza)[46]	0.6–1.8 mg SC per day	No dose adjustment Caution, limited practice
Amylinomimetics (injections)		
Pramlintide (Symlin)[47]	15–120 µg SC TID AC At initiation: ↓ mealtime insulin by 50%	eGFR <15 not studied

Abbreviations: AC, before meals; BID, 2 times per day; eGFR, estimated glomerular filtration rate; SC, subcutaneously; TID, 3 times per day.

Analgesics

Case 1: Meperidine

An 82-year-old Caucasian woman with known allergies to codeine and morphine was admitted to the hospital for a left hip replacement.[48] The patient had a history of GI bleeding, chronic obstructive pulmonary disease, back surgeries, and aortic aneurysm. Her medication list was not reported. Her baseline SCr ranged from 0.5 to

1.4 mg/dL, increased to 2.4 mg/dL on admission, and ranged from 1.2 to 2 mg/dL during her hospitalization. After surgery, meperidine 50 to 100 mg IV every 4 hours as needed was ordered for pain management. **Table 6** describes her clinical course.[48]

Table 6
Case 1: Meperidine clinical course

Hospital Day	Meperidine Daily Dose (mg)	Clinical Course
1	300	• Resting comfortably during the day • Overnight pain
2	450	• IV dose increased & patient resting comfortably
3	550	• Poor pain control • Patient-controlled analgesic begun infusion rate 15 mg/h • Patient seeing worms dancing on ceiling • MD states "just a side effect" • Later, patient pulling oxygen tubes and bed sheets
4	335	• Patient more disoriented and confused • Family requested to stop drug • Dose decreased → basal rate ↓ from 15 mg to 7.5 mg • Patient's visual hallucinations increased • Pump stopped at family's insistence
5	—	• Patient has jerky, seizurelike movements from 3:40 AM to late afternoon
6	—	• Symptoms resolved

Meperidine is 60% protein-bound and extensively metabolized by the liver to an active metabolite, normeperidine, which is renally eliminated.[48–50] Normeperidine as compared with meperidine has a half-life that is 5 to 10 times longer and thus is available for a significantly longer time in the bloodstream, contains 50% of the analgesic properties as meperidine, but has 2 to 3 times the CNS toxicity. Thus, meperidine (the parent drug) is less CNS toxic, is excreted faster, and is 50% more effective than the metabolite. Because both normeperidine and meperidine can accumulate in kidney dysfunction, meperidine warrants dose adjustments in patients with chronic kidney dysfunction according to the GFR. For the AKI patient, which the case patient displayed with the elevated SCr on the day of surgery, the SCr must be followed closely, and the dose of meperidine monitored frequently. The adverse neurologic effects demonstrated from improper dosing of meperidine and its metabolite in CKD include hallucinations, myoclonus, and seizures, all of which were experienced by this patient.

Case 2: Morphine
A 61-year-old African American man was admitted to the hospital for pain management related to a sickle cell crisis.[51] Past medical history included DM type 2, HTN, sarcoidosis, and CKD stage 3, although no medication list was available. On admission, the patient's CrCl was 24.8 mL/min, and he was initiated on tramadol and morphine. His clinical course is described in **Table 7**.[51]

Table 7
Case 2: Morphine clinic course

Hospital Day	Medications	Patient Clinical Course
1–5	Tramadol 50 mg 3×/d Morphine 5 mg SC q4–8h	• Pain controlled • Total daily morphine dose ≈ 20 mg

6	Pain medications
	  Tramadol 50 mg 3×/d
	  Morphine 5 mg SC
	    ×4 morphine infusion
	Resuscitation medications:
	  Naloxone
	  Epinephrine
	  Atropine
		• Pain controlled by morphine 5 mg × 2 doses
		• Noon pain ↑ morphine 5 mg/h, infusion started
		• Pain ↑ morphine 5 mg SC × 2 doses
		• Infusion ↑ 7 mg/h due to bolus doses
		• After 3 h, patient lethargic → infusion ↓ 3.5 mg/h
		• After 1.5 h patient ↑ lethargy → infusion stopped
		• Patient unresponsive 2.5 h later → cardiorespiratory arrest
		• Resuscitation fails, patient pronounced dead
		• Total morphine dose day 6 ≈ 39 mg

Abbreviation: SC, subcutaneous.

An autopsy was remarkable for ischemia in the cerebral cortex, suggesting respiratory arrest as the cause of death. Significant serum concentrations of morphine and its active metabolites morphine-3-glucoronide (M3G) and morphine-6-glucoronide (M6G) were found in postmortem serum samples, suggesting the patient's death was most likely the result of a toxic overdose elicited by morphine or its metabolites.[51]

The toxicity caused by morphine and its active metabolites, M3G and M6G, has been well established.[49] Morphine, like meperidine, is metabolized extensively in the liver into active metabolites, M3G and M6G, which are removed by the kidneys. Although morphine is hepatically metabolized via glucuronidation, studies have determined that plasma concentrations of morphine are higher in patients in CKD when compared with subjects with normal kidney function. Several phenomena may explain the accumulation of the parent drug morphine in CKD. Nonrenal metabolism has been shown to be reduced in CKD so that morphine may not be as readily glucuronidated. Both morphine and M6G cross the blood-brain barrier more easily in CKD, reducing the renal clearance of morphine. Most compelling is that due to a delay in kidney excretion, M3G and M6G may hydrolyze back to the parent drug.[51,52]

The decreased elimination of the metabolites contributes to the opioid toxicity. M6G is more potent than morphine, and M3G has been affiliated with the neuro-excitatory effects displayed during opioid intoxication.[52] Opioid toxicity is associated with respiratory depression, hypotension, and mental status changes.

Case 3: Gabapentin

A 75-year-old woman was admitted to the hospital for a fall with CNS changes. Two days before admission, the patient had been seen in clinic with complaints of increased severe left hip pain that was treated by increasing her gabapentin 300 mg from 2 to 3 times per day.[53] Her past medical history was significant for HTN, CKD stage 3 (baseline GFR 43 mL/min/1.73 m^2; admission GFR 34 mL/min/1.73 mL/min), left hip hemiarthroplasty, and osteoarthritis (OA).

Medication list:
• Diclofenac 75 mg twice daily
• Tramadol 50 mg 4 times daily

- Dihydrocodein 30 mg 4 times daily
- Amlodipine 5 mg daily
- Irbesartan 300 mg daily
- Gabapentin 300 mg 3 times daily
- Furosemide 80 mg daily

On admission, the patient was drowsy but easily aroused. Diclofenac 75 mg 2 times daily, irbesartan 300 mg daily, and furosemide 80 mg daily ("triple whammy" to be discussed later), which the patient was taking before admission, were discontinued due to worsening kidney function. The patient's medication and clinical course are delineated in **Table 8.**[53]

Table 8
Case 3: Gabapentin clinical course

Hospital Day	Pain Medication	Clinical Course
1–6	Gabapentin 300 mg 3×/d Tramadol 50 mg 4×/d Dihydrocodeine 30 mg 4×/d	On admission GFR 34 mL/min/1.73 m²
7	Gabapentin 300 mg 3×/d	Narcotics stopped due to ↑ lethargy, hypotension & ↓ kidney function: GFR 12 mL/min/1.73 m²
10	Gabapentin 300 mg 3×/d	Patient unresponsive & depressed respiratory rate; transferred to intensive care unit (ICU) Naloxone administered: suspected opioid toxicity Lethargy continued without improvement
11	—	Gabapentin stopped Continuous veno-venous hemofiltration (CVVH) started Improvement in cognitive & renal function
12–15	—	CVVH continued Cognitive and renal function return to baseline
16	—	Patient transferred from ICU → General medicine floor

Gabapentin is minimally metabolized and renally excreted primarily as an unchanged drug and therefore can accumulate when kidney function is reduced.[54] It is recommended the dose be decreased in patients with CKD and those over the age of 75, both of which were true for the case patient. The FDA package insert has a dosing chart. Accumulation of gabapentin due to improper dosing in diminished kidney function has been reported to cause CNS changes and myoclonic activity.[55,56] Discontinuation of the offending medication usually will allow the body to clear the gabapentin, although in severe cases of iatrogenic overdose, dialysis may be needed. Rhabdomyolysis due to gabapentin toxicity in both AKI and CKD has also been reported.

ANTICOAGULATION
Anticoagulation Case

A 69-year-old Hispanic male patient with a history of metabolic syndrome and CKD was admitted to the hospital for excessive nose bleeding, hyperkalemia, and AKI.[57] The patient's baseline SCr was 1.3 to 2 mg/dL (GFR 58–35 mL/min). It was noted dabigatran 150 mg twice daily was recently initiated for AFIB, and the patient had taken 9 doses before discontinuing the dabigatran due to bruising and bleeding. The patient received 2 units of packed red blood cells, vitamin K, desmopressin, a nonspecified treatment of hyperkalemia, and 7 HD procedures before he was discharged home with a SCr 1.8 mg/dL (GFR 40 mL/min). This case suggests the possibility of AKI due to dabigatran.

Dabigatran is an alternative to vitamin K antagonists, which require international normalized ratio (INR) monitoring.[57] Although dabigatran and other newer anticoagulant agents offer the convenience of less frequent monitoring, many are excreted by the kidney and have yet to be sufficiently studied in patients with CKD, particularly those with a GFR less than 30. Many of the novel agents require dose adjustments and monitoring in CKD (**Table 9**).[58–69]

Patients with CKD are more likely to succumb to morbidity and mortality associated with cardiovascular disease than to progress to ESRD.[70] Patients with CKD present a quagmire because the risk of thrombosis coexists with a predisposition to bleeding because of abnormal platelet aggregation and coagulation cascade in uremia.[71] Because of the increased risk of bleeding and opposing results in observational studies, anticoagulation in CKD patients continues to be a matter of controversy. A recent study suggested from subanalyses of 4 studies that the novel agents may reduce thrombotic events without increasing the risk of bleeding in patients with a GFR between 30 and 49 mL/min (see **Table 9**). However, the investigators noted that the patients with CKD in the general population, not preselected by a strict study protocol, may be more fragile than study subjects.

ANGIOTENSIN-CONVERTING ENZYME INHIBITORS, DIURETICS, AND NONSTEROIDAL ANTI-INFLAMMATORY DRUGS
The Case of the "Triple Whammy" and Acute Kidney Injury

A 67-year-old white woman presented to the ED because of a fall at home. Past medical history is significant for DM type 2, HTN, CKD (eGFR 28 mL/min/1.73 mL/min), mild OA, and dyslipidemia. Three days before presenting to ED, the patient had developed acute GI symptoms with fever, severe vomiting and diarrhea, night sweats, and tremor.

Medication list at time of GI illness:
- Metformin 500 mg by mouth twice daily
- Lisinopril/hydrochlorothiazide 20/12.5 mg by mouth once daily
- Naproxen 220 mg by mouth twice daily (patient self-started 3 days ago)
- Atorvastatin 40 mg by mouth once daily
- Furosemide 40 mg by mouth twice daily
- Glyburide 2.5 mg by mouth once daily

The patient continued to take all her medications despite her poor oral intake. The ED physical examination blood pressure showed hypotension (72/40), tachycardia (148 beats per minute) with poor skin turgor and pale color consistent with profound volume depletion. Blood and urine cultures were drawn and Gram stains were reported to be negative. Fractional excretion of sodium was 0.2%, consistent with prerenal disease thought by the practitioners to be hemodynamically (dehydration) mediated AKI.[72]

The most common cause of AKI on presentation in the ED is reduced glomerular capillary pressure caused by medications that affect kidney hemodynamics.[72] **Table 10** lists drugs associated with outpatient (or community-acquired or CA) versus inpatient (hospital acquired or HA) iatrogenic AKI. Three recurrent drug classes cited for AKI are renin-angiotensin-system inhibitors (RAAS), diuretics, and NSAIDS. In combination, these drugs have synergistic hemodynamic effects on the blood flow

Table 9
Anticoagulation medication dosing table

Drug	Dose	Renal Dosing (CrCl: mL/min)
Vitamin K Antagonist		
Warfarin (Coumadin)[58]	Individualized dosing. INR target 2–3	No dose adjustment
Direct Factor Xa Inhibitors		
Rivaroxaban (Xarelto)[59]	Nonvalvular AFIB: 20 mg daily with PM meal	Nonvalvular AFIB: CrCl 15–50: 15 mg daily with PM meal CrCl <15: Avoid DVT treatment or prophylaxis: CrCl <30: Avoid If AKI occurs: STOP
Apixaban (Eliquis)[60]	5 mg twice daily	Dose ↓ 2.5 mg twice daily when greater than 2 of the following apply: SCr >1.5 mg/dL ≥80 y/o Body weight ≤60 kg
Fondaparinux (Arixtra)[61]	<50 kg: 5 mg daily 50–100: 7.5 mg daily >100 kg: 10 mg daily	CrCl 30–50: use with caution CrCl <30: Avoid
Heparins		
Unfractionated heparin[62]	Individualized dosing	No dose adjustment
Dalteparin (Fragmin)[63]	Indication-dependent dose: 120–200 IU/kg/d SC Max dose: ≥10,000 IU	CrCl <30: 2500 or 5000 IU daily use caution, monitor anti-Xa Anti-Xa range 0.5–1.5 IU/mL
Enoxaparin (Lovenox)[64]	0.5–1 mg/kg SC twice daily	CrCl <30: 1 mg/kg SC once daily
Direct Thrombin Inhibitors		
Dabigaran (Pradaxa)[65]	150 mg twice daily	CrCl 15–30: 75 mg twice daily Stop 24 h before initiating warfarin/ parenteral anticoagulant CrCl <15 or dialysis: not studied
Argatroban[66]	IV infusion: 2 μg/kg/min Monitor aPTT Css: 1.5–3× baseline aPTT	Critically ill: 0.15–1.3 μg/kg/min, monitor aPTT Css: 1.5–3× baseline aPTT
Bivalirudin (Angiomax)[67]	IV bolus dose: 0.75 mg/kg IV infusion: 1.75 mg/kg/h	IV bolus dose: No dose adjustment CrCl 30–59: IV infusion: 1.75 mg/kg/h CrCl <30: IV infusion: 1 mg/kg/h Dialysis: IV infusion: 0.25 mg/kg/h Monitor: ACT
Desirudin (Iprivask)[68]	15 mg BID SC	CrCl 31–60: 5 mg BID SC CrCl <31: 1.7 mg BID SC Monitor aPTT & SCR daily, adjust dose
Lepirudan (Refludan)[69]	Bolus dose: 0.4 mg/kg IV infusion: 0.15 mg/kg/h	Bolus dose: 0.2 mg/kg CrCl 45–60: IV infusion 0.75 mg/kg/h CrCl 30–44: IV infusion 0.045 mg/kg/h CrCl 15–29: IV infusion 0.0225 mg/kg/h CrCl <15: Avoid

Abbreviations: ACT, activated clotting time; aPTT, activated partial thromboplastin time; Css, steady state; DVT, deep vein thrombosis.

Table 10
Nephrotoxic medications causing community-acquired acute kidney injury and hospital-acquired acute kidney injury

Drug	Mechanism of Nephrotoxicity[a]	Unique Risk Factors[a]	Clinical Features	Prevention/Monitoring[b]
CA-AKI				

NSAIDs	Inhibits prostaglandin-mediated vasodilation of the afferent arterioles[74]	1. Risk increases with:
		  a. Increasing doses
		  b. Increase duration of use[74]
			1. Weight gain (sodium retention and edema)[75]
			2. Reduced urine output
			3. History of concurrent illness that decreases intravascular volume (eg, gastroenteritis)
				1. Counsel high-risk patients to avoid over-the-counter use
				2. Avoid if possible in patients with hyperkalemia[74]
				3. Monitor serum potassium

ACEi ARBs Direct renin inhibitors (Aliskiren)	Efferent arteriole vasodilation leading to decreased glomerular capillary pressure[76] • This effect is beneficial at reducing stress on remnant nephrons in CKD, but large reductions in glomerular capillary pressure can induce CA-AKI	1. Overdiuresis 2. Volume depletion 3. Large reductions in sodium intake 4. Concomitant renin-dependent disease states (eg, cirrhosis, congestive heart failure) 5. Dual ACEi and ARB or aliskiren increases risk[77]	1. >30% increase in SCr not resolved by dose decrease[77] 2. Weight gain (edema) 3. Reduced urine output 4. History of concurrent illness 5. Hyperkalemia	1. Advise patient of sick day rules[78] 2. Evaluate temporal changes in SCr: 20%–25% increase is expected within 5–14 d of drug initiation[79] or any dose increase and drug should be continued in most clinical situations[80–82] a. >30% increase should be evaluated for CA-AKI

Diuretics
Loop diuretics:
Furosemide,
Bumetanide, Torsemide
Thiazide diuretics:
Chlorthalidone,
Hydrochlorothiazide,
Metolazone
	Reduce intravascular volume by increasing sodium and water excretion (natriuresis)[76]	1. If fluid overload (eg, CKD or congestive heart failure) use bumetanide or torsemide over furosemide due to erratic bioavailability of furosemide	Loops:
			1. Hypomagnesemia
			2. Hyperuricemia
			3. Loss of appetite
			4. Hypokalemia
			5. Hypotension
			6. Vertigo
			7. Phototoxicity
				1. Sick day rules
				2. Monitor weight
				  a. Establish a "dry" weight and take daily weights
				  b. Avoid overdiuresis
				Patient should contact provider if:
				  a. Gain 1 lb/d for several consecutive days
				  b. Gain 3–5 lbs in a week

(continued on next page)

Table 10
(continued)

Drug	Mechanism of Nephrotoxicity	Unique Risk Factors[a]	Clinical Features	Prevention/Monitoring[b]
			8. Increase in uric acid, glucose, and cholesterol with higher doses	
Fenofibrate	Proposed mechanisms: PPAR-related downregulation of cyclooxygenase-2 expression (decreased capacity to dilate afferent arteriole)[79] • Increased metabolic production of creatinine	1. Male 2. Non-Hispanic white 3. Long duration of DM 4. Pre-existing CKD 5. History of or clinical cardiovascular disease[80]	1. Increase in SCr levels (reversible)	1. Monitor SCr within 14 d of initiation and every 3–6 mo thereafter 2. Monitor around dose increases 3. Advise patient of sick day rules[78]
Rifampin	Tubulointerstitial nephritis (plasma cells, neutrophils, lymphocytes infiltration)[83]	1. Rifampin positive antibodies 2. Re-exposure to drug	1. Low-grade fever (30%–50%) 2. Maculopapular rash (33%–50%) 3. Eosinophilia (16%–33%) 4. Eosinophiluria (40%–90%) 5. Hematuria (48%–60%) 6. Proteinuria (16%–60%) 7. Pyuria (30%–50%)[84] 8. Red-orange discoloration of urine, feces, saliva, sweat, and tears	1. LFT (ALT and AST) before starting therapy and every 2–4 wk 2. Evaluate a bilirubin level, SCr, and a complete blood count (CBC; with platelets) before starting therapy and continue follow-up monitoring in patients with laboratory abnormalities 3. Evaluate patient history and adherence when initiating therapy
Licorice (Glycyrrhizic acid) Contained in: • Sweeteners	Inhibits 11β-hydroxysteroid-dehydrogenase	1. High cortisol levels 2. Cushing disease	1. Pseudo-aldosteronism a. Water retention	1. Blood pressure 2. Serum potassium 3. Serum bicarbonate

Medication	Mechanism	Clinical manifestations	Risk factors	Monitoring
• Flavorings • OTC supplements (cold sore treatment)	• This enzyme is responsible for the production of active cortisol and thus glucocorticoid access[85]	b. Increased blood pressure c. Hypokalemia d. Metabolic alkalosis e. Low renin activity 2. Rhabdomyolysis 3. Thrombocytopenia		4. Cortisol levels
HA-AKI				

Tenofovir	Transport by organic acid transporter into proximal tubule cells
	• Mitochondrial stress and apoptosis[86]
		1. Glycosuria
		2. Aminoaciduria
		3. Uric acid or phosphorus imbalances
		4. Renal tubular acidosis
		5. Decreased bone mass (due to phosphate wasting and calcitriol deficiency)
			1. Harvoni may increase risk
			  a. Coadministration may lead to supratherapeutic levels of tenofovir and further nephrotoxicity
			2. Lower body weights
			3. Tenofovir withdrawal
				1. Serum phosphorus
				  a. Phosphorus binds with calcium and can initiate or exacerbate vascular calcification (higher risk in CKD)
				2. Urinalysis biannually

Televancin	Proximal tubular vacuolation Mitochondrial damage to collecting duct Cholesterol uptake into proximal convoluted tubular cells[87]	1. Foamy urine 2. Hypokalemia	1. Higher body mass index (weight-based dosing) 2. Previous supratherapeutic vancomycin concentrations 3. Contrast dye 4. Fetal exposure a. Place pregnant women on risk management program to assess future risk for fetus (avoid if possible)[85]	1. Frequent monitoring of SCr and electrolytes 2. Urine electrolytes when indicated
Vancomycin	Direct tubular toxicity • Potential accumulation	1. Hypokalemia 2. Abdominal pain	1. Vancomycin exposure:	1. Escalating vancomycin trough

(continued on next page)

Table 10
(continued)

Drug	Mechanism of Nephrotoxicity	Unique Risk Factors[a]	Clinical Features	Prevention/Monitoring[b]
	Accumulation of crystalline degradation product[88]	a. Prolonged trough >15 µg/mL b. Large exposure/area under the curves[89–93] c. Prolonged duration 2. Host-related factors	3. Hypotension leading to severe facial flushing ("red man syndrome")	2. CBC with differential 3. Auditory function with excessive IV doses
Aminoglycosides	Saturable accumulation of aminoglycosides in S1 and S2 segments of the proximal tubule leading to inhibition of phospholipases and cell death	1. Previous episodes of severe dehydration/hemodynamic instability 2. Concomitant diuretics such as furosemide 3. Sulfa allergy a. Contains sodium metabisulfate	1. Hypo-osmolar urine 2. Proteinuria 3. Electrolyte wasting (potassium and magnesium)	1. Maintain target trough concentrations for traditional or high-dose once-daily regimens 2. Aminoglycoside concentrations may rise before SCr 3. Microscopic urinalysis for proteinuria or cases 4. Microscopic analysis for proteinuria or cases (NAG)

Abbreviations: AST, aspartate aminotransferase; ALT, alanine aminotransferase; LFT, liver function test; PPAR, peroxisome proliferator-activated receptor.
[a] Common risk factors for all drugs listed are: CKD, heart failure, age, severe liver disease, nephrotoxins (diuretics, contrast media, nephrotoxic antibiotics).
[b] Prevention and monitoring that are applicable to all above drugs are: blood urea nitrogen, serum creatinine elevation from baseline.

to the glomerulus, ultimately reducing glomerular capillary pressure. This combination has been referred to as the "triple whammy."[73]

RAAS medications, which include ACEIs and ARBs, lower glomerular capillary pressure by a vasodilator effect on the efferent (or exit) arterioles. Diuretics, such as furosemide, decrease intravascular volume by increasing the amount of water and sodium excretion by the kidneys. NSAIDS inhibit vasodilation of the afferent arterioles by interfering with prostaglandins. The National Kidney Disease Education Program has developed a 2-minute, very easy-to-understand instructional animation to show the interaction of these medications on glomerular capillary pressure (https://www.youtube.com/watch?v=J2YaULhMx5g).

Several recent analyses have sought to further clarify the risk associated with the "triple whammy" on AKI risk.[72,73,94] Lapi and colleagues[73] retrospectively evaluated a cohort of more than 487,000 users of antihypertensive medications from the United Kingdom's Clinical Practice Research Datalink to determine whether the combination of diuretic and RAAS use increased the risk of AKI with the addition of NSAID. The investigators approached the analysis conservatively excluding patients with a previous CKD diagnosis who represent a significant high-risk population with current use of both diuretic and RAAS therapy. The investigators found that the use of NSAIDS with only a diuretic or an RAAS was not associated with risk of AKI. When NSAIDS therapy was given concomitantly with diuretics and RAAS to a non-CKD population, a 31% higher rate of AKI was observed (relative risk [RR] 1.31, 95% confidence interval [CI] 1.12–1.53).

An analysis of the French Pharmacovigilance Database aimed to evaluate serious adverse kidney events among patients taking combinations of RAAS, diuretics, and NSAIDS using a case/noncase approach.[72] The use of 1-, 2-, or 3-drug combinations of NSAIDS, RAAS, or diuretics (eg, RAAS + RAAS or RAAS + diuretic, or RAAS + NSAIDS or any combination of the these) was associated with increasing risk of AKI with reported odds ratios of 2.19, 5.27, and 16.46, respectively.

The most recent analysis evaluating the risk of AKI with addition of NSAID therapy to RAAS or diuretics sought to overcome limitations of previous analyses that limited AKI case identification to hospital coding by expanding the definition of AKI to a 50% increase in SCr from baseline.[76] Using anonymous data from residents of Tayside, the investigators found an increased AKI risk with NSAIDS use. This AKI risk was increased in patients who took both double and triple combinations with RAAS and all classes of diuretics (RR 1.66 95% CI 1.40–1.97). Acute exposure to NSAIDS was associated with higher risk compared with chronic treatment (RR 3.40 vs 1.32), indicative of the importance of education surrounding any new NSAID prescription given to a patient presently taking RAAS or diuretic therapy. CKD was identified as an associated risk factor even when GFR was relatively preserved (>60 mL/min/1.73 m^2).

The risk of CA-AKI increases when the patient has a concomitant illness that results in volume depletion (eg, gastroenteritis). Recent analyses have shown that the incidence of CA-AKI is higher than of HA-AKI, with 80% rates of AKI (as evidenced by ICD-9 [International Classification of Diseases-9] code) occurring at the time of admission.[95] Although duration of hospitalization and mortality are lower among CA-AKI patients than in those with HA-AKI, recovery of renal function is incomplete, and similar long-term outcomes on kidney function are apparent, with nearly 40% developing new-onset or progression of CKD.[72,96]

Importantly, many cases of dehydration (prerenal) AKI can be avoided if patients are aware of these risks and take steps to stop their usual medications with innocuous acute illnesses. The British National Health System (NHS) has developed sick day rules aimed at reducing preventable episodes of AKI.[97] These sick day rules

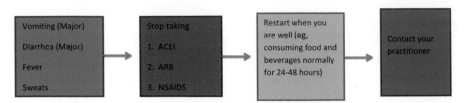

Fig. 1. Sick day rules guide. (*Adapted from* Salford CCG sick day rules. National Institute for Health Research. 2015. Available at: http://clahrc-gm.nihr.ac.uk/salford-sick-day-rules/. Accessed June 18, 2015.)

instruct patients to stop nephrotoxic medications (defined as ACEI/ARB/NSAIDS) on development of fever, diarrhea, or vomiting (**Fig. 1**). Patients are instructed to replace fluids by drinking water or having some sugar and salt. Medications can be restarted once the patient begins to feel better, approximately 1 to 2 days later (for most patients). The utilization of sick day rules in patients at high risk for AKI could reduce preventable hospitalizations. The NHS has created a simple index card that can be explained by a provider and given to patients at high risk for AKI. Incidentally, the NHS sick day guidelines also recommend that the metformin be discontinued due to potential risk of lactic acidosis in the face of the unknown magnitude of acute GFR decline.[27,29]

SUMMARY

Recognizing the risk for medication errors and reporting patient outcomes associated with improper medication dosing in patients with CKD or at risk for AKI is a fundamental step to decreasing the number of medication errors. The complexities associated with adjusting medications for kidney dysfunction require an enhanced recognition and adherence by patients and prescribers alike. The dosing guidelines for CKD patients by either GFR or CrCl are found in the FDA package inserts and are vital to reducing the morbidity and mortality incidence associated with medication errors in this very fragile population.

REFERENCES

1. Stevens LA, Li S, Wang C, et al. Prevalence of CKD and comorbid illness in elderly patients in the United States: results from the Kidney Early Evaluation Program (KEEP). Am J Kidney Dis 2010;55(3 Suppl 2):S23–33.
2. Weir MR, Fink JC. Safety of medical therapy in patients with chronic kidney disease and end-stage renal disease. Curr Opin Nephrol Hypertens 2014;23(3): 306–13.
3. Long CL, Raebel MA, Price DW, et al. Compliance with dosing guidelines in patients with chronic kidney disease. Ann Pharmacother 2004;38:853–8.
4. Farag A, Garg AX, Li L, et al. Dosing errors in prescribed antibiotics for older persons with CKD: a retrospective time series analysis. Am J Kidney Dis 2014;63(3): 422–8.
5. Taché SV, Sönnichsen A, Ashcroft DM. Prevalence of adverse drug events in ambulatory care: a systematic review. Ann Pharmacother 2011;45:977–89.
6. Gurwitz JH, Field TS, Harrold LR, et al. Incidence and preventability of adverse drug events among older persons in the ambulatory setting. JAMA 2003; 289(9):1107–16.

7. Arnoff GR, Arnoff JR. Drug prescribing in kidney disease: can't we do better? Am J Kidney Dis 2014;63(3):382–3.
8. Jones SA, Bhandari S. The prevalence of potentially inappropriate medication prescribing in elderly patients with chronic kidney disease. Postgrad Med J 2013;89:247–50.
9. Hoskote SS, Annapureddy N, Ramesh AK, et al. Valacyclovir and acyclovir neurotoxicity with status epilepticus. Am J Ther 2014. [Epub ahead of print].
10. Asahi T, Tsutsui M, Wakasugi M, et al. Valacyclovir neurotoxicity: clinical experience and review of the literature. Eur J Neurol 2009;16:457–60.
11. Valtrex [package insert]. Research Triangle Park, NC: GlaxoSmithKline; 2008.
12. Acyclovir. Micromedex healthcare series. DRUGDEX system [database online]. Greenwood Village (CO): Truven Health Analytics; 2014. Available at: http://www.thomsonhc.com/. Accessed June 8, 2014.
13. Valacyclovir oral. Drug facts and comparisons. Facts & comparisons [database online]. St Louis (MO): Wolters Kluwer Health Inc; 2013. Accessed June 8, 2014.
14. Valacyclovir. Micromedex healthcare series. DRUGDEX system [database online]. Greenwood Village, CO: Truven Health Analytics; 2014. Available at: http://www.thomsonhc.com/. Accessed June 8, 2014.
15. Levaquin [package insert]. Guarbo, Puerto Rico: Janssen Ortho LLC; 2008.
16. Friedrich LV, Dougherty R. Fatal hypoglycemia associated with levofloxacin. Pharmacotherapy 2004;24(12):1807–12.
17. Parekh TM, Raji M, Lin YL, et al. Hypoglycemia after antimicrobial drug prescription for older patients using sulfonylureas. JAMA Intern Med 2014;174(10):1605–12.
18. Saul P. Special report acute kidney. Practitioner 2013;257(1765):23–6.
19. Cox ZL, McCoy AB, Matheny ME, et al. Adverse drug events during AKI and its recovery. J Am Soc Nephrol 2013;8(7):1070–8.
20. Hellman N. Bactrim & elevated creatinine. Available at: http://renalfellow.blogspot.com/2008/12/bactrim-elevated-creatinine.html. Accessed June 1, 2015.
21. Bactrim [package insert]. Philadelphia, PA: Mutual Pharmaceutical. Available at: http://www.accessdata.fda.gov/drugsatfda_docs/label/2003/17377slr057_bactrim_lbl.pdf. Accessed June 1, 2015.
22. Fraser TN, Avellaneda AA, Graviss EA, et al. Acute kidney injury associated with trimethoprim/sulfamethoxazole. J Antimicrob Chemother 2012;67:1271–7.
23. Antoniou T, Gomes T, Juurlink DN, et al. Trimethoprim-sulfamethoxazole-induced hyperkalemia in patients receiving inhibitors of the renin-angiotensin system: a population-based study. Arch Intern Med 2010;170(12):1045–9.
24. Seaquist E. Cases in hypoglycemia. University of Minnesota 28th Annual ADA Clinical Conference May 2013. Available at: http://professional.diabetes.org/admin/UserFiles/4-CC%20PowerPoints/D4-Seaquist%20hg%20cases%202013%20orlando.pdf. Accessed June 25, 2015.
25. Micronase [package insert]. New York, NY: Pfizer; 2010.
26. Verbeek RK, Musuamba FT. Pharmacokinetics and dosage adjustment in patients with renal dysfunction. Eur J Clin Pharmacol 2009;(65):757–73.
27. Kidney Disease: Improving Global Outcomes CKD Work Group. KDIGO 2012 clinical practice guideline for evaluation and management of chronic kidney disease. Kidney Int Suppl 2013;3:1–150.
28. Rajpathak SN, Chunmay FU, Brodovicz K, et al. Sulfonylurea monotherapy and emergency room utilization among elderly patients with type 2 diabetes. Diabetes Res Clin Pract 2015;109(3):507–12.

29. Metformin [package insert]. US Department of Health and Human Services, US Food and Drug Administration. Available at: www.fda.gov/ohrms/dockets/dailys/02/May02/053102/800471e6.pdf. Accessed June 21, 2015.
30. Glucotrol [package insert]. New York, NY: Pfizer; 2013.
31. Amaryl [package insert]. Bridgewater, NJ: Sanofi-Aventis U.S. LLC; 2013.
32. Starlix [package insert]. East Hanover, NJ: Novartis; 2013.
33. Prandin [package insert]. Princeton, NJ: Novo Nordisk; 2011.
34. Avandia [package insert]. Triangle Park, NJ: GlaxoSmithKline LLC; 2014.
35. Actos [package insert]. Thousand Oaks, CA: Physician Partner; 2010.
36. Precose [package insert]. Wayne, NJ: Bayer HealthCare Pharmaceuticals; 2011.
37. Glyset [package insert]. New York, NY: Pfizer; 2014.
38. Invokana [package insert]. Titusville, NJ: Janssen Pharmaceuticals; 2011.
39. Jardiance [package insert]. Ridgefield, CT: Boehringer Ingelheim Pharmaceuticals; 2014.
40. Januvia [package insert]. Whitehouse Station, NJ: Merck & Co., Inc; 2010.
41. Onglyza [package insert]. Mount Vernon, IN: Bristol-Meyers Squibb; 2012.
42. Tradjenta [package insert]. Ridgefield, CT: Boehringer Ingelheim Pharmaceuticals; 2014.
43. Nesina [package insert]. Deerfield, IL: Takeda Pharmaceuticals America; 2014.
44. Byetta [package insert]. San Diego, CA: Amylin Pharmaceuticals; 2009.
45. Bydureon [package insert]. Wilmington, DE: AstraZeneca Pharmaceuticals LP; 2015.
46. Victoza [package insert]. Princeton, NJ: Novo Nordisk; 2015.
47. Symlin [package insert]. San Diego, CA: Amylin Pharmaceuticals; 2014.
48. Seifert CF, Kennedy S. Meperidine is alive and well in the new millennium: evaluation of meperidine usage patterns and frequency of adverse drug reaction. Pharmacotherapy 2004;24(6):776–83.
49. Yaksh TL, Wallace MS. Chapter 18. Opioids, analgesia, and pain management. In: Brunton LL, Chabner BA, Knollmann BC, editors. Goodman & Gilman's the pharmacological basis of therapeutics. 12 edition. New York: McGraw-Hill; 2011. Available at: http://accesspharmacy.mhmedical.com/content.aspx?bookid=374&Sectionid=41266224. Accessed June 25, 2015.
50. Demerol [package insert]. Laval, Quebec: Sanofi-Aventis; 2014.
51. Lagas JS, Wagenaar JF, Huitema AD, et al. Lethal morphine intoxication in a patient with a sickle cell crisis and renal impairment: case report and a review of the literature. Hum Exp Toxicol 2011;30(9):1399–403.
52. Hemstapat K, Monteith GR, Smith D, et al. Morphine-3-glucuronide's neuroexcitatory effects are mediated via indirect activation of N-methyl-D-aspartic acid receptors: mechanistic studies in embryonic cultured hippocampal neurones. Anesth Analg 2003;97(2):494–505.
53. Miller A, Price G. Gabapentin toxicity in renal failure: the importance of dose adjustment. Pain Med 2009;10(1):190–2.
54. Neurontin [package insert] New York, NY: Pfizer; 2015.
55. Kaufman KR, Parikh A, Chan L, et al. Myoclonus in renal failure: two cases of gabapentin toxicity. Epilepsy Behav Case Rep 2014;2:8–10.
56. Bilgir O, Calan M, Bilgir F, et al. Gabapentin-induced rhabdomyolysis in a patient with diabetic neuropathy. Intern Med 2009;48(12):1085–7.
57. Pazmino P. Dabigatran associated acute renal failure. Am J Kidney Dis 2012; 59(4):B63.
58. Coumadin [package insert]. Princeton, NJ: Bristol-Meyers Squibb; 2011.
59. Xarelto [package insert]. Titusville, NJ: Janssen Pharmaceuticals; 2011.

60. Eliquis [package insert]. Princeton, NJ: Bristol-Meyers Squibb; 2011.
61. Arixtra [package insert]. Triangle Park, NC: GlaxoSmithKline LLC; 2013.
62. Heparin sodium injection [package insert]. Kirkland, Quebec: Pfizer; 2014.
63. Fragmin [package insert]. Kirkland, Quebec: Pfizer; 2014.
64. Lovenox [package insert]. Bridgewater, NJ: Sanofi-Aventis U.S. LLC; 2013.
65. Pradaxa [package insert]. Ridgefield, CT: Boehringer Ingelheim Pharmaceuticals, Inc; 2015.
66. Argatroban [package insert]. Triangle Park, NC: GlaxoSmithKline LLC; 2014.
67. Angiomax [package insert]. Parsippany, NJ: The Medicines Company; 2013.
68. Iprivask [package insert]. Northbrook, IL: Marathon Pharmaceuticals, LLC; 2014.
69. Refludan [package insert]. Berlex, NJ: Berlex; 2004. Available at: http://www.accessdata.fda.gov/drugsatfda_docs/label/2006/020807s011lbl.pdf. Accessed June 29, 2015.
70. Bargman JM, Skorecki K. Chronic kidney disease. In: Kasper D, Fauci A, Hauser S, et al, editors. Harrison's principles of internal medicine. 19 edition. New York: McGraw-Hill; 2015. Available at: http://accessmedicine.mhmedical.com.proxy.cc.uic.edu/content.aspx?bookid=1130&Sectionid=79746512. Accessed June 30, 2015.
71. Khai P, Edwards NC, Lip GYH, et al. Atrial fibrillation in CKD: balancing the risks and benefits of anticoagulation. Am J Kidney Dis 2013;62(3):615–32.
72. Schissler MM, Zaidi S, Kumar H, et al. Characteristics and outcomes in community-acquired versus hospital-acquired acute kidney injury. Nephrology (Carlton) 2013;18(3):183–7.
73. Lapi F, Azoulay L, Yin H, et al. Concurrent use of diuretics, angiotensin converting enzyme inhibitors, and angiotensin receptor blockers with non-steroidal anti-inflammatory drugs and risk of acute kidney injury: nested case-control study. BMJ 2013;346:e8525.
74. Huerta C, Castellsague J, Varas-Lorenzo C, et al. Nonsteroidal anti-inflammatory drugs and risk of ARF in the general population. Am J Kidney Dis 2005;45(3):531–9.
75. Gooch K, Culleton BF, Manns BJ, et al. NSAID use and progression of chronic kidney disease. Am J Med 2007;120(3):280.e1–7.
76. Dreischulte T, Morales DR, Bell S, et al. Combined use of nonsteroidal anti-inflammatory drugs with diuretics and/or renin-angiotensin system inhibitors in the community increases the risk of acute kidney injury. Kidney Int 2015;88(2):396–403.
77. St Peter WL, Odum LE, Whaley-Connell AT. To RAS or not to RAS? The evidence for and cautions with renin-angiotensin system inhibition in patients with diabetic kidney disease. Pharmacotherapy 2013;33(5):496–514.
78. Sick day rules in kidney disease. Drug Ther Bull 2015;53:37.
79. Parving HH, Brenner BM, McMurray JJ, et al. Cardiorenal end points in a trial of aliskiren for type 2 diabetes. N Engl J Med 2012;367(23):2204–13.
80. Fried LF, Emanuele N, Zhang JH, et al. Combined angiotensin inhibition for the treatment of diabetic nephropathy. N Engl J Med 2013;369:1892–903.
81. Bonds DE, Craven TE, Buse J, et al. Fenofibrate-associated changes in renal function and relationship to clinical outcomes among individuals with type 2 diabetes: the Action to Control Cardiovascular Risk in Diabetes (ACCORD) experience. Diabetologia 2012;55(6):1641–50.
82. Attridge RL, Frei CR, Ryan L, et al. Fenofibrate-associated nephrotoxicity: a review of current evidence. Am J Health Syst Pharm 2013;70:1219–25.

83. Chiba S, Tsuchiya K, Sakashita H, et al. Rifampicin-induced acute kidney injury during the initial treatment for pulmonary tuberculosis: a case report and literature review. Intern Med 2013;52:2457–60.
84. Pai AB, Mason DL. Acute kidney injury. In: Tisdale JE, Miller DA, editors. Drug-induced diseases, prevention detection and management. 2nd edition; 2010. p. 853–4.
85. Allard T, Wenner T, Greten HJ, et al. Mechanisms of herb-induced nephrotoxicity. Curr Med Chem 2013;20(22):2812–9.
86. Fernandex B, Montoya-Ferrer A, Sanz AB. Tenofovir nephrotoxicty: 2011 update. AIDS Res Treat 2011;2011:354908.
87. Polyzos KA, Mavros MN, Vardakas KZ. Efficacy and safety of telavancin in clinical trials: a systematic review and meta-analysis. PLoS One 2012;7(8):e41870.
88. Carreno JJ, Kenney RM, Lomaestro B. Vancomycin-associated renal dysfunction: where are we now? Pharmacotherapy 2014;34(12):1259–68.
89. Patel N, Pai MP, Rodvold KA, et al. Vancomycin: we can't get there from here. Clin Infect Dis 2011;52(8):969–74.
90. Stella VJ, Quanren H. Cyclodextrins. Toxicol Pathol 2008;36(1):30–42.
91. KDIGO clinical practice guideline for acute kidney injury. Kidney disease improving global outcomes. Kidney International 2012;2 Suppl(1):1–141.
92. Nderitu P, Doos L, Strauss VY, et al. Analgesia dose prescribing and estimated glomerular filtration rate decline: a general practice database linkage cohort study. BMJ Open 2014;4:1–10.
93. Krishman N, Perazella MA. Drug-induced acute interstitial nephritis: pathology, pathogenesis, and treatment. Iran J Kid Dis 2015;9(1):3–13.
94. Lapi F, Azoulay L, Yin H, et al. Concurrent use of diuretics, angiotensin converting enzyme inhibitors, and angiotensin receptor blockers with non-steroidal anti-inflammatory drugs and risk of acute kidney injury: nested case-control study. BMJ 2013;346:e8525.
95. Der Mesropian PJ, Kalamaras JS, Eisele G, et al. Long-term outcomes of community-acquired versus hospital-acquired acute kidney injury: a retrospective analysis. Clin Nephrol 2014;81(3):174–84.
96. Wonnacott A, Meran S, Amphlett B, et al. Epidemiology and outcomes in community-acquired versus hospital-acquired AKI. Clin J Am Soc Nephrol 2014;9(6):1007–14.
97. Salford CCG sick day rules. National Institute for Health Research. 2015. Available at: http://clahrc-gm.nihr.ac.uk/salford-sick-day-rules/ Accessed June 18, 2015.

Food for Thought
Diet and the Kidney

 CrossMark

Arlene Keller Surós, MSHS, RD, PA-C

KEYWORDS

- Renal diet • Potassium • Protein • Bicarbonate • Supplementation • Antioxidants

KEY POINTS

- Adherence to kidney diet guidelines is an inexpensive way to promote kidney health and decrease morbidity.
- The most impactful dietary changes in patients with chronic kidney disease (CKD) are limiting sodium and increasing bicarbonate.
- Increasing dietary fiber in patients with CKD can decrease serum urea and serum creatinine, which slows the progression of the disease.

The kidney diet has been the bane and the promise of patients with kidney disease for decades. From the original 1945 dietary guidelines from the Food and Nutrition Board of the National Academy of Sciences exhorting children to drink 8 glasses of water per day to the present knowledge that overconsumption of water can be dangerous, the renal diet has been adjusted, enhanced, and debated.[1–3] Nephrology continues to develop, especially with regard to the relationship between nutrition and chronic kidney disease (CKD). There has been an influx of data published since the turn of the century as well as dietary guidelines developed by the kidney community both in the United States and internationally. Because it is difficult to keep up with evolving theories, beliefs, and the most recent research, many practitioners will follow what they learned in training. This article serves as a dietary primer for the non-nephrology PA by outlining the peer-reviewed, best practices that are available and encouraged for your patients with kidney disease in 2016.

MODIFICATION OF DIET IN RENAL DISEASE STUDY

Protein is acknowledged as an early marker of nephrotic syndrome. The belief that managing protein would slow kidney disease was the basis of a long-term research study of patients with kidney disease in the United States and Canada, the Modification of Diet in Renal Disease, more commonly known by its acronym the MDRD study.[4] In the early 1990s, nephrology asked the following question: does protein restriction

No disclosures.
The Hospitalist Group, Virginia Hospital Center, 1625 North George Mason Drive, Suite 425, Arlington, VA 22205, USA
E-mail address: arlene@suros.com

Physician Assist Clin 1 (2016) 77–100
http://dx.doi.org/10.1016/j.cpha.2015.09.010
physicianassistant.theclinics.com
2405-7991/16/$ – see front matter © 2016 Elsevier Inc. All rights reserved.

matter? In what is now a landmark study, 840 patients with an elevated serum creatinine were enrolled in a randomized, multicenter National Institute of Health–sponsored study to answer exactly that question.[5] In this study, patients were given either a usual-protein diet (1.3 g/kg/d) or a low-protein diet (0.58 g/kg/d). For the next 2 to 5 years, the rate of decline of kidney function was followed; it was found that there was little difference between the groups. This finding started the long discussion and debate in the kidney community about dietary protein.

PROTEIN

The MDRD study results set off multiple secondary analyses of the same data.[6] In a meta-analysis of the data as reviewed by multiple experts, Levey and colleagues[6] stated that many investigators thought there was no correlation between protein restriction and the progression of kidney disease. However, after reviewing the data themselves, Levey and colleagues[6] concluded that there was some justification in recommending a low-protein diet. They specified 0.6 g/kg/d as the optimum protein restriction for patients with kidney disease. This recommendation was taught throughout the medical community, and many professors and instructors still teach this to their students. However, since that publication in 1999, new data have emerged challenging this recommendation.

Realistically, many patients cannot calculate or restrict protein in their diets. Furthermore, many of the same patients who have kidney disease also have diabetes whereby higher protein intake is often recommended. Patients on dialysis, either hemodialysis or peritoneal dialysis, are told to increase protein intake as studies have shown that supplementing patients on dialysis with protein will increase survival.[7] However, admitting practitioners in hospitals will often order a renal diet for patients on dialysis, which may, depending on the institution, includes a protein restriction. Dietitians have addressed this issue with computerized order sets that include various subsets of renal diets: the dialysis renal diet does not include protein restriction.

That said, recent guidelines suggest that patients with CKD with a glomerular filtration rate (GFR) less than 60 mL/min still should have some protein restriction. In 2012, Kidney Disease Improving Global Outcomes (KDIGO), an international group of kidney experts (including those in the United States), looked at data and research from around the world. These experts developed a set of guidelines for the management of patients with CKD.[8] Included are guidelines for known complications (**Table 1**). As this is the most robust set of guidelines available, they are accepted as the final word on protein for patients with CKD at this time and are considered standard of care.

Table 1
Incidence of complications with progression of CKD from stage 1 to stage 5

GFR (mL/min)	>90	60–89	45–59	30–44	<30
Anemia (%)	4	5	125	23	51
Hypertension (%)	18	41	72	78	82
Vitamin D deficiency (%)	14	9	11	11	27
Acidosis (%)	11	8	9	18	31
Hyperphosphatemia (%)	7	7	9	9	23
Hypoalbuminemia (%)	1	1	3	9	7
Hyperparathyroidism (%)	5	9	23	44	72

Adapted from Kidney Disease: Improving Global Outcomes (KDIGO) CKD Work Group. KDIGO 2012 Clinical Practice Guideline for the Evaluation and Management of Chronic Kidney Disease. Kidney inter Suppl 2013;3:1–150.

- They suggest lowering protein intake to 0.8 g/kg/d in adults with diabetes or those without diabetes but with a low GFR (below 30 mL/min) along with appropriate education.
- They suggest avoiding high-protein intake (>1.3 g/kg/d) in adults with CKD at risk of progression.

SODIUM

The next biggest issue for patients with CKD is salt. As many patients have cardiac issues in addition to kidney disease, guidelines were developed with this group in mind. Data collected nationwide note that most adults consume more than the recommended amount of salt. In fact, the average daily salt intake for an American is 3.1 to 3.9 g for men and 2.4 to 3 g for women.[9] This consumption is at a time when the general recommendation for salt intake for Americans is 2.3 g/d.[10] In other words, many regular Americans, that is, nonkidney patients, are already eating almost 2 times the recommended doses of salt each day; we are asking patients with kidney disease to cut this amount by another 30% to 40%. Thus, we are asking patents with kidney disease to lower salt in their diet by more than 60% each day.

Although often difficult to follow, dietary sodium restriction is vital for patients with CKD. Sodium restriction not only lowers blood pressure but it also decreases proteinuria, cardiac end points, and albuminuria and can slow progression of kidney disease.[9,11,12] Thus, KDIGO has developed peer-reviewed, outcome-driven guidelines on salt for patients with CKD.[8]

- They recommend lowering salt intake to less than 90 mmol (<2 g) per day of sodium (corresponding to 5 g of sodium chloride) in adults, unless contraindicated.
- For the special population who loses salt or who are prone to hypotension, sodium restriction is contraindicated.

As patients age, taste bud loss means they are prone to heavier salt use.[13] However, encouraging salt substitutes may actually substitute one problem for another. Many over-the-counter salt substitutes exchange potassium chloride (KCl) for sodium chloride or salt. This substitution can be problematic for those patients with CKD who are prone to hyperkalemia, those who are on a medication that can increase potassium retention (ie, angiotensin converting enzyme [ACE-I] or angiotensin receptor blockers [ARBs]), or those who are trying to increase their fruit and vegetable intake. Some manufacturers have realized this and use herbs and spices rather than KCl as the main ingredient in their products.[14] One of the most famous patients with kidney disease is the late Chef Paul Prudhomme of Louisiana who developed an entire series of seasonings that are not only safe for patients with kidney disease but also have great flavors for those patients losing their taste sensation.[15]

POTASSIUM

Most patients with kidney disease are on an ACE-I or ARBs, which are the classes of antihypertensive medications recommended by every guideline for CKD. However, this means that hyperkalemia is a real and present danger for patients with kidney disease. Thus salt substitutes must be carefully chosen, and potassium in the diet must be monitored and adjusted.

The Academy of Nutrition and Dietetics has developed guidelines that are distributed through the National Government Guidelines Program.[16]

- For adults with CKD (stages 3–5 including those who have a kidney transplant) who exhibit hyperkalemia, limit daily potassium intake to less than 2.4 g with adjustments based on the following:
  - Serum potassium level
  - Blood pressure
  - Medications
  - Kidney function
  - Hydration status
  - Acidosis
  - Glycemic control
  - Catabolism
  - Gastrointestinal (GI) issues: vomiting, diarrhea, constipation, and GI bleed
- Dietary and other therapeutic lifestyle modifications are recommended as part of a comprehensive strategy to reduce cardiovascular disease risk in adults with CKD. The degree of hypo or hyperkalemia can have a direct effect on cardiac function, either of which have potential for cardiac arrhythmia and sudden death.

For those patients with CKD following a potassium-restricted diet, high-potassium foods should be avoided and portion sizes of medium-potassium foods should be limited (**Table 2**).

Hyperkalemia is a fact of life for patients with CKD, especially those who are hemodialysis dependent. However, patients on dialysis can and do live at higher serum potassium levels. Often this is because of the thrice-weekly dialysis schedule and the transient hyperkalemia that occurs on the off-dialysis days. In a bizarre turn of events, this means that patients who are dialysis dependent are often allowed a more liberal dietary potassium restriction than nondialysis patients. In fact, in peritoneal dialysis there is typically a complete absence of potassium restriction and often patients must take potassium supplements.[17]

Table 2 Potassium in foods			
	Low Potassium (<150 mg/serving)	**Medium Potassium (150–250 mg/serving)**	**High Potassium (>250 mg/serving)**
Fruit	Applesauce	Apple	Apricot
	Blueberries	Apple juice	Banana
	Cranberries	Cherries	Cantaloupe
	Cranberry juice	Fruit cocktail (canned)	Coconut
	Grapes	Grapefruit (one-half)	Dates
	Grape juice	Peach	Dried fruit
	Lemon	Pear	Figs
	Lime	Plum	Guava
	Pineapple	Strawberries	Honeydew melon
		Tangerine	Kiwi fruit
		Watermelon	Mango
			Nectarines
			Orange
			Orange juice
			Papaya
			Plantain
			Pomegranate
			Prunes
			Prune juice
			Raisins

(continued on next page)

Table 2 (continued)			
	Low Potassium (*<150 mg/serving*)	**Medium Potassium** (*150–250 mg/serving*)	**High Potassium** (*>250 mg/serving*)
Vegetables	Alfalfa sprouts	Broccoli	Acorn squash
	Bamboo shoots	Cauliflower	Artichoke
	Bean sprouts	Celery	Asparagus
	Cabbage	Collard greens	Avocado
	Corn	Green peas	Beets
	Cucumber	Kale	Beans (kidney,
	Eggplant	Mushrooms	lima, navy, pinto)
	Green beans	Mustard greens	Black-eyed peas
	Green pepper	Spinach	Brussels sprouts
	Lettuce	Turnips	Lentils
	Onion	Turnip greens	Okra
	Radish	Yellow squash	Parsnips
	Wax beans	Zucchini	Potato
			Pumpkin
			Rutabaga
			Sweet potato
			Swiss chard
			Tomato
			Tomato juice
			Tomato sauce
Other	—	—	Almonds
			Bran
			Carob
			Cashews
			Chocolate
			Molasses
			Peanut butter
			Peanuts
			Potato chips
			Walnuts
			Wheat bran

PHOSPHORUS

Although there is much discussion on the most appropriate goal for patients with CKD with regard to serum phosphorus levels, most kidney experts agree that it is necessary to monitor and lower serum phosphorus in patients with CKD. This necessity is exponentially more difficult as kidney function is lost and dialysis starts, but the discussion of phosphorus should occur at the earlier stages of CKD.

As one loses kidney function, one loses the ability to excrete phosphorus.[18] Early in CKD, this is less of an issue, as the tubules in the kidney will compensate by decreasing reabsorption of phosphorus. However, as the severity of kidney disease progresses, these tubules are damaged and are, thus, unable to decrease reabsorption further leading to elevation in serum phosphorus. As phosphorus is found in many protein-rich foods, if patients with CKD decrease dietary protein intake, they potentially can decrease dietary phosphorus. However, phosphorus is the hidden ingredient in many foods and beverages.

Phosphorus is commonly added to food as a preservative and, thus, is found in many items one would not expect (**Table 3**). Interestingly, fresh fruits, vegetables, and animal proteins contain organic phosphorus, which has a lower absorption rate

Table 3
Food high in phosphorus

Dairy	Nuts & Seeds	Grains	Dried Beans	Protein	Additives	Other
Cheese	Almonds	Baking mixes	Black-eyed peas	Carp	Calcium phosphate	Caramel
Cottage cheese	Brazil nuts	Biscuits	Kidney	Fish roe	Disodium dihydrogen pyrophosphate	Chocolate
Cream soups	Cashews	Bran	Lentils	Halibut	Disodium phosphate	Cocoa
Custard	Peanuts	Bran flakes	Lima	Mussels	Monopotassium phosphate	Cola
Ice cream	Peanut butter	Cornbread	Navy	Organ meats	Monosodium phosphate	Dates
Milk	Pecans	Muffins	Pinto	Oysters	Phosphoric acid	Dried fruit
Pudding	Pumpkin seeds	Oatmeal	Soybeans (edamame)	Pork	Pyrophosphate polyphosphates	Molasses
Yogurt	Sunflower seeds	Raisin bread	—	Processed meats	Sodium hexametaphosphate	Pepper-type sodas
	Walnuts	Whole-wheat breads	—	Salmon	Sodium tripolyphosphate	Raisins
	—	Wheat germ	—	Sardines	Tetrasodium pyrophosphate	—
	—	—	—	Scallops	Tricalcium phosphate	—
	—	—	—	Swordfish	—	—
	—	—	—	Veal	—	—

than the inorganic phosphorus found in additives and preservatives.[18] Fresh meat, fruits, vegetables and bakery products sold in grocery stores are sometimes treated with an inorganic phosphorus-containing preservative in order to make the food look more appetizing and have a longer shelf life. Therefore, consider telling your patients with CKD that growing their own fruit and vegetables and paying close attention to ingredient labeling is the healthiest way to go.

VITAMIN D

Vitamin D supplementation is a hotly contested topic among the nephrology community, and both sides of the debate are well documented and supported by data. Vitamin D comes in 2 forms: activated (1, 25 dihydroxyvitamin D) and inactivated (25 hydroxyvitamin D). The kidney contains an enzyme (1-alpha-hydroxylase) that converts the inactive form of vitamin D to the active form. As the kidney fails, so does the production of 1-alpha-hydroxylase; thus, active vitamin D levels decrease.[19] Therefore, oral supplements of the active form of vitamin D are administered as the kidney fails and patients get closer to dialysis. Although both sides of the debate agree on the merits of vitamin D supplementation, the controversy resides over when to begin and at what dose.

Cardiac events prove to be the most common cause of death in patients with CKD. These cardiac events are mainly related to the calcification of blood vessels and not the cholesterol emboli that are seen in patients with usual cardiac diseases.[20] As vitamin D and calcium are interrelated, the concept of decreasing calcification of blood vessels by manipulating vitamin D levels is extremely appealing. However, this has been difficult to prove with case-controlled studies. A review by Inda Filho and Melamed[21] published in 2013 highlighted the continuing uncertainty by concluding: "More research is needed to determine whether Vitamin D supplementation can reduce cardiac events and mortality in CKD patients."[21]

Because kidney experts are unable to agree, the Academy of Nutrition and Dietetics has stepped in with a consensus recommendation[16]:

- In adults with CKD (including after kidney transplant), vitamin D supplementation should occur if the serum level of 25-hydroxyvitamin D is less than 30 ng/mL (75 nmol/L).

CALCIUM

Although vitamin D is a topic of controversy, calcium is not. It is well accepted that calcification of vessels causes detrimental cardiac end points and that patients with CKD develop cardiovascular disease at a higher rate than the general population.[22] Thus, it is theorized that if calcium is controlled, calcification of vessels will decrease and the goal of decreasing mortality and morbidity in the CKD population could

Table 4
Over-the-counter orthopedic supplements

Name	Source	Common Uses	Safe for CKD
Glucosamine	Corn or wheat sugar	Joint pain	Probably
Chondroitin sulfate	Polysaccharide	Osteoarthritis	Probably

Data from Barrett S. Glucosamine and chondroitin for arthritis: benefit is unlikely. Kidlington, Oxford: Quackwatch; 2010; and Uebelhart D, Malaise M, Marcolongo R, et al. Intermittent treatment of knee osteoarthritis with oral chondroitin sulfate: a one-year, randomized, double-blind, multicenter study versus placebo. Osteoarthritis Cartilage 2004;12(4):269–76.

Table 5
Functions, food sources, and recommended dietary allowances of vitamins and minerals

Vitamin/Mineral	Functions	Sources	Recommended Dietary Allowance	Extra Needed in CKD
Vitamin A	Promotes vision, growth, bone development, proper immune function, development and maintenance of epithelial tissue	Apricot Broccoli Cantaloupe Carrots Collard greens Endive Fortified milk Kale Mango Mustard greens Pumpkin Red pepper Romaine lettuce Spinach Sweet potato Swiss chard	700–900 µg/d	No
Vitamin D	Promotes absorption of calcium and phosphorus, regulates parathyroid hormone	Catfish Fortified milk Halibut Herring Mackerel Salmon Sardines Shrimp Tuna	15–20 µg/d	Probably; supplementation should be determined by vitamin D, calcium, phosphorus, and PTH levels

	Function	Sources	Amount	
Vitamin E	Protects cell membranes of oxidation and free radicals	Almonds, Avocado, Brazil nuts, Corn oil, Hazelnuts, Milk, Peanuts, Peanut butter, Pistachio nuts, Soybean oil, Sunflower oil	15 mg/d	No
Vitamin K	Synthesis of proteins essential for blood clotting	Broccoli, Cauliflower, Kale, Spinach, Turnip greens	90–120 µg/d	No
Vitamin B$_1$ (thiamin)	Carbohydrate metabolism and energy production, essential for proper nerve conduction	Enriched bread, Enriched cereals, Enriched rice, Lean pork, Legumes/dried beans, Pasta, Potatoes	1.1–1.2 mg/d	Yes
Vitamin B$_2$ (riboflavin)	Energy production and growth	Cheese, Eggs, Enriched bread, Enriched cereals, Lean beef, Lean pork, Milk, Spinach, Yogurt	1.1–1.3 mg/d	Yes

(continued on next page)

Table 5 (*continued*)

Vitamin/Mineral	Functions	Sources	Recommended Dietary Allowance	Extra Needed in CKD
Vitamin B$_3$ (niacin)	Carbohydrate and protein metabolism, aids in fat synthesis and tissue respiration	Enriched bread Enriched cereals Fish Lean meat Peanuts Peanut butter Poultry	14–16 mg/d	Yes
Vitamin B$_6$ (pyridoxine)	Protein synthesis, heme production, essential for normal brain and nervous system development and function	Avocado Banana Beef Fish Oatmeal Pork Potatoes Poultry	1.3–1.7 mg/d	Yes
Folate (folic acid)	Production and maturation of red and white blood cells	Asparagus Avocado Broccoli Eggs Legumes/dried beans Nuts Spinach/dark green leafy vegetables	400 µg/d	Yes

Vitamin B$_{12}$	Growth, development, and proper function of cells, especially those in the nervous system; aids folate in production of red blood cells	Beef Cheese Eggs Fish Milk Pork Poultry Yogurt	2.4 µg/d	Yes
Vitamin C	Aids in iron absorption, essential for collagen production and wound healing, promotes immune function	Broccoli Brussels sprouts Cauliflower Citrus fruits Collard greens Kiwi Mango Melon Papaya Peppers Strawberries Sweet potato	75–90 mg/d	Yes[a]
Vitamin B$_7$ (biotin)	Aids in fat, protein, and carbohydrate metabolism	Eggs Oatmeal Organ meats Peanuts Peanut butter Poultry Walnuts Wheat bran	30 µg/d	Yes

(continued on next page)

Table 5
(continued)

Vitamin/Mineral	Functions	Sources	Recommended Dietary Allowance	Extra Needed in CKD
Vitamin B₅ (pantothenic acid)	Essential for fat, carbohydrate, and protein metabolism	Chicken Eggs Lean beef Milk Organ meats Salmon Yogurt	5 mg/d	Yes
Iron	Heme production, normal immune function, aids in synthesis and proper function of neurotransmitters	Baked potato (with skin) Broccoli Dried fruit Lean beef Legumes/dried beans Liver Molasses Oysters Poultry Shellfish Spinach Tofu	8–18 mg/d	Yes

Abbreviation: PTH, parathyroid hormone.
a Avoid total intake (including food and supplements) greater than 100 to 200 mg/d because of risk for oxalosis and kidney stone formation.

Table 6
Base foods and potassium

Base-Producing Food	Low Potassium	Medium Potassium	High Potassium
Apple	—	✔	—
Apricot	—	—	✔
Carrots	—	—	✔
Cauliflower	—	✔	—
Eggplant	✔	—	—
Lettuce	✔	—	—
Orange	—	—	✔
Peach	—	✔	—
Pear	—	✔	—
Potatoes	—	—	✔
Raisins	—	—	✔
Spinach	—	✔	—
Strawberries	—	✔	—
Tomato	—	—	✔
Zucchini	—	✔	—

possibly be achieved. Practitioners taking care of elderly, osteoporotic patients often encourage calcium supplementation. However, for patients with CKD, this may increase detrimental cardiac end points. The Academy of Nutrition and Dietetics reminds us that patients with CKD are a special population[16]:

- For adults with CKD (GFR <60 mL/min, including after kidney transplant), the daily calcium intake (including dietary calcium, calcium supplementation, and calcium-based phosphate binders) should not exceed 2000 mg/d.

Bisphosphonates are renally cleared and, thus, must be renally dosed.[23] There are few clinical trials addressing bisphosphonate use in the CKD population. That said, it seems that bisphosphonates are safe in patients with CKD with a GFR greater than 30 mL/min. However, for those patients with severe kidney disease, bisphosphonates must be used with caution. Although few practitioners will start patients with CKD with a GFR less than 30 mL/min on a bisphosphonate, it is common that patients lose kidney function and the medication is inadvertently continued. Caution must be exercised in the CKD population, and frequent medication reviews are vital to keep a practitioner from overlooking this preventable complication.

VITAMINS AND ANTIOXIDANTS

Clinicians are often asked if vitamin supplements are beneficial in treating CKD. Although mega doses of vitamins and minerals are not encouraged, some degree of supplementation may be warranted for patients with concomitant conditions. Many patients with CKD are also diabetic, and neuropathy is a common complaint. Vitamin B_{12} can help with neuropathy, but the extent of how much is undetermined.[24]

High homocysteine levels are often found in patients with CKD.[25] High homocysteine is known to be a risk factor for increased cardiovascular events. B vitamins

Box 1
High-fiber foods

Grains

Brown rice

Oatmeal or oat bran

Rye bread

Wheat germ

Whole-grain breads

Whole-grain or bran cereals

Whole-grain crackers

Whole-wheat pasta

Fruit

Apple

Apricot

Banana

Berries

Dried fruit

Grapefruit

Mango

Orange

Peach

Pear

Pineapple

Vegetables

Asparagus

Bean sprouts

Broccoli

Brussels sprouts

Cabbage

Carrots

Cauliflower

Celery

Corn

Green beans

Peas

Potato (with skin)

Spinach

Other

Almonds

Brazil nuts

Cashews

Garbanzo beans

Kidney beans

Lentils

Lima beans

Navy beans

Pinto beans

Popcorn

Sesame seeds

Split peas

Sunflower seeds

Walnuts

can mediate high homocysteine. Although B vitamin supplementation has been hypothesized to be a simple and inexpensive way to decrease cardiac end points in patients with CKD, it has not been proven to be cardioprotective in this population.[26]

That said, vitamin B_{12} supplementation is useful for both diabetic neuropathy and for the anemia that accompanies CKD. Accordingly, the Academy of Nutrition and Dietetics encourages B vitamin supplementation in anemia[16]:

- In adults with CKD (including after kidney transplant), vitamin B_{12} and folic acid supplementation should be given if the MCV is more than 100 ng/mL and serum levels of these nutrients are less than normal values.

As B vitamins are water soluble, they are leached from the blood during dialysis. Therefore, replacement of B vitamins is vital for both hemodialysis and peritoneal dialysis patients. For this reason, renal-specific multivitamins contain higher amounts of B vitamins compared with standard multivitamins. In fact, the military developed a protocol to give patients who are dialysis dependent a prenatal vitamin

---

Box 2
Criteria for use as probiotic

1. Organism fully identified

2. Organism safe for consumption
   a. Not pathogenic, not toxic to GI mucosa
   b. No antibiotic resistance genes

3. Organism survives GI transit

4. Organism colonizes GI tract via adherence (may be transient)

5. Organism shows positive health effects
   a. Antagonizes pathogenic bacteria
   b. At least one phase 2 study showing benefit

6. Organism stable for processing and storage

Adapted from Borchers AT, Selmi C, Meyers FJ, et al. Probiotics and immunity. J Gastroenterol 2009;44(1):26–46.

Table 7
Common herbs

Herb	Plant Parts	Common Medicinal Uses/Efficacy	Mechanism of Action Precautions	Use in CKD
Yohimbe (*Pausinystalia yohimbe*)	Evergreen bark teas, capsule, tablets	Aphrodisiac Erectile dysfunction	Alpha-2 receptors antagonist Associated with hypertension Interaction with MAO inhibitors	No
Saw palmetto (*Serenoa repens, Sabal serrulata*)	Dried, whole berries, tablets, capsules, teas	Mild efficacy for BPH Bladder disorders, prostate cancer: insufficient evidence for efficacy	Unknown Mild stomach discomfort	Unknown
American/Canadian ginseng (*Baie rouge*)	Root	Possible effective: URI	May affect insulin levels, alter immune system Adverse effect: diarrhea, itching, insomnia, hypertension, heart rate changes	No
Siberian ginseng (*Eleutherococcus senticosus, Acanthopanax senticosus*)	Root extract	Possibly effective: herpes simplex 2 Insufficient evidence for blood pressure management or CKD	Affects brain, immune system; often contains adulterants (eg, silk vine) Multiple drug interactions; avoid in heart disease, high blood pressure, schizophrenia	No
Asian/Chinese ginseng (*Panax spp*)	Root extract	Common cold remedy Possible improvement in concentration Effects may be augmented by gingko leaf coadministration	High mislabeling rate Adverse effect: insomnia Many drug interactions Avoid in autoimmune diseases and transplant patients Anticoagulant effect, long-term use has hormonal effects (>3 mo)	No
Echinacea (*Echinacea purpura, Angustifolia pallida*)	Aboveground parts of plant and root; fresh, dried, teas, extracts	Possibly effective for colds, influenza, URI	Activates immune response Cross allergy to daisy family Adverse effects: rash, asthma, GI; caution with immunosuppressant medications	No

Name	Parts/forms	Effectiveness	Notes/precautions	
Horse chestnut (*Aesculus hippocastanum*)	Seeds, bark, flower, leaves	Possibly effective for varicose veins and pain	Anticoagulant; Reduces venous and capillary permeability; Death if raw seed, bark, flower or leaf is eaten; Kidney damage possible	No
Gingko (*Gingko biloba*)	Tree leaves: capsule, tablet, teas, extract	No memory improvement effect	Carcinogenic in mice; Potential drug interactions	No
Aloe vera (*Aloe barbadensis*)	Plant leaf gel, FDA approved as natural food flavoring	Mildly effective: wound healing; Some effectiveness as laxative	Topical use safe; Oral use: rat carcinogen; Adverse effects of diarrhea and alteration of blood glucose	No; Topical: yes
Green tea, Chinese tea, Japanese tea (*Camellia sinensis*)	Leaves, dried extracts, capsules, teas	Mixed effectiveness: cancer treatment, mental alertness	Safe in moderate amounts; Concentrated extract: liver damage; Caution with warfarin	No
St. John's wort, Klamath weed, goatweed (*Hypericum perforatum*)	Flowers, teas, tablets, capsules, extracts	Mixed results: depression, anxiety	Reduces cyclosporine levels; Anticoagulant effect; Sunlight sensitivity	No
Garcinia cambogia (sold as: HCA [hydroxycitric acid, 50%]).	Rinds of fruit extract	Weight loss	Appetite suppressant: blocks adipocyte formation; No data available on precautions	No
Valerian or setwall (*Valerianae radix*, roots: *officinalis* species)	Roots, rhizomes, stolon; Teas, extracts, tinctures, capsules	Putative effectiveness for insomnia and sedation	Many chemical constituents, include valerenic acid, iridoids; Mechanism not known; Long-term safety not studied; Adverse effects: headaches, pruritus, GI disorders, dizziness	No
Chayote or mirliton (*Sechium edule*) Cucurbitaceae fruit family	Stem, tuber root, young leaves	Insufficient evidence for kidney stones, hypertension, arteriosclerosis, or CKD cure	No specific precautions	Unknown

(continued on next page)

Table 7
(continued)

Herb	Plant Parts	Common Medicinal Uses/Efficacy	Mechanism of Action Precautions	Use in CKD
Triphala formula	Indian herbal, 3 fruits: harada, *Amia*, bihara Tablets, teas	Vegetarian laxative	Antiinflammatory, high in vitamin C Adverse effect: diarrhea	Unknown
Kelp: sold as solgar by Nature Way Vitamin Shoppe Yang supplement	Dried seaweed, sea plant	Trace mineral supplement: copper, zinc, manganese, chromium, iron High calcium, sodium, iodine source	Purity variability, contaminated with toxic metals: mercury, arsenic Caution: high calcium, salts; adverse effect: hypothyroidism	No
Acai berry	Juices, powders, tablets, capsules	No evidence: weight loss or antiinflammatory properties	Mechanism unknown May affect MRI tests	Unknown
Cat's claw (*Uncaria tomentosa*)	Capsules, tablets, tinctures, elixirs, teas	Boost immune system, arthritis remedy, cancer, AIDS-related symptoms (insufficient evidence)	Tannins: antioxidant Adverse effects: rash, hypotension, possible kidney damage, interaction with anticoagulants, antirejection meds, and autoimmune disease	No

Abbreviations: BPH, benign prostatic hyperplasia; FDA, Food and Drug Administration; MAO, monoamine oxidase; meds, medications; URI, upper respiratory infection.

Table 8
Common Navajo herbals

Name	Common Use	Use in CKD	Preparation
American mistletoe (*Phoradendron flavescens*)	Antihypertensive Sedative	Unsafe (USDA)	Tea
Bearberry (*Arctostaphylos uva-ursi*)	Bladder, kidney, liver RX Diuretic, back sprains Venereal disease	Safe in early CKD	Tea
Big sagebrush (*Artemisia tridentate*)	Stomach gas/problems Colds, sore eyes, headache Diarrhea, sore throat, vomiting	Safe in early CKD	Hair tonic Bug repellant
Bindweed (*Convolvulus sepium*)	Laxative Gallbladder remedy	Safe in early CKD	Tea from stems, roots and leaves dried/crushed
Broom snakeroot (*Gutierrezia purshiana*)	Bee, wasp, ant stings Nausea, rheumatism Malaria	Safe in early CKD	Chewed poultice
Cascara sagrada (*Rhamnus purshiana*)	Laxative	Safe in early CKD	Aged dried bark boiled
Dandelion (*Taraxacum officinale*)	GI problems Laxative	Safe in early CKD	Tea
Juniper (*Juniperus communis*)	Stomach aches Hemorrhage, relief of gas, cystitis, diuretic	Safe in early CKD	Tea from berries
Mormon tea (*Ephedra nevadensis*)	Decongestant, asthma Sunburn lips	Safe in early CKD	Tea Chewed twig
Aspen	Fever Mild pain from arthritis	Safe in early CKD	Tea from bark
Indian tobacco (*Lobelia inflata*)	Asthma, lung ailments	Poisonous (USDA)	Tea
Peyote (*Lophophora williamsii*)	Sacrament of Native American church Psychotomimetic properties	Illegal in United States	Tea

Abbreviation: RX, prescription.

when renal vitamins are not available.[27] Prenatal vitamins also contain higher amounts of the vitamins and minerals required by patients on dialysis: B vitamins and iron.[28]

Antioxidants are a popular topic in the general literature read by many patients and their families. In a Cochrane Review, multiple studies of antioxidant therapy in patients with CKD were reported.[29] Data are available from more than 10 high-level, placebo-controlled studies including 1900 patients with CKD and/or kidney transplant. Interventions included vitamin E, coenzyme Q, acetylcysteine, bardoxolone methyl, and human recombinant superoxide dismutase were compared with placebo. Studies showed no decrease in cardiovascular events in the high-risk CKD population. Thus, antioxidants are not shown to help patients with CKD. That said, patients will often take these supplements on their own. Aside from the financial strain of purchasing these antioxidant supplements, there is no evidence to show that they are dangerous to the CKD population. In addition to antioxidants, many over-the-counter supplements are taken for joint pain (**Table 4**). Those listed have been tested in patients with CKD.

Other than the B vitamins and iron, there is little need for further supplementation for patients with CKD (**Table 5**). That said, there is little downside of vitamins in this cohort. However, the cost should be a consideration, especially for those patients who think specialty vitamins are superior.

BICARBONATE

Decreasing metabolic acidosis is another intervention that we can do to slow progression of CKD.[30] It is woefully underutilized and underacknowledged outside of the kidney community. Keeping the blood from becoming more acidotic protects the kidney and decreases the rate of loss of kidney function. This can be accomplished through sodium bicarbonate supplements (tablets, liquids or off-the-shelf baking soda) or through dietary changes. Increasing consumption of base foods will decrease acidosis.[31] Many of these base foods are also high in potassium; thus, care must be taken when encouraging increased intake of these foods. By selecting lower-potassium foods with high base content, patients with CKD can decrease acidosis without contributing to hyperkalemia (**Table 6**).

FLUIDS

For all the discussion in the lay literature of fluid management and the kidneys, there are actually very little peer-reviewed data published. Much of the information involves the interaction of the cardiorenal system and the use of diuretic therapy. That said, the Institute of Medicine (IOM) has published an opinion regarding daily intake of fluids. The IOM suggests that 3 L/d of fluid for men and 2.2 L/d for women is adequate fluid intake to survive and thrive.[32] Three liters translates into twelve 8-oz cups per day or 8 average-size cans of soda per day.

As kidney disease progresses, fluid restriction is needed, as fluid can overwhelm the poorly functioning kidney. When one gets to dialysis, fluid restriction is the norm. In the early stages of CKD, fluids can protect the kidney from infection, medication adverse effects, and kidney stones.[32] However, fluid overload can cause congestive heart failure for patients with a poorly functioning heart. Thus, the recommendations for fluid intake depend not only on the CKD stage but also on cardiac output.

FIBER

Many medications given to patients with CKD can cause constipation. Additionally, patients with CKD are often sedentary, increasing the incidence of constipation. Although exercise is commonly recommended for those patients with diabetes, obesity, and CKD, it is often not followed by typical patients. Fiber or laxative use is common in patients with CKD.

In addition to preventing constipation, high-fiber intake has been shown to decrease mortality.[33] It is thought that this is related to the decrease in inflammation that occurs with the higher-fiber diet. A recent meta-analysis showed that high-fiber intake in patients with CKD decreased serum urea and serum creatinine.[34] A randomized controlled trial showed increasing dietary fiber for 6 weeks decreased uremic solutes in hemodialysis patients.[35] These studies indicate that increasing dietary fiber can slow the progression of CKD (**Box 1**).

PROBIOTICS

Probiotics are defined by the World Health Organization as "live organisms which when administered in adequate amounts confer a health benefit on the host."[36] Specific criteria must be met to be listed as a probiotic (**Box 2**). As long as preparation is pure and in accordance with the US Department of Agriculture (USDA) quality controls, probiotics are safe for patients with CKD. However, many patients take these in tablet form instead of eating foods containing naturally occurring probiotics. The issue of contamination is important to patients with CKD, as toxicity for these patients is a true risk.

HERBALS

Herbal supplements are both a promise and a bane of patients with CKD. Many patients think that herbals make them feel better, but some of these supplements have caused morbidity and mortality in this fragile population.[37] One of the most well-researched herbals with toxic kidney effects is aristolochic acid (AA).[38] AA is used by Chinese herbalists for weight loss. Because of an increased risk of kidney injury, AA has been banned in the United States. However, it is still available via the Internet and patients may still inquire about it.

As reported in a recent article in the *Journal of the American Medical Association*, the manufacturing of herbal supplements is not well controlled or regulated and products often contain banned substances.[39] Thus, despite data on the safety of some herbals in the CKD population (**Table 7**), one cannot recommend the over-the-counter herbal supplements with a high degree of confidence. Often what is listed on the bottle is not what is actually in the bottle as *Consumer Reports* found in a recent review of commonly purchased supplements.[40]

The Native American and Latino populations often use medicine men and women to make and distribute herbal supplements (**Table 8**). Contrary to commercially manufactured herbal supplements, these tribal medications have been used for centuries; as the actual practitioner makes them, they are often pure and, therefore, may be safer in the CKD population. However, it is important to consider that many of these medications have not been sufficiently tested for safety.

SUMMARY

The kidney diet has evolved as Americans have changed their eating habits. Home-cooked meals have been increasingly replaced by takeout and frozen prepackaged meals, which has subsequently increased the sodium, potassium, and phosphorus load for many of our patients. The size of a standard plate has increased from 9 in in 1960 to 11 in in 2015, and the serving size has increased along with it. Our patients are both eating and drinking more and exercising less. This behavior has led to the explosion in the incidence of diabetes and hypertension, which substantially influences the development and progression of CKD. Following the evidence-based dietary guidelines and recommendations discussed in this article can help slow the rate of progression of kidney disease. If practitioners and patients collaborate to make proactive dietary changes, CKD does not have to lead to kidney failure.

REFERENCES

1. Tsindos S. What drove us to drink 2 litres of water a day? Aust N Z J Public Health 2012;36(3):205–7.
2. Negoianu D, Goldfarb S. Just add water. J Am Soc Nephrol 2008;19:1041–3.
3. McCartney M. Waterlogged? BMJ 2011;343:d4280.
4. Levey AS, Adler S, Caggiula AW, et al. Effects of dietary protein restriction on the progression of advanced renal disease in the Modification of Diet in Renal Disease Study. Am J Kidney Dis 1996;27(5):652–63.
5. Klahr S, Levey AS, Beck GJ, et al. The effects of dietary protein restriction and blood-pressure control on the progression of chronic renal disease. Modification of Diet in Renal Disease Study Group. N Engl J Med 1994; 330:877–84.
6. Levey AS, Greene T, Beck GJ, et al. Dietary protein restriction and the progression of chronic renal disease: what have all of the results of the MDRD study shown? Modification of Diet in Renal Disease Study Group. J Am Soc Nephrol 1999;10(11):2426–39.
7. Lacson E Jr, Wang W, Zebrowski B, et al. Outcomes associated with intradialytic oral nutritional supplements in patients undergoing maintenance hemodialysis: a quality improvement report. Am J Kidney Dis 2012;60(4): 591–600.
8. Kidney Disease: Improving Global Outcomes (KDIGO) CKD Work Group. KDIGO 2012 clinical practice guideline for the evaluation and management of chronic kidney disease. Kidney Int 2013;3(Suppl):1–150.
9. Wright JA, Cavanaugh KL. Dietary sodium in chronic kidney disease: a comprehensive approach. Semin Dial 2010;23(4):415–21.
10. U.S. Department of Agriculture and U.S. Department of Health and Human Services. Dietary guidelines for Americans, 2010. 7th edition. Washington, DC: U.S. Government Printing Office; 2010.
11. Jones-Burton C, Mishra SI, Fink JC, et al. An in-depth review of the evidence linking dietary salt intake and progression of chronic kidney disease. Am J Nephrol 2006;26(3):268–75.
12. Vegter S, Perna A, Postma MJ, et al. Sodium intake, ACE inhibition, and progression to ESRD. J Am Soc Nephrol 2012;23(1):165–73.
13. Boyce JM, Shone GR. Effects of ageing on smell and taste. Postgrad Med J 2006; 82(966):239–41.
14. Available at: http://www.mrsdash.com/. Accessed June 7, 2015.
15. Available at: https://www.chefpaul.com/site.php. Accessed June 7, 2015.
16. American Dietetic Association. Chronic kidney disease evidence-based nutrition practice guideline. Chicago: American Dietetic Association; 2010.

17. Tucker K. Nutritional requirements of peritoneal dialysis, International Society for Peritoneal Dialysis. Available at: ISPD.org. Accessed June 14, 2015.
18. González-Parra E, Gracia-Iguacel C, Egido J, et al. Phosphorus and nutrition in chronic kidney disease. Int J Nephrol 2012;2012:597605.
19. Melamed ML, Thadhani RI. Vitamin D therapy in chronic kidney disease and end stage renal disease. Clin J Am Soc Nephrol 2012;7(2):358–65.
20. Baigent C, Landray MJ, Reith C, et al. The effects of lowering LDL cholesterol with simvastatin plus ezetimibe in patients with chronic kidney disease (Study of Heart and Renal Protection): a randomised placebo-controlled trial. Lancet 2011; 377(9784):2181–92.
21. Inda Filho AJ, Melamed ML. Vitamin D and kidney disease: what we know and what we do not know. J Bras Nefrol 2013;35(4):323–31.
22. West SL, Swan VJ, Jamal SA. Effects of calcium on cardiovascular events in patients with kidney disease and in a healthy population. Clin J Am Soc Nephrol 2010;5(Suppl 1):S41–7.
23. Toussaint N, Elder G, Kerr P. Bisphosphonates in chronic kidney disease; balancing potential benefits and adverse effects on bone and soft tissue. Clin J Am Soc Nephrol 2009;4:221–33.
24. Talaei A, Siavash M, Majidi H, et al. Vitamin B12 may be more effective than nortriptyline in improving painful diabetic neuropathy. Int J Food Sci Nutr 2009; 60(Suppl 5):71–6.
25. Gonin JM, Nguyen H, Gonin R, et al. Controlled trials of very high dose folic acid, vitamins B12 and B6, intravenous folinic acid and serine for treatment of hyperhomocysteinemia in ESRD. J Nephrol 2003;16(4):522–34.
26. Nursalim A, Siregar P, Widyahening IS. Effect of folic acid, vitamin B6 and vitamin B12 supplementation on mortality and cardiovascular complication among patients with chronic kidney disease: an evidence-based case report. Acta Med Indones 2013;45(2):150–6.
27. Zuber K. Pregnancy and CKD. Oral presentation NKF spring clinical meetings. Dallas, TX, April 2015. Accessed March 27, 2015.
28. McKeating A, Farren M, Cawley S, et al. Maternal folic acid supplementation trends 2009-2013. Acta Obstet Gynecol Scand 2015;94(7):727–33.
29. Jun M, Venkataraman V, Razavian M, et al. Antioxidants for chronic kidney disease. Cochrane Database Syst Rev 2012;(10):CD008176.
30. Goraya N, Wesson DE. Does correction of metabolic acidosis slow chronic kidney disease progression? Curr Opin Nephrol Hypertens 2013;22(2):193–7.
31. Goraya N, Simoni J, Jo CH, et al. A comparison of treating metabolic acidosis in CKD stage 4 hypertensive kidney disease with fruits and vegetables or sodium bicarbonate. Clin J Am Soc Nephrol 2013;8(3):371–81.
32. National Kidney Foundation. Six tips to be water wise for healthy kidneys. Available at: https://www.kidney.org/content/6-tips-be-water-wise-healthy-kidneys. Accessed May 1, 2015.
33. Krishnamurthy VM, Wei G, Baird BC, et al. High dietary fiber intake is associated with decreased inflammation and all-cause mortality in patients with chronic kidney disease. Kidney Int 2012;81(3):300–6.
34. Chiavaroli L, Mirrahimi A, Sievenpiper JL, et al. Dietary fiber effects in chronic kidney disease: a systematic review and meta-analysis of controlled feeding trials. Eur J Clin Nutr 2015;69(7):761–8.
35. Sirich TL, Plummer NS, Gardner CD, et al. Effect of increasing dietary fiber on plasma levels of colon-derived solutes in hemodialysis patients. Clin J Am Soc Nephrol 2014;9(9):1603–10.

36. Guidelines for the evaluation of probiotics in food: Joint FAO/WHO Working Group meeting. London, Ontario, Canada, April 30–May 1, 2002.
37. Jha V. Herbal medicines and chronic kidney disease. Nephrology (Carlton) 2010; 15(Suppl 2):10–7.
38. Lai MN, Lai JN, Chen PC, et al. Increased risks of chronic kidney disease associated with prescribed Chinese herbal products suspected to contain aristolochic acid. Nephrology (Carlton) 2009;14(2):227–34.
39. Cohen PA, Maller G, DeSouza R, et al. Presence of banned drugs in dietary supplements following FDA recalls. JAMA 2014;312(16):1691–3.
40. Cooper L. What's wrong with herbal remedies? They might not contain what they claim—and probably don't work, either. Yonkers, NY: Consumer Reports; 2015.

Before Crossing the Red Line

Surgery and Chronic Kidney Disease

April Crunk, PA-C[a],*, Catherine G. Brown, CRNP, MSN[b]

KEYWORDS

- Surgery • Anesthesia • Metabolites • CKD • Diabetes mellitus • Kidney patient

KEY POINTS

- Patients with kidney disease have higher rates of surgical procedures.
- Extra caution should be exercised in the preoperative, perioperative, and postoperative periods.
- Medication dosing requires adjustments for the kidney patient.
- The physician assistant often sees the patient in all phases of the surgical experience.

THE SURGICAL CHRONIC KIDNEY DISEASE PATIENT
The Scene: Operating Theater Circa 1830

Dr Robert Liston, famed British surgeon, enters the operating theater. The audience includes aspiring surgeons, medical students, and assorted bystanders who came to watch the spectacle and to time the surgeon famous for his lightning fast amputations.

The patient is brought in, although dragged in is more descriptive. The assistants are primarily strong men whose job it is to hold the patient down. The forerunners of first surgical assistants are ready with tourniquets, needle, and thread for the procedure.

The great Dr Liston approaches the pale and sweating patient. The first assistant ties a tourniquet tightly around the thigh and in less than a minute, thanks to Dr Liston's skill, the mangled left leg lies on the ground and the assistants commence to tie off the blood vessels and sew the flap shut.

With the patient's screams still echoing in the room, Dr Liston rinses his hands in a basin and goes off to lunch with little attention to the blood spattered on his clothes. The bystanders who have timed the master are pleased with the show.

Disclosures: None.
[a] Department of Interventional Radiology, University of Alabama at Birmingham, NHB H 623, 619 19th Street S, Birmingham, AL 35249-6830, USA; [b] Hospitalist Service, University of Alabama at Birmingham, 619 19th Street South, Birmingham, AL 35294, USA
* Corresponding author.
E-mail address: acrunk@uabmc.edu

Physician Assist Clin 1 (2016) 101–113
http://dx.doi.org/10.1016/j.cpha.2015.09.011 physicianassistant.theclinics.com
2405-7991/16/$ – see front matter © 2016 Elsevier Inc. All rights reserved.

The patient likely became septic and died; had he lived, he would have been ever haunted by the memory, an early case of posttraumatic stress disorder.

In the 1840s this all changed. A paper describing painless dentistry via a secret formula now known to contain ether transformed surgery forever. Although initially dismissed by Liston and other surgeons as a needless luxury, a few demonstration procedures using anesthesia made believers out of the skeptics. Liston fully embraced anesthesia, although he continued his rapid surgical style.

Antisepsis took longer to take hold. In 1847, Ignaz Semmelweiss promoted hand washing in the maternal wards to decrease infection and was largely ignored. In 1867, the renowned Joseph Lister published an article in *The Lancet* promoting the use of carbolic acid to reduce sepsis in wounds. Although he was largely ignored, by the turn of the 20th century, both anesthesia and antiseptic techniques were becoming common place.[1]

Fast forward to the 21st century. The operating room is no longer a theater. The patient comes in voluntarily. Usually there is some anesthesia on board. The assistants are gowned and gloved, having scrubbed before entering. Instead of cries for mercy and screams of excruciating pain, the hiss and whir of equipment with sounds of the surgeon's favorite compact disk fill the air.

In the 21st century, surgery is common. Virtually no part of the human anatomy is off limits. Surgeons are known for their precision and skill as well as speed. Yet none of this would be possible without anesthesia, ranging from a regional block to full intubation. None of it is possible without the anesthetist who oversees it all, and the provider who manages preoperative and postoperative evaluation and care.

SURGERY AND THE CHRONIC KIDNEY DISEASE PATIENT

In addition to procedures experienced by the general public, chronic kidney disease (CKD) patients also have procedures particular to kidney disease. These include both peritoneal and hemodialysis accesses for dialysis along with procedures to correct or salvage the access.

Even under the best of circumstances, surgery is a stressful event for any patient. For the CKD patient, even those in early stages (glomerular filtration rate [GFR] >30 mL/min), surgery can be a considerable insult to organ systems. To ensure the patient optimal chances for a smooth perioperative and postoperative course, pertinent past medical history and comorbidities should be evaluated and managed. This includes evaluation for appropriate preoperative screening, and preoperative and perioperative medication for optimization of the medical therapy being received.

FOCUS ON THE STORY

It is well-accepted that a thorough history can be your most valuable medical tool. Begin gathering past medical history with a strong attention given to known previous history of kidney disease. In patients with known kidney dysfunction, it is important to quantify the severity of impairment by identifying the stage of disease[2] (**Fig. 1**).[2] Baseline data of previous blood urea nitrogen, creatinine, GFR, and urinalysis (with special attention to evidence of albuminuria) should be gleaned from past medical records when available. Those medical conditions that are known to impact kidney patients should also be evaluated. These include, but are not limited to:

- Coronary artery disease,
- Cardiomyopathy,
- Previous cerebral vascular accident,

Prognosis of CKD by GFR and Albuminuria Categories: KDIGO 2012			Persistent albuminuria categories Description and range		
			A1	A2	A3
			Normal to mildly increased	Moderately increased	Severely increased
			<30 mg/g <3 mg/mmol	30–300 mg/g 3–30 mg/mmol	>300 mg/g >30 mg/mmol
GFR categories (mL/min/ 1.73 m²) Description and range	G1	Normal or high ≥90			
	G2	Mildly decreased 60–89			
	G3a	Mildly to moderately decreased 45–59			
	G3b	Moderately to severely decreased 30–44			
	G4	Severely decreased 15–29			
	G5	Kidney failure <15			

Fig. 1. Prognosis of CKD by GFR and albuminuria category. (*From* KDIGO 2012 clinical practice guideline for the evaluation and management of chronic kidney disease. Kidney Int Suppl 2013;3: p. 1-150; with permission. Available at: http://www.kdigo.org/clinical_practice_guidelines/pdf/CKD/KDIGO_2012_CKD_GL.pdf.)

- Diabetes mellitus,
- Hepatic diseases (ie, cirrhosis),
- Lupus,
- Dementia, and
- Chronic pain.

Each of these comorbidities is a "red flag" for disease states that may contribute to decreased cardiac output resulting in diminished blood flow to the kidneys and subsequent worsening of function.

An accurate medication history is also critical in the preoperative evaluation. Recent use of nephrotoxic agents can acutely impair kidney health. Examples include:

- Antibiotics,
- Nonsteroidal antiinflammatory drugs, and
- Contrast dye.

If the patient is already on dialysis, the clinician should consider if hemodialysis is needed preoperatively to clear nephrotoxins before surgery. It is important to consider if radiologic studies will be performed that will include contrast dye. Many radiologists feel that dialysis needs to be done within 24 hours of a procedure, although there are no studies showing this makes any difference for the dialysis-dependent patient. It does make a difference if the patient is not yet on dialysis and postcontrast hemodialysis should be considered to reduce the incidence of contrast induced nephropathy.[3] That said, if it is decided that the patient needs temporary access for short-term dialysis, a vascular catheter or "vascath" may be placed. One must ensure the benefit of this procedure outweighs the risks of central venous catheter placement (bleeding, infection, trauma to the vessel). This can be determined by discussions between the proceduralist and kidney practitioner.

A medication history should include current use of narcotic agents in preparation for the patient's postoperative care. Many narcotic agents have a prolonged half-life and, in patients with a decreased creatinine clearance, clinicians should be alert to potential overaccumulation of these agents which may lead to CNS and respiratory depression (See Gilmartin C, Pai AB, Hughes D, et al: Risky Business: Lessons from Medication Misadventures in Chronic Kidney Disease, in this issue).[4] Knowledge of what agents the patient may already have chronically "on board" is critical to the perioperative and postoperative periods. A thorough social history is also vital as this can be used as a tool to tease out any past medical concerns that the patient does not vocalize. Social history can also provide clues to underlying undiagnosed diabetes mellitus, coronary artery disease, and cirrhosis. Patients with a sedentary life style and/or morbid obesity are at increased risk for diabetes mellitus. Those with a history of intravenous (IV) drug use or heavy alcohol use are at increased risk for cirrhosis. If these are positive on the social history, further exploration of the potential for underlying undiagnosed disease must be initiated.

PREOPERATIVE EVALUATION WITH OBJECTIVE TESTS AND ALGORITHMS

If the surgical need is not emergent, CKD patients should have the following testing:

- Complete metabolic profile,
- GFR calculations,
- Urine albumin to creatine ratio,[5] and
- Baseline electrocardiograph.

A baseline electrocardiograph is recommended by the American College of Cardiology/American Heart Association (ACC/AHA) Task Force Report as a screening tool for potentially serious underlying cardiac disease before surgery.[6] It should be remembered that CKD patients are high risk for cardiac disease simply because they have kidney dysfunction.[2]

Risk assessment tools can be valuable in assessing the patient's postoperative risk of morbidity and mortality. These tools are readily available to all practitioners as online or smartphone apps (www.uptodate.com/contents/evaluation-of-cardiac-risk-prior-to-noncardiac-surgery#H2 and www.qxmd.com). Tools such as the Eagle's Cardiac Risk Assessment, the Goldman Revised Cardiac Risk Index (RCRI), and Detsky's Modified Cardiac Risk Index allow for the calculation of major, intermediate, and minor cardiovascular risk to the patient. Eagle's Cardiac Risk Assessment is the tool recommended by the ACC/AHA Task Force Report.[6] More recent studies by the American College of Surgeons find that the National Surgical Quality Improvement Program Surgical Risk Calculator considers more detailed patient history and surgical procedure risk.[7] It uses Current Procedural Terminology codes to target the procedure involved and the inherent risk with such procedures. This tool includes 22 criteria that allow for a more accurate prediction of death, total complication rate, and serious complication rate. This tool is not only valuable in assessing the risk for the procedure itself, but also sheds light on where the clinician may be proactive in intervening for optimal outcomes.

OPTIMIZING MEDICAL MANAGEMENT

Knowing that comorbid conditions place all patients at increased risk, and some certainly increase the risk specifically for CKD patients those comorbidities should have medical therapy optimized before a planned procedure. This cannot always be managed in the case of an emergent surgery. The comorbidities of greatest concern are those conditions that can cause deterioration of kidney disease:

- Hypertension,
- Hypotension,
- Overall volume status,
- Electrolyte imbalance, and
- Cardiac health.

Hypertension should be acutely controlled and surgery postponed unless the procedure is emergent. Hypotension must be addressed quickly because prolonged hypotension will lead to further kidney injury.[8] The patient's overall volume status should be maintained in a euvolemic state as much as possible and dialysis (either hemodialysis and peritoneal dialysis if the patient is dialysis dependent) should be arranged in coordination with the posted surgical time. Electrolyte imbalances should be corrected before surgery unless the procedure is emergent. Electrolyte imbalances can lead to cardiac arrhythmias which have the potential to decrease cardiac output thus resulting in decreased blood flow to the kidneys and subsequent further injury.[8] Although reversal of chronic cardiac disease is not likely to occur before surgery, cardiac health can be improved by the administration of aspirin therapy, statin therapy, or beta-blockade. Beta-blockade is known to lower postoperative mortality and, if the patient is not hypotensive, therapy should be initiated.[6]

Preoperative antibiotic dosing has been a subject of controversy. There is no evidence to support administering antibiotics to CKD patients as prophylaxis. CKD patients are at no increased risk for infection in specific relation to their CKD. However, many CKD patients have diabetes mellitus as a comorbidity and these patients most certainly have increased postoperative infection rates. The use of antibiotics both preoperatively and postoperatively should be considered thoughtfully with regard to the actual surgical case and the potential for infection in relation to the procedure rather than in relation to CKD. Prescribing antibiotics without this consideration can expose the CKD patient to unnecessary doses of nephrotoxic agents causing further kidney damage.[9]

ENTER ANESTHESIA

Preoperative evaluation for anesthesia requires an interview with the patient to obtain pertinent medical, anesthesia, and surgical histories. Appropriate physical examination, review of laboratory indices, electrocardiogram, radiologic imaging, and previous progress notes or consultations may be necessary to provide accurate assignment of the American Society of Anesthesiologists (ASA) physical status classification (**Table 1**). The ASA ranks risk from 1 to 6, ranging from healthy, minimum risk to the brain dead organ donor patient.

All patients should, at a minimum, receive clinical assessment of the airway, and cardiac and pulmonary systems during the preanesthetic examination. The airway examination includes assessment measurements determining the ease of intubation, prognathic condition (relationship of jaws to head), dentition, neck circumference, body mass index, and beard status. Cardiac and pulmonary examinations confirm or establish comorbid conditions that increase ASA classification status. Review of

Table 1		
ASA physical status classification		
ASA Classification	**Description**	**Examples**
I	Normal healthy patient	Nonsmoker
II	Patient with mild systemic disease	Smoker, well-controlled HTN, Diabetes, CKD
III	Patient with severe systemic disease	COPD, ESRD, poorly controlled diabetes or HTN, implanted pacemaker, cardiac stent, ejection fraction <40%
IV	Patient with severe systemic disease that is a threat to life	Recent MI, CVA, TIA, or cardiac surgery, sever valve dysfunction, ejection fraction <25%
V	Moribund patient not expected to survive without surgery	Ruptured thoracic or abdominal aneurysm, ischemic bowel with cardiac pathology
VI	Patient who is dead	Organ donor

The Addition of an 'E' to the ASA staging indicates emergency surgery.

Note that the staging does not include age of patient, type of anesthesia (local vs general), pregnancy, type of surgery.

Abbreviations: ASA, American Society of Anesthesiologists; CKD, chronic kidney disease; COPD, chronic obstructive pulmonary disease; CVA, cerebrovascular accident; ESRD, end-stage renal disease; HTN, hypertension; TIA, transient ischemic attack.

From ASA Physical Status Classification System. American Society of Anesthesiologists. Available at: https://www.asahq.org/resources/clinical-information/asa-physical-status-classification-system. Accessed May 02, 2015.

recent laboratory indices provides valuable information about the physiologic functional status of the heart, lungs, kidney, and blood.

The anesthesiologist can also use the RCRI to determine perioperative risk. This correlates patient and surgical perioperative risk for patients with a history of ischemic heart disease, heart failure, cerebrovascular disease, insulin-dependent diabetes, and decreased kidney function. The RCRI can also be used for those patients with active comorbidities.

The anesthesia, medical, and surgical histories are the bedrock of the preoperative evaluation. Medications, allergies, and pertinent family history are included. For example, in the hypertensive patient, it is essential to note if the blood pressure is controlled; the ejection fraction, if available; and any previous adverse experiences with medications.

Of particular concern with all patients is avoiding acute kidney injury (AKI). Approximately 18% patients develop AKI after cardiac surgery and 2% to 6% will require dialysis. Those who develop AKI have prolonged intensive care stays, increased hospital costs, and a greater risk of death. Selection of vasopressors, IV fluids, and close monitoring of hemoglobin perioperatively are essential to decrease the incidence of AKI.[10]

Postoperative Care

The pearls of preoperative and perioperative management should remain the guiding factor for postoperative care. Volume status should remain in a euvolemic state if possible. Fluid intake and output should be matched through close monitoring. For those patients who are admitted to the hospital in either an inpatient or observation status and are at risk of AKI, chemistry laboratory tests should be followed to evaluate for worsening kidney function. Close monitoring of risks for kidney insult is imperative with special attention being given to hypertension, hypotension, postoperative ischemia, and the use of nephrotoxic agents.

Pain Management

Postoperative pain should be anticipated and managed aggressively with certain caveats. Patients with CKD have an impaired ability to clear narcotics and if additional renal insult occurs during or after surgery, these drugs have the propensity to accumulate in the patient's system. Drugs such as meperidine should be avoided because the metabolite (normeperidine) has a long half-life and can cause both central and respiratory depression. When one attempts to reverse the effects with naloxone, a paradoxic reaction may occur resulting in enhanced sedation. Caution should be exercised with the use of morphine owing to its prolonged sedative effect. However, morphine is used for some hemodialysis patients because it is removed during dialysis. Fentanyl is the opioid of choice given that it is well-tolerated, does not lower blood pressure, and has a short half-life. Oxycodone has been used successfully in CKD patients and acetaminophen is a safe agent that should be added to augment other pain modalities. Nonsteroidal antiinflammatory drugs should be strictly avoided given their nephrotoxicity.[4]

Postoperative care should focus on getting patients moving as soon as is feasible. It is well-accepted that early movement decreases morbidity and mortality. Movement decreases risks of venous thromboembolism and the risk of health care–associated pneumonia. Mobility also improves mobilization of total fluid volume, gut motility, and overall cardiac and pulmonary health.

Dose all prescriptions for the kidney patient according to GFR dosing as noted in the Food and Drug Administration package insert. For the AKI patient with a moving GFR (either up or down), dosing of medications is significantly more complicated and may require a consult with the pharmacist. Often the pharmacist can be the best reference for the practitioner to consult when there are questions of medication choice and/or dosing regimens.[11]

The Reality of the Situation

If CKD progresses to end-stage renal disease, renal replacement therapy in the form of dialysis or kidney transplantation can be considered. If a transplant is not available, and with more than 100,000 patients on the waiting list, most likely it is not, dialysis access is a necessity. This is true for either peritoneal dialysis or hemodialysis.

Kidney failure patients will need an access point. The dialysis access is the lifeline. These are often placed in the intervention suite or by the vascular surgeon.

Go with the Flow

Vein preservation for the CKD patient is imperative and this starts early in the lifespan of the CKD patient. IVs proximal to the wrist should be avoided if at all possible. When the GFR is less than 30 mL/min/1.73 m^2, peripherally inserted central catheters are no longer an option for long-term IV needs. Because upper extremity arteriovenous fistulas and arteriovenous grafts are the most common (and preferred) accesses for dialysis, internal jugular vein catheters (not subclavian vein) are the preferred choice for central venous access.[2]

Preprocedure Outpatient Care for the Kidney Patient

What about other outpatient procedures planned for the CKD patient? Because periprocedural morbidity and mortality rates are increased with renal impairment, our attention should be focused on lowering surgical and procedural risks. Common red flags include hyperkalemia, increased bleeding possibility, anemia, hypertension, hyperglycemia, and hypoglycemia. As stated, without question, a good history and physical should be performed. Aside from this, standard laboratory tests before a procedure should include a renal panel (sodium, potassium, chloride, blood urea nitrogen, creatinine, calcium, bicarbonate, GFR, CO_2, P_{CO_2}, pH, complete blood count), coagulation studies (prothrombin time, partial thromboplastin time, International Normalized Ratio), arterial blood gas (if bicarbonate level is <18 mEq/L) and possibly a chest x-ray to evaluate for fluid status. Serum does not lie. Treat what is seen.

Hyperkalemia
General endotracheal anesthesia should be avoided if possible if the serum potassium is greater than 5.5 mEq/L. The use of oral or enema-delivered polysterene-binding resins, a combination of insulin and IV dextrose, IV bicarbonate can reduce serum potassium levels if the surgery is emergent.[12]

Increased bleeding possibility
Uremia is a clinical syndrome associated with fluid, electrolyte, and hormone imbalances as well as metabolic abnormalities that develop when kidney function declines. Uremia can cause platelet dysfunction, which can lead to increased bleeding perioperatively. For the patient with end-stage renal disease, dialysis may be performed before any procedure to reduce uremic complications. Antiplatelet agents should be held for 72 hours before a procedure. This can become problematic in patients with cardiac conditions or valve replacements and often the cardiologist or hospitalist will admit the patient for heparin dosing before a planned procedure. However, with the newest data showing that this anticoagulation "bridging" is not needed for atrial fibrillation patients, this practice likely will be severely curtailed in the future.[13] Diphenhydramine, nonsteroidal antiinflammatory drugs, chlordiazepoxide, and cimetidine theoretically may increase the risk of intraprocedural bleeding; thus, consideration for holding these drugs before the procedure should be discussed between the practitioner and the proceduralist.

Anemia
The kidneys produce the hormone erythropoietin, which stimulates the bone marrow to produce red blood cells. CKD patients may experience low hemoglobin (Hct vol dependent) levels requiring administration of blood products. CKD patients function at a lower hemoglobin and transfusion will increase their antibody loads and, thus, unless the anemia is critical and symptomatic, most CKD patients should not be transfused simply for a number.[14]

Hypertension
Hypertension is a common cause and effect of CKD. All hypertensive medications should be taken before the procedure even if the patient is NPO (nothing by mouth). A short-acting drug like hydralazine 5 mg IV may be used intraprocedurally if necessary to lower blood pressure. The accumulation of fluid may be attributing to the increase in blood pressure, so consideration of diuretics may be the answer to getting blood pressure under control if the patient makes urine. Loop diuretics can be used at all stages of CKD and are the diuretic of choice for the CKD patient. In the anuric patient, a loop diuretic can be used to expand pulmonary vasculature.[15]

Hypoglycemia
Hypoglycemia most commonly happens in patients with diabetes who are made NPO before the procedure. Keep an eye on glucose levels preoperatively, intraoperatively,

and postoperatively. Inadvertent preprocedure hypoglycemia can be avoided with a low-dose infusion of dextrose. Catecholamine release for mobilization of glycogen stores may lead to hypertension.[15]

Hyperglycemia

Patients with uncontrolled glucose should be treated with sliding scale insulin on the day of the procedure. Each surgical practice has its own protocols as developed by the anesthesia department.[12]

Contrast-Enhanced Study

For the patient with a contrast allergy who needs enhanced studies, a preprocedure dose of one of the following is recommended:

- Methylprednisolone, one 32-mg tablet, PO at 12 and 2 hours before the study and
- Prednisone, one 50-mg tablet PO q 13 hours, 7 hours, and 1 hour before the contrast-enhanced study.[16]

If the patient had a previous moderate or severe reaction to contrast or one that included a respiratory component, an alternative study, such as ultrasonography or MRI, should be considered. Otherwise, the following may be used:

- H1 antihistamines; diphenhydramine, one 50-mg tablet 1 PO q 1 hour before the study;
- H2-histamine receptor blockers (optional) cimetidine, 300 mg 1 PO q 1 hour before the study; and/or
- Ranitidine 50 mg PO q 1 hour before the procedure.

Note: cimetidine and/or ranitidine are optional additions to the diphenhydramine medication to cover both histamine 1 and histamine 2 type reactions.

Creatinine Clearance

Creatinine is a breakdown product of creatine, which is an important part of muscle. The creatinine clearance is often used interchangeably with the GFR to determine kidney function. Although it is not exactly the same, it is close enough to use for medication dosing. The Food and Drug Administration identifies medication dosing by the GFR.[17] Recommendations are drug specific and may need to be given before, supplementally during, or after hemodialysis or peritoneal dialysis.

Preprocedure Antibiotics

The potential benefit of preprocedure antibiotic prophylaxis is determined by:

- Patient factors,
- Procedure factors, and
- The potential morbidity of infection.

When the potential benefit may outweigh the risks and anticipated costs (ie, expense of agent and administration, risk of allergen, other adverse reactions, and induction of bacterial resistance), preprocedural antibiotics should be considered. Wound classifications may help in the decision-making process regarding the potential need for preprocedure antibiotics.

Almost all wounds fall into 1 of these 4 classes:

- Clean,
- Clean contaminated,

- Contaminated, or
- Dirty.

Most outpatient procedures will fall into clean and clean contaminated categories[18] (see wound classification **Table 2**[19]).

If antibiotics are indicated, the dose should be given within 1 hour of the procedure or just before the procedure occurs, that is, "on call to the procedure room."

Parenteral cephalosporins are the most commonly used prophylactic antibiotics, usually given as IV bolus or fast drip within 15 to 60 minutes before surgical procedures. Prophylaxis using vancomycin or gentamicin is given as slow drip for 1 hour, within 1 to 2 hours before surgery. Antibiotic prophylaxis may be continued up to 24 hours after surgery. To determine the type of appropriate antibiotics for prophylaxis, some experts categorize them based on the type of surgery. Type I surgery only involves skin, excluding other tracts of the body; therefore, the target pathogens are *Staphylococcus*. Type II involves both skin and other tracts, thus target pathogens include *Staphylococcus*, gram-negative, and anaerobic pathogens (see procedure/antibiotic choice **Table 3**[20]).

Table 2 Wound classification			
Clean	**Clean Contaminated**	**Contaminated**	**Dirty**
Class I	Class II	Class III	Class IV
75% of all wounds Elective procedures; little inflammation; no preruptune of membranes before procedure	Wounds to be opened for drainage; procedure does not cause a lot of trauma to the tract	Wounds containing a foreign object inside of it	Wounds containing purulence, or presence of a perforated viscus
Does not involve digestive, urinary or respiratory tracts	Can involve digestive, urinary and/or respiratory tracts; organ or body part has experienced a sudden burst	Bullet, dislodged wood or metal, etc; wound contains more inflammation around the site, and often a large amount of fluid (blood, bile, etc) present	Includes anything purulent in any body area
Angioplasty, mechanical thrombectomy, eye surgery, small skin incisions, dental prophylaxis and restoration, neurologic procedures	Infected ear, pin, or wire removal from previous surgery, caesarean section that has a rupture of membranes before procedure performed, dental extraction	Foreign body retrieval, penetrating injuries, surgical wounds that are a side effect of a mistake in technique, including those that become infected with bodily fluids, that is, bile spill from cholecystectomy	Old, traumatic wounds, devitalized tissue, existing infection or perforation, that is, ruptured appendicitis, necrotic tissue

Adapted from Zinn J, Swofford V. Quality improvement initiative: classifying and documenting surgical wounds. Wound Care Advisor 2014;3(1):34.

Table 3
Procedure/antibiotic choice

Type of Operation	Antibiotic Choice	Alternative
Type I		
Cardiovascular surgery, orthopedic surgery, cranial surgery, vascular graft	Cefazolin 1 g <80 kg Cefazolin 2 g >80 kg	Cefuroxime
If allergic to penicillin or high risk for MRSA	Vancomycin 15 mg/kg	—
Type II		
Colorectal surgery, hysterectomy, appendectomy	Cefazolin (dose based as listed above) plus metronidazole 15 mg/kg IV infused over 30–60 min and completed about 1 h before surgery	Cefoxetan, cefoxitin or ampicillin-sulbactam
If allergic to penicillin	—	Metronidozole plus gentamicin or quinolone

Please note, the above listed pre-medication antibiotics should be dosed based upon the GFR.
Abbreviation: MRSA, methicillin-resistant *Staphylococcus aureus*.
Adapted from Setiawan B. The role of prophylactic antibiotics in preventing perioperative infection. Acta Med Indones 2011;43:4.

Dental Visits

Patients with CKD and those on dialysis are more likely to have periodontal disease and other oral health problems than found in the general population. Diabetes, cardiovascular disease and osteoporosis are risk factors in oral health care issues for both the CKD and non-CKD patient. This increases the need for regular dental checkups to reduce inflammation and infection of the oral cavity. Buildup of bacteria in the mouth can cause infection. CKD patients have weakened immune systems, making them more susceptible to infection. Something as easily controllable as gingivitis (inflammation of the gums), if not treated, can lead to periodontitis and (inflammation around the teeth) periodontal disease. In periodontitis, gums pull away from the teeth and form spaces (called "pockets") that become infected. The body's immune system fights the bacteria as the plaque spreads and grows below the gum line. However, with their already compromised immune system, CKD patients are less able to combat the bacteria. Bacterial toxins and the body's natural response to infection start to break down the bone and connective tissue that hold teeth in place. If not treated, the bones, gums, and tissue that support the teeth are destroyed. As CKD progresses, the kidneys are less able to remove phosphate. Higher than normal phosphate levels, plus the underlying kidney disease, reduce the kidney's ability to make active vitamin D (1,25 D[OH]$_2$). Active vitamin D is needed to maintain bone in the oral cavity (and throughout the body) leading to possible tooth loss.[21]

If a dental abscess occurs, a course of amoxicillin (or clindamycin for the penicillin-allergic patient) is given, using GFR to dose (and all dosing is oral):

- GFR greater than 30 mL/min: amoxicillin 1 g day 1, then 1 g 3 times a day for 10 days
- GFR 10 to 30 mL/min: amoxicillin 1 g every 12 hours
- GFR < 10 mL/min: give amoxicillin 1 g every 24 hours
- For the peritoneal dialysis patient: amoxicillin 250 mg every 12 hours[21]

According to the American Dental Association in coordination with the AHA, an expert panel was formed in 2014 to develop antibiotic prophylaxis for dental procedures. Antibiotics are now only recommended in 2 groups of patients:

- Those with heart conditions that may predispose them to infective endocarditis, and
- Those who have prosthetic joints for the first 6 months after the procedure.

The current guidelines support premedication for a smaller group of patients than previous versions. The changes were based on a review of scientific evidence showing the risk of adverse reactions to antibiotics outweighing the benefits of prophylaxis for most patients. Concern about the development of drug-resistant bacteria also was a factor.

Should a patient forget to premedicate at home before their appointment, the recommendation states the antibiotic should be given before the procedure. This is important because it allows the antibiotic to reach adequate blood levels.

However, the guidelines to prevent infective endocarditis also note: "If the dosage of antibiotic is inadvertently not administered before the procedure, the dosage may be administered up to 2 hours after the procedure."[22] If a patient requires prophylaxis and is already taking antibiotics for another condition, it is recommend the dentist select an antibiotic from a different class than the one the patient is already taking.[21] The CKD patient should speak with the dentist before the appointment to ensure proper coordination of care.[1]

SUMMARY

The CKD patient comes with a complicated collection of chronic diseases that all interact to make surgery more of a challenge. However, careful scrutiny of the preprocedural laboratory studies correlated with a thorough history and physical will decrease perioperative risks. Postoperatively, the practitioner must be vigilant to identify AKI as well as metabolic or electrolyte abnormalities. With heightened awareness of the fragility of the CKD patient, operative risks can be reduced significantly.

REFERENCES

1. Gawande A. Two hundred years of surgery. N Engl J Med 2012;366:1716–7.
2. Kidney Disease: Improving Global Outcomes (KDIGO) CKD Work Group. KDIGO 2012 Clinical practice guideline for the evaluation and management of chronic kidney disease. Kidney Int Suppl 2013;3:1–150.
3. Deray G. Dialysis and iodinated contrast media. Kidney Int 2006;69:S25–9. Available at: www.nature.com/ki/journal/v69/n100s/full/5000371a.html.
4. Dean M. Opioids in renal failure and dialysis patients. J Pain Symptom Manage 2004;28:497–504.
5. Available at: http://nkdep.nih.gov/resources/quick-reference-uacr-gfr.shtml. Accessed May 10, 2015.
6. Eagle K, Berger PB, Calkins H, et al. Guidelines for perioperative cardiovascular evaluation for noncardiac surgery: report of the American College of Cardiology/ American Heart Association Task Force on practice guidelines (Committee on Perioperative Cardiovascular Evaluation for Noncardiac Surgery). J Am Coll Cardiol 1996;27:910–48.
7. Bilimoria K, Liu K, Paruch JL, et al. Development and evaluation of the universal ACS NSQIP surgical risk calculator: a decision aid and informed consent tool for patients and surgeons. J Am Coll Surg 2013;217(5):833–42.

8. Kidney Disease: Improving Global Outcomes (KDIGO) CKD Work Group. KDIGO 2012 Clinical Practice Guideline for the Evaluation and Management of Chronic Kidney Disease. Kidney inter. Suppl. 2013;3:1–150.
9. Verbeeck RK, Musuamba FT. Pharmacokinetics and dosage adjustment in patients with renal dysfunction. Eur J Clin Pharmacol 2009;65(8):757–73.
10. Thiele R, Isbell J, Rosner M. AKI associated with cardiac surgery. Clin J Am Soc Nephrol 2015;10:500–14.
11. Matzke G, Aronoff GR, Atkinson AJ, et al. Drug dosing consideration in patients with acute and chronic kidney disease—a clinical update from kidney disease: improving global outcomes (KDIGO). Kidney Int 2011;80:1122–37.
12. Krishnan M. Preoperative care of patients with kidney disease. Am Fam Physician 2002;66(8):1471–7.
13. Douketis J, Spyropoulos AC, Kaatz S, et al, BRIDGE Investigators. Perioperative bridging anticoagulation in patients with atrial fibrillation. N Engl J Med 2015; 373(9):823–33.
14. Singh A, Szczech L, Tang KL, et al, CHOIR Investigators. Correction of anemia with Epoetin Alfa in chronic kidney disease. N Engl J Med 2006;355:2085–98.
15. Greenberg A, Cheung A. NKF primer on kidney disease. 5th edition. Elsevier.
16. Society of Interventional Radiology. Published SIR clinical practice guidelines by service line as of Mar 1, 2015. Available at: www.sirweb.org/clinical/svclines. shtml#B. Accessed May 23, 2015.
17. Zuber K, Liles AM, Davis J. Medication dosing in patients with chronic kidney disease. J Am Acad Physician Assist 2013;26(10):19–25.
18. Venkatesan AM, Kundu S, Sacks D, et al. Practice guideline for adult antibiotic prophylaxis during vascular and interventional radiology procedures. J Vasc Interv Radiol 2010;21(11):1611–30.
19. Zinn J, Swofford V. Quality improvement initiative: classifying and documenting surgical wounds. Wound Care Advisor 2014;3(1):34. Available at: http:// woundcareadvisor.com/quality-improvement-initiative-classifying-and-documenting-surgical-wounds_vol3-no1/.
20. Setiawan B. The role of prophylactic antibiotics in preventing perioperative infection. Acta Med Indones 2011;43:4.
21. Sollecito TP, Abt E, Lockhart PB, et al. The use of prophylactic antibiotics prior to dental procedures in patients with prosthetic joints. J Am Dent Assoc 2015; 146(1):11–6.e8.
22. Wilson W, Taubert KA, Gewitz M, et al. Prevention of infective endocarditis: guidelines from the American Heart Association. J Am Dent Assoc 2008;139(Suppl): 3–24. Available at: www.ada.org/en/member-center/oral-health-topics/antibiotic-prophylaxis.

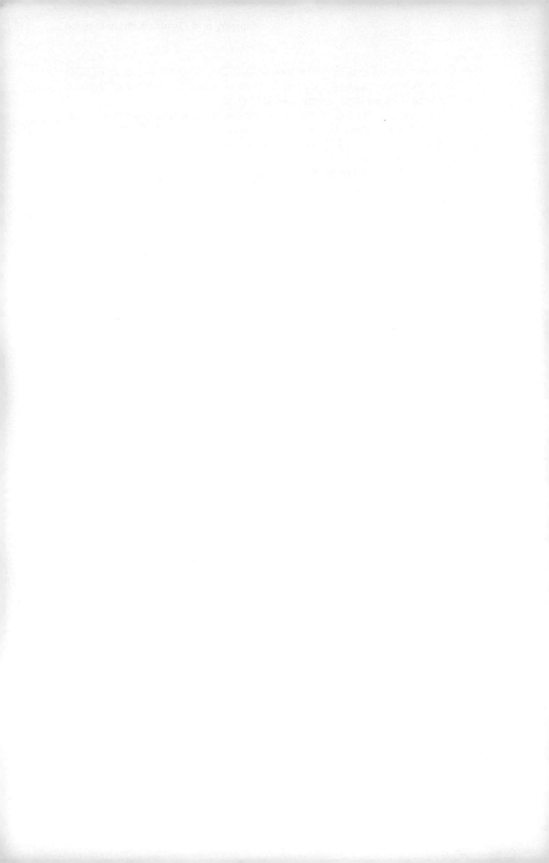

Cardiorenal Disease
The Pump and the Filter

Laura Troidle, PA

KEYWORDS

- Cardiorenal • Acute • Chronic • AKI • CHF

KEY POINTS

- There are 5 different types of cardiorenal disease, with the disease being a result of either an acute or cardiac event.
- One organ, either the heart or the kidney, is affected as a reaction to a pathologic disruption in the other organ.
- The diagnosis and treatment of cardiorenal disease depends on the cause of the initial insult.

Mrs XX is a 61-year-old woman with a history of an ischemic cardiomyopathy with a known ejection fraction of 35% to 40% as well as severe aortic stenosis, moderate mitral regurgitation, pulmonary hypertension, biventricular implantable cardioverter-defibrillator, right nephrectomy for a renal cell cancer, and severe peripheral vascular disease who presented to the hospital with marked dyspnea on exertion, orthopnea, and pedal edema and was found to have an increase in her serum creatinine.

Her baseline creatinine was 1.2 mg/dL. It had increased to 1.8 mg/dL before admission. It was noted to be 2.4 mg/dL on presentation to the emergency department. Her furosemide had been put on hold when her creatinine was first noted to be increasing from her baseline. Her weight was 179 lb on presentation, and a chest radiograph revealed pulmonary edema. She was admitted for diuresis. On discharge, her weight decreased to 149 lb. She was also started on lisinopril and maintained on furosemide with a stable creatinine of 1.5 mg/dL.

DEFINITION

Cardiorenal syndrome (CRS) refers to a whole host of insults that alter the function of either the kidney or the heart, thereby physiologically altering the balance of the base-line kidney-heart relationship. These insults may be acute or chronic. They may

Disclosure: The author has nothing to disclose.
Metabolism Associates, 136 Sherman Avenue, Suite 405, New Haven, CT 06511, USA
E-mail address: kltroidle@sbcglobal.net

Physician Assist Clin 1 (2016) 115–125
http://dx.doi.org/10.1016/j.cpha.2015.09.002
2405-7991/16/$ – see front matter © 2016 Elsevier Inc. All rights reserved.

physicianassistant.theclinics.com

originate within the kidney or the heart. But, together, these insults alter the ability of either organ to maintain homeostasis.

Given that there exist many manners by which an alteration in the kidney/heart relationship may occur, Ronco and colleagues[1] defined 5 types of CRS based on acute or chronic injury to either the heart or the kidney (**Table 1**). Type 1 CRS refers to acute cardiac events leading to kidney disease. Type 2 refers to chronic cardiac events leading to kidney disease. Type 3 refers to acute kidney injury (AKI) leading to heart failure (HF). Type 4 refers to chronic kidney disease (CKD) leading to HF. Type 5 refers to systemic secondary causes that lead to both kidney and cardiac failures.

- CRS is a group of diseases that either acutely or chronically alter the cardiorenal homeostasis. CRS may occur from an independent systemic source that leads to both kidney and cardiac failure.

PREVALENCE

It is a well-appreciated observation that HF is common, with patients greater than 45 years old having a lifetime risk of HF of approximately 20%.[2] HF is the most common cause of death among patients with end-stage renal disease (ESRD). As CKD worsens, the percentage of patients with cardiovascular disease (CVD), including HF, increases as well as patient morbidity and mortality.[3] In fact, patients with stage 3 CKD, with a glomerular filtration rate (GFR) of 30 to 60 mL/min, are more likely to die of CVD than to progress to ESRD.

It is estimated that kidney dysfunction is present in approximately 30% to 60% of patients with HF.[4] Patients treated for acute or chronic HF often have changes in kidney function (in about 20% to 30% of patients).[5]

Thus, CVD is common; its role with acute or chronic changes in the GFR cannot be underestimated and neither can the role of kidney disease in the development of acute or chronic changes to the heart (**Box 1**).

A COMPLEX PHYSIOLOGY

Dr Arthur Guyton[6] eloquently describes how the accepted pathophysiology of hypertension is much more than mere increased total peripheral resistance. His work with

Table 1
Types of CRS and clinical scenarios

	Clinical Example
Type 1: Acute cardiac events that lead to worsening of kidney disease	May be seen in patients with acute myocardial infarction who develop AKI
Type 2: Chronic cardiac events that lead to worsening of kidney disease	May be seen in patients with chronic systolic dysfunction who has increase in creatinine over time with no other explanations
Type 3: An acute change to heart function caused by AKI	May be seen in patients who develop AKI and develop an arrhythmia or an ischemic event as a result
Type 4: Development of worsening HF from CKD	May be seen in any patient with CKD who develops a cardiac consequence, such as cardiac hypertrophy or other cardiovascular event
Type 5: Systemic causes affecting both the kidney and the heart	May be seen in patients developing sepsis or vasculitis

Box 1
CVD information
CVD is common among all patient types, including ESRD populations.
The percentage of patients with CVD increases as CKD stage worsen.
Thirty percent to 60% of patients with HF have evidence of kidney injury.
Treatment of HF results in changes to kidney function in 20% to 30% of patients.

Dr Thomas Coleman and a computer model revealed the important effect that a high arterial pressure had on increasing urinary output as well as the converse, a decreased urinary output when the arterial pressure was low so as to maintain euvolemia and normotension.

For how simple can a principle be? It is elemental that if the arterial pressure is too low for the kidneys to eliminate all the fluid entering the body, then fluid will accumulate until the pressure does rise high enough; but the pressure will not rise any higher because at higher pressures more output than intake would occur, and the pressure would fall again to the same exact level required for fluid balance. How much simpler could a principle be?[6]

What happens when there is an imbalance of the process Dr Guyton eloquently describes as a simple phenomenon?

What links both the heart and the kidney together is an elaborate circulatory system that is designed to keep blood moving in its intended direction. It is best to take a moment and review the key physiologic components of the circulatory system with regard to the heart and kidney so that the pathophysiology, diagnosis, and treatment of each subtype of CRS may be better understood.

The circulatory system has many key deliveries to make, including oxygen, carbon dioxide, nutrients, waste products, medications, components of the immune system, as well as many other substrates that are key to maintaining homeostasis. Key features of the circulatory system include volume, pressure, and flow. An alteration in any element has the potential to affect systemic or local hemodynamics that are part and parcel to the various types of CRS.

Any circulatory system must maintain an adequate, constant pressure to ensure an adequate blood flow to and through local tissues to make these deliveries possible. Blood flow is regulated centrally through the autonomic nervous system with sympathetic and parasympathetic pathways. Catecholamines, such as norepinephrine, stimulate the sympathetic side, while acetylcholine works on the parasympathetic arm. Additionally, angiotensin II, a product of the central renin-angiotensin-aldosterone system (RAAS), acts as a humoral agent to stimulate the autonomic system.

Peripherally, local hormones contribute to blood flow across precapillary and postcapillary beds. These hormones include prostaglandins and bradykinins that act as vasodilators and enhance blood flow through these beds. And angiotensin II acts as a vasoconstrictor to increase the pressure across the exchange system (**Fig. 1**).

It is worth focusing on the RAAS component, as this important regulatory pathway of volume is an area of focus in the 5 types of CRS. The RAAS system is designed to regulate blood pressure via control of fluid and sodium.[7] Briefly, renin is a hormone released from the juxtaglomerular cells at the afferent arterioles of the glomerulus in response to changes in renal perfusion, changes in sodium delivery to the distal tubule, and sympathetic nerve stimulation. Renin is inhibited via negative feedback

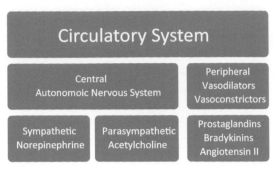

Fig. 1. Circulatory system.

from angiotensin II. Once released, renin stimulates the production of angiotensin I that becomes hydrolyzed by angiotensin-converting enzyme (ACE) to angiotensin II. Angiotensin II, the product of the RAAS system, then causes vasoconstriction both locally within the kidney as well as systemically to increase blood pressure. It also increases cardiac contractility, increases renal tubular sodium reabsorption, stimulates the sympathetic nervous system (catecholamines), and stimulates the adrenal glomerulosa cells to release another hormone, aldosterone. Aldosterone causes distal tubular sodium reabsorption and potassium loss. Dysregulation of these events contributes to the development of CRS (**Fig. 2**).

It is important to keep in mind the basic physiology and homeostatic mechanisms at play between the heart and the kidney. Each type of CRS has different pathophysiologic features that, when understood, can possibly be used to both prevent and treat a patient with CRS (**Fig. 3**).

TYPE 1 CARDIORENAL SYNDROME
Acute Heart Failure Leading to Acute Kidney Injury

Type 1 CRS may occur from any acute cardiac injury that leads to renal insult.[1] The insult may be a result of an acute coronary event, acute tamponade, a nonischemic event, or complications from cardiac surgery, for example. Patients developing type 1 CRS may have varying degrees of volume expansion, with some patients being

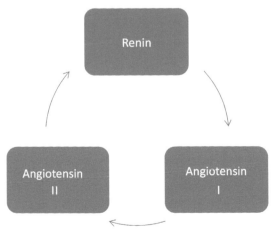

Fig. 2. RAAS system cycle.

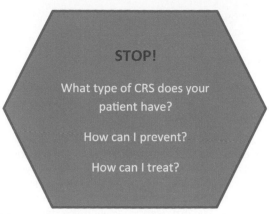

Fig. 3. Using physiology to understanding the approach to patients.

intravascularly deplete and other patients with significantly more volume expansion, including volume overload. The common link for all of these patients is that the renal arterial blood flow is compromised.

The systemic response to acute HF results in a decreased cardiac output leading to venous congestion from poor forward flow. This congestion, in turn, leads to increased systemic vascular resistance (SVR) and the activation of RAAS and the sympathetic nervous system. The sympathetic nervous system activates RAAS. Renin is stimulated and, in turn, stimulates angiotensin II that leads to catecholamine release and aldosterone stimulation. Renal blood flow is maintained across the glomerular capillary bed via the constriction of the efferent arteriole that occurs with angiotensin II stimulation. The catecholamines stimulate reactive oxygen species and decrease nitric oxide leading to endothelial dysfunction (**Box 2**).

Determination of the reason for the decline in renal arterial blood flow and then restoring its flow are essential for optimal management of patients with type I CRS. Loop diuretics may be used to reduce venous congestion by lowering filling pressures and unloading the heart to allow for improved pump function. Volume, on the other hand, may restore forward cardiac flow for patients with restrictive heart disease. Treatment of cardiac tamponade may result in a rapid improvement of the cardiac output. Cessation of the use of ACE inhibitors (ACEIs) or angiotensin receptor blockers (ARB) may allow the efferent arteriole to pursue its vasoconstrictor role to maintain pressure across the glomerular capillary bed. Nonsteroidal antiinflammatory drugs must be avoided to allow for dilation of the afferent arterioles as well. It is important to make a prompt assessment and take measures to prevent or treat patients with CRS type I as the severity of the AKI may lessen any response.

Box 2
Summary of physiologic events of type 1 CRS

Decreased cardiac output and venous congestion → increased SVR

RAAS and SNS activation

Renin → angiotensin II (AII) → aldosterone

Catecholamine release

Type I cardiorenal syndrome
  Acute HF → AKI
    Considerations:
    • Why is renal arterial blood flow compromised?
    • How can the heart be helped to improve renal arterial blood flow?
    • Are there any offending agents or events contributing?

TYPE II CARDIORENAL SYNDROME

Type II CRS refers to chronic HF leading to alterations in kidney function.[1] In order for this diagnosis to be considered it is necessary to identify the coexistence of both HF and CKD as well as linking the HF with the development or worsening of underlying kidney disease. A common scenario is a patient who develops an injury to left ventricular function and the patient subsequently develops kidney injury at the same time. Recurrent episodes of HF are also associated with the development of CKD and its progression.

The systemic response is similar to the response noted among patients with type I CRS in that there is a decrease in cardiac function and an increase in venous congestion. But because of the chronicity of this subtype of CRS, there exist large amounts of renin and angiotensin II leading to chronic efferent arteriole vasoconstriction. However, in contrast to type I CRS, these chronically RAAS-activated patients are volume expanded. Treatment of these patients, therefore, is targeted at blocking RAAS, although the benefit may be one sided with improvements in HF mortality yet progression of CKD. Aldosterone inhibitors may also be of benefit.

Type II CRS
  • Patients typically volume expanded with chronic HF
  • Chronic renin, angiotensin II, and aldosterone stimulation
  • Consider ACEI, ARB, or aldosterone inhibitors→ better HF survival, worsen CKD?
  • Left ventricular assist devices

TYPE III CARDIORENAL SYNDROME

Type III CRS refers to the development of AKI that leads to the development of acute cardiac decompensation.[1] The effect on the heart from the kidney dysfunction may be a direct effect of the AKI when patients develop a metabolic disorder, such as hyperkalemia or metabolic acidosis. Drug pharmacokinetics may also be altered with AKI and impact the heart; or the negative effect on cardiac function may occur indirectly from an inflammatory process via cytokines, for example. The sympathetic nervous system may also be hyperactive in patients developing AKI leading to the activation of RAAS, which can lead to myocardial cell apoptosis and impaired coronary circulatory responses (**Box 3**).

TYPE IV CARDIORENAL SYNDROME

Type IV CRS refers to the development of HF among patients with any stage of CKD.[1] The link of cardiac disease among patients with CKD or ESRD is not a surprise as it is the most common cause of death among this population. An example of this type of patient is a patient with any stage CKD who develops hypertension due to chronic volume expansion and then develops left ventricular hypertrophy, or this may occur in patients with CKD with hyperphosphatemia who develops decompensated HF.

| Box 3 |
| Type III CRS summary |
| AKI→ acute HF |
| Direct effects: metabolic, pharmacologic→ release has negative cardiac effect |
| Indirect effects: cytokines, mediate inflammation and negative cardiac effect |

Patients with CKD have several pathophysiologic events that occur with their disease that contribute to the development of HF. Expanded volume leads to the activation of RAAS that leads to hypertension and subsequent left ventricular hypertrophy and cardiac fibrosis. Vascular calcification may occur as a result of secondary hyperparathyroidism and the complex interactions of calcium, phosphorus, parathyroid hormone, and fibroblast growth factor-23 (FGF-23). Uremia in and of itself may also have negative cardiac effects (**Box 4**).[1]

TYPE V CARDIORENAL SYNDROME

Type V CRS refers to patients who develop simultaneous AKI and acute cardiac decompensation as a result of a systemic process.[1] Sepsis is a common example of such a systemic event leading to an acute tubular necrosis as well as a septic cardiomyopathy with significant myocardial stunning. Sepsis activates both the autonomic nervous system: catecholamines and RAAS. Further aggravating the situation is the development of metabolic abnormalities, such as metabolic acidosis that further suppress cardiac function and the poor kidney perfusion from the reduced cardiac ejection fraction. Other systemic illnesses that may simultaneous cause AKI and acute HF include hepatorenal syndrome and vasculitis. Treatment is aimed at addressing the underlying disease, such as sepsis, and providing supportive care to both organs by optimizing blood pressure via the use of blood pressure support agents, treating metabolic acidosis, optimizing volume status via the use of intravenous fluids, or diuretics. Some studies have shown that RAAS activation during sepsis is associated with endothelial dysfunction and mortality. Blockade of the RAAS system may be beneficial (**Box 5**).

Thus, there exist many different unions of the kidney with the heart. The relationship is more of a 2-way street than one way in that it is not as simple an ideology that the heart fails to pump and the kidney has diminished blood flow. That said, it is often difficult to determine which type of CRS a particular patient may be experiencing. The clinician is expected to obtain an accurate timeline of events and determine the pathophysiology that best fits the story. Therapeutic interventions are then aimed at the proposed pathophysiology. But can we do better?

BIOMARKERS AND CARDIORENAL SYNDROME

Biomarkers are substances that may be measured to indicate the possibility of a disease process or to predict outcomes. Specifically, the National Institutes of Health

| Box 4 |
| Type IV CRS summary |
| CKD→ chronic, worsening heart disease |
| CKD→ volume expansion→ hypertension → left ventricular hypertrophy |
| CKD→ secondary hyperparathyroidism→ HF |

Box 5
Type V CRS summary
Simultaneous AKI and HF from systemic event
Sepsis, hepatorenal syndrome, vasculitis
Treat underlying disease
Optimize effects

defines a biomarker as a "characteristic that is, objectively measured and evaluated as an indicator of normal biological processes, pathogenic processes, or pharmacologic responses to a therapeutic intervention."[8] These substances are surrogate end points to provide information that may not be clinically evident. Biomarkers may include a commonly measured chemistry, such as potassium, calcium, phosphorus, or lesser-known substances for which there are limited assays available to measure (**Box 6**).

Biomarkers come in all shapes and forms. Based on the definition of biomarkers, this refers to a whole host of easily measurable substances as well as less common substances. Many clinicians may measure these substances and treat the highs and lows without giving much thought as to the cascade of consequences that affect the kidney and heart relationship. It is important for the clinician to understand the role that abnormal concentrations of these biomarkers may have. The information may also be used to educate patients and possibly increase medical compliance.

Table 2 identifies several bone mineral substances that meet the biomarker criteria and are each abnormal in patients with CRS.[9] FGF-23, as the primary regulator of phosphorus and vitamin D homeostasis (which contributes) to bone homeostasis, is linked with several factors that are often abnormally high or low in patients with CKD. These factors include phosphorus, 1, 25 $(OH)_2$ vitamin D, and parathyroid hormone. Abnormalities in any bone mineral biomarker are linked with the development and/or progression of either cardiac or kidney elements. It is unknown if each directly or indirectly effects the cardiovascular system; but each substance, when abnormal, is associated with cardiovascular mortality.

Urinary albumin excretion is an example of another easily measured substance that may be altered in patients with CKD. Excess albumin remaining in the Bowman space makes it difficult for the proximal tubular cells to perform reabsorption, which leads to cell death and worsening of underlying CKD. Albuminuria is also associated with the development of HF.[10] Whether the effect of albuminuria on the heart is direct or indirect remains to be established.

There are other lesser-known biomarkers associated with CRS. **Table 3** identifies these biomarkers[11] and is intended to provide a small reference list of substances that have been identified with various physiologic or pathophysiologic processes

Box 6
Biomarkers as indicators
Biomarkers are indicators of
Biological process
Pathogenic process
Pharmacologic response

Table 2
Bone mineral biomarkers

Biomarker	Effect	Treatments
Phosphorus	Hyperphosphatemia contributes to vascular calcification and decreases active 1, 25(OH)$_2$ vitamin D production → RAAS activation.	Phosphorus-lowering agents, such as sevelamer, lower phosphorus levels.
Active 1, 25 (OH)$_2$ vitamin D	Low levels stimulate RAAS. Replacing 1, 25 (OH)$_2$ vitamin D is associated with lower mortality.	Provide 1, 25 (OH)$_2$ vitamin D, but this will increase FGF-23 levels.
Parathyroid hormone	Elevated levels stimulate FGF-23.	Lower PTH levels with cinacalcet.
FGF-23	It regulates vitamin D and phosphorus metabolism to maintain homeostasis. FGF-23 increases with CKD. Hyperphosphatemia and increased parathyroid hormone levels increase FGF-23.	Sevelamer lowers FGF-23 levels; or, because FGF-23 activates RAAS, inhibitors of RAAS, such as ACEIs or ARBs, may be beneficial.

Table 3
Biomarkers

Biomarker	Effects	Other
KIM-1	Detected in urine. Upregulated in ischemic kidney injury and shed by proximal tubule cells. Possible role in kidney recovery and tubular regeneration	It is commercially available. It may be limited in ability to distinguish a patient with an injury versus a patient who is starting to turn around.
Interleukin-18	Detected in the urine. Proinflammatory cytokine: plays a role in the inflammatory stage of AKI	Targeting this cytokine may lessen the inflammatory processes.
Liver-type fatty acid-binding protein	Detected in urine. Detected immediately postoperatively in patients who develop AKI. Renoprotective protein	It may be used to guide clinical intervention in patients in whom it is elevated. Example: Optimize the volume in postoperative cardiac patients by aggressively and quickly intervening in patients who have a low central venous pressure and seem hypovolemic.
Angiotensinogen	Detected in the urine. When elevated, linked to length of hospital stay, need for dialysis, death	It may be able to identify patients who may benefit from RAAS inhibition, including the optimal time to administer the ACEI or ARB.
Neutrophil gelatinase-associated lipocalin	Detected in urine and plasma. Prognostic marker. Upregulated after ischemic or nephrotoxic injury. May enhance kidney's ability to recover	Like KIM-1, its use may be limited in ability to distinguish injury phase from recovery phase.

Abbreviation: KIM-1, kidney injury molecule.

that occur in patients developing CRS. Although these substances do not distinguish a patients with type 1 CRS from a patient with type 3 CRS, per say, each may have predictive value of AKI that, when identified early, before clinically obvious, a change in management may be offered to alter the predicted course in a more positive direction.

Biomarker data are at best very encouraging and have the potential to identify novel ways to manage patients with AKI. However, the usefulness in patients with CRS is currently difficult to understand. Depending on the time the biomarker is detected, the biomarker may either be a marker of injury or a marker of recovery. Much more data need to be determined.

Considerations:
- Identify patient with cardiac and/or renal insults.
- Can you measure a biomarker that may accurately predict your patient may develop CRS?
- If so, can you intervene to thwart the predicted course?

SUMMARY

The kidney and the heart coexist. So it is a similar extension that kidney disease and HF must coexist. There are 5 different types of CRS that represent the kidney-heart relationship and, when identified, may lead to an appropriate and effective treatment that may improve outcomes for patients. Both disease processes ignite a cascade of pathophysiologic events that upset this natural relationship. It is important to recognize this and use this knowledge to optimize the approach to these complicated patients.

REFERENCES

1. Ronco C, McCullough P, Anker SD, et al. Cardio-renal syndromes: report from the consensus conference of the Acute Dialysis Quality Initiative. Eur Heart J 2010; 31:703–11.
2. Lloyd-Jones DM, Larson MG, Leip EP, et al. Lifetime risk for developing congestive heart failure: the Framingham Heart Study. Circulation 2002;106:3068–72.
3. Thompson S, James M, Wiebe N, et al, for the Alberta Disease Network. Cause of death in patients with reduced kidney function. J Am Soc Nephrol 2015;26: 2504–11.
4. Adams KF, Fonarow GC, Emerman CL, et al. Characteristics and outcomes of patients hospitalized for heart failure in the United States: rationale, design, and preliminary observations from the first 100,000 cases in the Acute Decompensated Heart Failure National Registry (ADHERE). Am Heart J 2005;149:209–16.
5. Forman DE, Butler J, Wang Y, et al. Incidence, predictors at admission, and impact of worsening renal function among patients hospitalized with heart failure. J Am Coll Cardiol 2004;43:61–7.
6. Guyton AC. The surprising kidney-fluid mechanism for pressure control-its infinite gain. Hypertension 1990;16:725–30.
7. Atlas SA. The renin-angiotensin aldosterone system: pathophysiological role and pharmacologic inhibition. J Manag Care Pharm 2007;13(8 Suppl B):S9–20.
8. Biomarkers Definition Work Group. Biomarkers and surrogate endpoints: preferred definitions and conceptual framework. Clin Pharmacol Ther 2001;69: 89–95.
9. Kovesdy CP, Quarles LD. The role of fibroblast growth factor-23 in cardiorenal syndrome. Nephron Clin Pract 2013;123:194–201.

10. Blecker S, Matsushta K, Kottgen A, et al. High-normal albuminuria and risk of heart failure in the community. Am J Kidney Dis 2011;58:47–55.
11. Alge JL, Arthur JM. Biomarkers of AKI: a review of mechanistic relevance and potential therapeutic implications. Clin J Am Soc Nephrol 2015;10:147–55.

Rolling Stones
The Evaluation, Prevention, and Medical Management of Nephrolithiasis

Harvey A. Feldman, MD, FACP

KEYWORDS

- Nephrolithiasis • Kidney stones • Hypercalciuria • Hyperoxaluria • Hyperuricosuria
- Medical expulsive therapy

KEY POINTS

- Nephrolithiasis, an increasingly prevalent and costly ailment, is a heterogeneous phenotype influenced by both genetics and multiple environmental factors.
- Nearly 80% of kidney stones are composed of calcium and are due to idiopathic hypercalciuria; uric acid and struvite (infection) stones are the next most common.
- A focused history and physical examination along with laboratory and imaging studies are necessary to identify risk factors that can be addressed with directed therapy.
- All patients should consume enough fluids to generate more than 2 L of urine daily. For calcium stones, normal calcium intake with reduced sodium and animal protein is preventative for stone formation.
- Drug therapies include thiazide diuretics, potassium citrate and allopurinol. The effectiveness of medical expulsive therapy to facilitate passage of stones under 10 mm is uncertain.

INTRODUCTION

Kidney stones have plagued mankind since the beginnings of recorded history. Stones were found in an Egyptian mummy dating back nearly 7000 years. The word lithotomy comes from ancient Greek and stones are mentioned in the Hippocratic Oath.[1,2] Fortunately, through the centuries great advances have been made in our understanding of this affliction. The intent of this review is to present current information on the epidemiology, risk factors, evaluation, medical management, and prevention of the most common causes of nephrolithiasis in adults. Information on rare genetic causes

Disclosures: None.
Physician Assistant Program, Nova Southeastern University, 3200 South University Drive, Terry Building 1258, Ft. Lauderdale, FL 33028-2018, USA
E-mail address: hfeldman@nova.edu

Physician Assist Clin 1 (2016) 127–147
http://dx.doi.org/10.1016/j.cpha.2015.09.008
2405-7991/16/$ – see front matter © 2016 Elsevier Inc. All rights reserved.

of nephrolithiasis and surgical management can be found in Edvardsson and colleagues[3] and Bird and associates.[4]

EPIDEMIOLOGY
Incidence and Prevalence Rates in the United States

Nephrolithiasis is a common affliction that can strike at any age, including childhood. Among adults, the incidence of a first symptomatic stone begins to increase after age 20, peaks between ages 30 and 50, and then declines but never disappears.[5] The lifetime risk of developing at least 1 kidney stone is 19% in men and 9% in women.[6] Once a person has had a kidney stone, the chance of future stones progressively increases with each episode.[7]

The prevalence of kidney stones has been increasing over the past several decades[6] (**Fig. 1**). According to data from the National Health and Nutrition Examination Survey (NHANES), the prevalence has increased dramatically from 3.2% between 1976 and 1980 to 8.8% between 2007 and 2010.[6] These numbers tell only part of the story; the prevalence rates vary by sex, age, and race. Although males have always had a higher prevalence of stones than females, the ratio of males to females has narrowed over this time frame. Moreover, women now comprise a majority of hospital admissions for management of nephrolithiasis.[8] Along with the overall increase in stone prevalence, there has been a trend of increasing prevalence with age, both in the United States and in several other countries worldwide.[9] NHANES data also reveal significant differences in stone prevalence by race, with non-Hispanic blacks showing the lowest rates, Caucasians the highest rates, and Hispanics and other racial groups falling in the middle[6] (**Fig. 2**).

The cost of nephrolithiasis has also escalated in recent decades and is now more than $5 billion per year, including the costs of hospitalization, surgery, and time lost from work.[10] Contributing to the increasing costs of health care since the 1990s is the near doubling of emergency department visits for kidney stones and the tripling

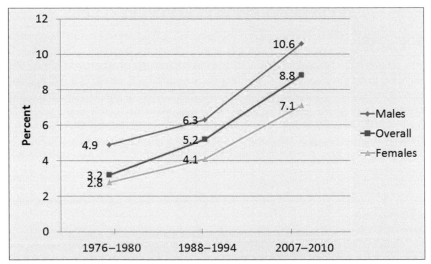

Fig. 1. Prevalence rates of kidney stones according to data from the National Health and Nutrition Examination Surveys. (*Data from* Scales CD, Smith AC, Hanley JM, et al. Prevalence of kidney stones in the United States. Europ Urol 2012;62:160–5.)

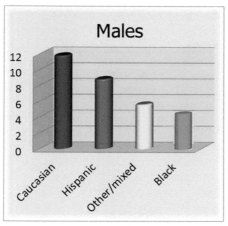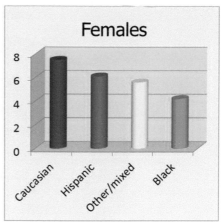

Fig. 2. Prevalence rates of kidney stones by sex and race based on data from the National Health and Nutrition Examination Survey, 2007 to 2010. (*Data from* Scales CD, Smith AC, Hanley JM, et al. Prevalence of kidney stones in the United States. Europ Urol 2012;62:160–5.)

of the use of computed tomography in that setting.[11] The increasing prevalence of stones with age has also affected costs. Older patients are more likely to experience morbidity from their stones and to require hospitalization for surgical intervention, whereas younger patients are usually treated in the less costly outpatient setting.[5,12,13]

Prevalence of Specific Types of Kidney Stones

The frequencies of specific stone types vary among reported series. However, by far, calcium-containing stones are the most common types, accounting for about three-quarters of all stones. Idiopathic hypercalciuria is the most common abnormality contributing to calcium stones, comprising at least 50% of cases. Pure calcium oxalate (CaOx) stones make up 60% or more of all calcium stones with the remainder being calcium phosphate and mixed stones (eg, CaOx/uric acid, CaOx/calcium phosphate). Uric acid stones and struvite stones (also known as infection or triple phosphate stones), are the next most common types, and cystine and other rare genetic stone types and drug-related stones make up 1% or less of the total[5,14,15] (**Fig. 3**).

RISK FACTORS FOR NEPHROLITHIASIS

Five categories of risk factors for nephrolithiasis are discussed in this review:

- Ambient temperature
- Genetics
- Diet
- Systemic disorders
- Urinary

Ambient Temperature

Three lines of evidence link ambient temperature to kidney stone risk.[16]

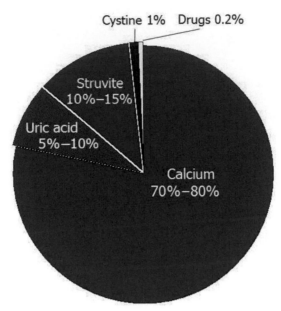

Fig. 3. Prevalence rates of specific kidney stone types. The percentages reflect calculated weighted averages of stone types derived from 12 case series reported in Ref.,[15] plus data from Refs.[5,14] (*Data from* Refs.[5,14,15])

Geographic

In the United States, there is a North-to-South trend as well as a West-to-East trend in kidney stone prevalence, with the highest rates in the Southeast, the so-called "stone belt."[17] However, the West-to-East correlation is less well-explained by ambient temperature alone. Across all states, as well as internationally, the association of ambient temperature with nephrolithiasis is stronger in men than in women.[18] In addition, kidney stones are uncommon among the Black populations of Nigeria and South Africa but very high in Arab populations in Kuwait and Saudi Arabia, despite similar ambient temperatures.[19]

Seasonal

Within single geographic areas, higher stone rates occur during summer months when temperatures are higher and sun exposure is greater.[19,20] Also, a correlation may exist between global warming and the increasing trend in kidney stone prevalence. It is predicted that by 2095, global warming may place 70% of the US population at risk of nephrolithiasis.[21]

Occupational

Work exposure to high ambient temperatures is associated with higher rates of kidney stones.[16] Also, military deployment to hot desert climates associates with increased risk.[16,22] Occupations that prevent frequent fluid intake or access to toilets (eg, taxi drivers) also predispose to nephrolithiasis.

The pathophysiologic explanation for the association of ambient temperature with nephrolithiasis is that heat induces sweating and body fluid loss that, if not fully replaced, leads to decreased urine volume and increased concentration of stone-forming urinary constituents. However, multiple confounding variables mitigate establishing a firm causal relationship between ambient temperature and nephrolithiasis in specific individuals or groups of individuals. **Box 1** lists these competing factors.

Box 1
Factors influencing the ambient temperature: kidney stone link

Fluid loss from sweating

Humidity ($\uparrow$ fluid loss in arid climates)

Sunlight exposure ($\uparrow$ vitamin D exposure)

Regional dietary variations

Migration trend to urban areas (cities warmer than rural areas)

Regional genetic variations (including gender and race)

Regional socioeconomic variations

Data from Fakheri RJ, Goldfarb DS. Ambient temperature as a contributor to kidney stone formation: implications of global warming. Kidney Int 2011;79:1178–85.

Genetic Factors

Evidence supporting a genetic component in the risk of developing kidney stones comes from 3 sources.

Family clustering

Between 25% and 40% of patients with a kidney stone report a family history of stones.[7,23] Compared with men without a family history of stones, those with a family history have a 2- to 3-fold greater risk of forming a stone.[23]

Ethnic differences

As noted, the prevalence of stones is less among blacks, especially compared with Caucasians.[6] There may be a genetic difference in urinary excretion patterns among races. Black post menopausal non-stone forming women have a higher urine pH and citrate compared to white menopausal women. White women have higher urinary calcium, phosphorus and relative supersaturation of CaOx and calcium phosphate.[24] A cross-sectional study of calcium stone formers in Toronto, Canada, revealed marked differences in prevalence rates of stones between different ethnic groups not explained by environmental factors, suggesting genetic differences in stone risk between these groups.[25]

Twin studies

Monozygotic twins have higher concordance rates for stones than dizygotic twins. In the Vietnam Era Twin Registry study, the concordance rate for stones between monozygotic twins was nearly twice that for dizygotic twins. Heredity accounted for 56% of the risk with unique environmental factors comprising most of remaining risk.[26]

Except for rare monogenic disorders such as cystinuria or primary hyperoxaluria, nephrolithiasis is a complex polygenic disorder, manifested most commonly by the urinary phenotype of hypercalciuria, and significantly influenced by multiple environmental factors.

Dietary Factors

Among environmental factors, diet most significantly influences kidney stone formation. The major dietary factors are as follows.

Fluid intake

Low fluid intake causes low urine volume and supersaturation of stone-forming urinary constituents.[10] Increasing fluid intake is essential in the prevention of kidney stones (see Prevention section).

Calcium

Contrary to conventional wisdom, a low calcium diet actually promotes calcium stone formation compared with a normal intake of approximately 1000 to 1300 mg/d, especially in patients with hypercalciuria.[7] The results of 1 randomized controlled trial[7] and 3 prospective observational studies[27–29] are summarized in **Table 1**.

The mechanism by which low dietary calcium intake promotes nephrolithiasis is shown in **Fig. 4**.[7,30] Calcium binds to oxalate in the intestines and forms an insoluble complex, which is excreted in the stool. This process frees up oxalate for intestinal absorption and increases supersaturation of CaOx in the urine.

In contrast, calcium supplements, when taken apart from oxalate-containing meals, may increase risk for stones.[28] If taken with dietary oxalate, however, there is no impact on oxalate excretion.[29]

Oxalate

Dietary oxalate has a limited effect on urinary oxalate excretion and CaOx stone formation.[31,32] In 3 large prospective cohort studies that used food frequency questionnaires (Nurses' Health Study I and II [NHS I and II] and Health Professionals Follow-up Study [HPFS]), the mean oxalate intake and oxalate excretion were similar in participants with and without a history of kidney stones.[30,33] Although postprandial spikes in urinary oxalate might have an impact on CaOx stone formation,[34] endogenous factors contribute more substantially to urinary oxalate excretion. These factors are summarized in **Box 2**.

Fructose

Fructose, a monosaccharide that is widely consumed in the form of high fructose corn syrup and is also a metabolic product of sucrose, has been linked to an increased risk

---

Table 1
Studies comparing effect of low versus normal dietary calcium on risk of kidney stones

Reference	Sex	Participants Age Range (y)	Dietary Calcium (mg) Low	Normal	Follow-up (y)	Relative Risk Normal vs Low Calcium
Borghi et al,[7] 2002[a]	Males	34–56	400	1200	5	0.49
Curhan et al,[27] 1993 HPFS[b]	Males	40–75	516	1326	4	0.66
Curhan et al,[28] 1997 NHS I[b]	Females	34–59	<488	>1098	12	0.65
Curhan et al,[29] 2004NHS II[b]	Females	27–44	525	1357	8	0.73

Abbreviations: HPFS, Health Professionals Follow-up Study; HPSF, male health professionals ages 40 to 75; NHS I and II, Nurses' Health Study I and II; NHS I, female nurses ages 34 to 59; NHS II, female nurses ages 27 to 44 at baseline.
[a] The normal calcium group was also placed on a reduced sodium and animal protein diet, which also contributed to lower relative risk of stones.
[b] Results were adjusted for other dietary factors and confounders related to stone risk.

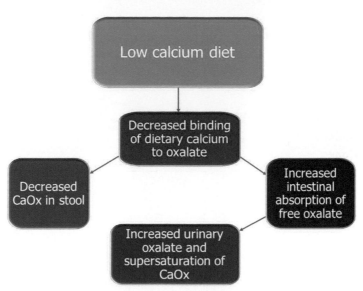

Fig. 4. Mechanism by which low calcium intake causes hyperoxaluria. Less calcium in the intestinal tract reduces the amount of calcium available to form insoluble complexes with oxalate. This leaves more unbound oxalate available for absorption, which leads to hyperoxaluria. CaOx, calcium oxalate. (*Data from* Borghi L, Schanchi T, Meschi T, et al. Comparison of two diets for the prevention of recurrent stones in idiopathic hypercalciuria. N Engl J Med 2002;346:77–84.)

for kidney stones. Results from the NHS I and II and HPFS cohorts show a linear correlation between fructose intake and stone risk[35] (**Fig. 5**). The mechanisms for this association are not fully known. Studies show variable effects of fructose on lithogenic urinary constituents, including calcium, oxalate, and uric acid.[32,35,36] Fructose also increases uric acid production and thus may be linked to nephrolithiasis via the metabolic syndrome and diabetes (see below).

Sodium
High sodium intake inhibits renal tubular reabsorption of calcium. This increases calcium excretion, leading to hypercalciuria and calcium stones.[32,37] In contrast, potassium decreases urine calcium and reduces stone risk.[38]

Box 2
Factors influencing urinary oxalate excretion

Dietary oxalate intake and bioavailability

Endogenous oxalate production

Vitamin C intake

Variable intestinal oxalate absorption
   Genetic variation
   Dietary calcium intake
   Amount of oxalate-degrading bacteria (eg, *Oxalobacter formigenes*)

Variable intestinal oxalate secretion

Data from Refs.[30–33]

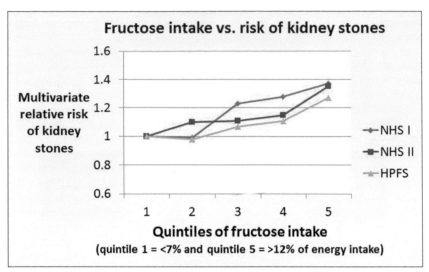

Fig. 5. High fructose intake increases the risk of kidney stones. HPFS, Health Professionals Follow-up Study; NHS, Nurses' Health Study. (*Data from* Taylor EN, Curhan GC. Fructose consumption and the risk of kidney stones. Kidney Int 2008;73:207–12.)

Protein
A high intake of animal protein (excluding dairy) has multiple lithogenic effects. It promotes hypercalciuria by inhibiting renal calcium reabsorption and by causing bone resorption through the generation of metabolic acid. The acid load also decreases urine citrate, an important inhibitor of stone formation. Because animal protein is a source of purines, high intake causes hyperuricosuria, which is a risk factor for calcium stones.[32]

The combination of high sodium and high animal protein produces greater perturbations in urinary calcium and citrate excretion than either alone.[39] These effects provide the rationale for combining low sodium and low protein with normal calcium intake to prevent stones.[7]

Citrate
The reduction in stone risk from citrate is multifactorial. (1) Dietary citrate decreases calcium absorption in the intestine. (2) Citrate forms soluble complexes with calcium in the urine. (3) By alkalinizing the urine, citrate also inhibits uric acid and cystine stones. (4) Systemically, alkalinization from citrate inhibits bone dissolution and increases renal calcium reabsorption.[32,40] Therefore, hypocitraturia is a risk factor for nephrolithiasis.

Vitamins C and D
Vitamin C (ascorbic acid) is metabolized to oxalate. After ingestion of at least 1 g of vitamin C supplementation, urinary oxalate increases and crystallization of CaOx is promoted in calcium stone formers.[41] In the HPSF cohort, vitamin C intake above the recommended daily allowance (90 mg/d) was correlated positively with risk for symptomatic stones.[38] Vitamin D supplementation sufficient to increase the serum 25-hydroxyvitamin D level to 20 to 100 ng/mL has no significant association with kidney stone incidence.[42]

Systemic Disorders

Table 2 lists systemic disorders and renal anatomic abnormalities that predispose to nephrolithiasis. It is beyond the scope of this review to discuss all of these in detail. However, because of growing importance, the relationships between nephrolithiasis and bariatric surgery and the spectrum of obesity, the metabolic syndrome, and diabetes will be discussed.

Bariatric surgery

Jejunoileal bypass surgery, introduced in the 1970s, was associated with a 23% incidence of nephrolithiasis, 11% symptomatic.[43] Because of this and many other adverse consequences, this procedure is no longer done. However, the current Roux-en-Y gastric bypass procedure is also associated with increased risk of nephrolithiasis. Matlaga and colleagues[44] reported a stone incidence of 7.65% over a 4- to 5-year period compared with 4.63% in matched controls. The cause is an increase in urinary oxalate and supersaturation of CaOx brought about by fat malabsorption. Fatty acids bind dietary calcium, leaving free oxalate available for intestinal absorption.[45] An increase in urinary calcium and a decrease in urine volume have also been found after gastric bypass.[45]

The obesity–metabolic syndrome–diabetes spectrum

Obesity and weight gain increase the risk of nephrolithiasis, especially in women.[46] Data from NHANES III (1988–1994) showed a progressive increase in risk of nephrolithiasis with increasing number of metabolic syndrome traits. Those with 4 or 5 traits had twice the risk of those without any trait.[47] In a cross-sectional study of NHANES 2007 to 2010, participants with prediabetes and type 2 diabetes were more likely to have kidney stones compared with nondiabetic participants and the risk of nephrolithiasis increased with the severity of hyperglycemia.[48]

In the pathogenetic path linking obesity, the metabolic syndrome, and diabetes with kidney stones, insulin resistance and low urine pH play central roles (**Fig. 6**). At a urine pH of less than 5.5 (the pKa of uric acid), the poorly soluble undissociated form of uric acid predominates, favoring uric acid stones. Indeed, the proportion of uric acid stones was found to be 3 times greater in patients with type 2 diabetes than in nondiabetic patients (35.7% vs 11.3%), and conversely, patients with uric acid stones were 4 times more likely to have type 2 diabetes than patients with calcium stones (27.8% vs 6.9%).[49]

Urinary Factors

Table 3 lists the major urinary factors that promote stones and their corresponding stone types. A few points are worth noting. (1) The abnormal values reported by

Table 2		
Systemic and renal disorders associated with nephrolithiasis		
		Calcium Oxalate and Uric Acid
Increased Calcium Excretion	**Renal Anatomic Abnormalities**	**Stones**
Hyperparathyroidism	Polycystic kidney disease	Inflammatory bowel disease
Sarcoidosis	Medullary sponge kidney	and other malabsorptive
Vitamin D intoxication	Horseshoe kidney	states
Paget's disease	Ureteropelvic junction	Bariatric surgery
Cushing's syndrome	obstruction	Obesity, the metabolic
Hyperthyroidism		syndrome, and diabetes
Malignant tumors		Gout
Distal renal tubular acidosis		

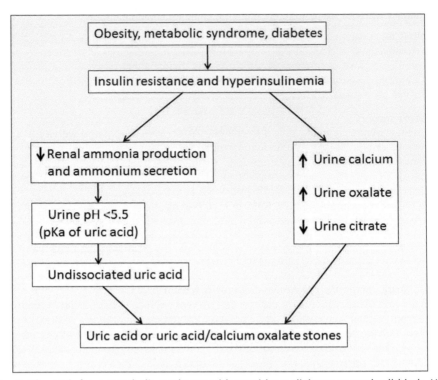

Fig. 6. The path from metabolic syndrome with or without diabetes to nephrolithiasis. Hyperinsulinemia, resulting from insulin resistance, decreases urinary pH and alters urinary constituents that leads to uric acid or mixed uric acid/calcium stones. (*Data from* Ref.[46–49])

laboratories for these urinary constituents are misleading. They assume a dichotomous cutoff when, in fact, these are continuous biological variables with risk rising even within the "normal" ranges.[50] (2) Multiple factors may combine to promote stone formation, whereas individually each might not be sufficient. (3) The opposing effects of stone-inhibiting factors in urine can mitigate the lithogenicity of stone-promoting factors. Of these, urinary citrate is the best studied and has been shown to be effective therapeutically.[51,52]

Table 3
Urinary factors that promote stones and their association with specific stone types

Promoters of Stones	Stone Type
Low urine volume	All stones
Low urine citrate	Calcium oxalate
Calcium	Calcium oxalate, calcium phosphate
Oxalate	Calcium oxalate
pH	
Low (<5.5)	Uric acid
High (>6.2)	Calcium phosphate, struvite
Infection with urease-producing bacteria (eg, Proteus mirabilis)	Struvite

CLINICAL PRESENTATION OF ACUTE RENAL COLIC

Stones that remain in the renal collecting system, even if large, may be asymptomatic if they do not cause obstruction, infection, or hematuria. However, when a stone passes down the ureter, it causes spasm and obstruction resulting in acute onset of severe pain referred to as renal colic. The term is a misnomer because the pain is not intermittent but rather continuous in a waxing–waning pattern. Stones may become lodged anywhere between the ureteropelvic junction and the ureterovesical junction. Once in the bladder, stones usually pass through the urethra without difficulty. Each site of obstruction creates a somewhat different pattern of pain with a corresponding set of differential diagnoses (**Table 4**). Nausea, vomiting, and gross or microscopic hematuria usually accompany the pain. Fever is absent unless infection is present. Older patients tend to present more commonly with symptoms of urinary tract infection, atypical pain, and gastrointestinal symptoms.[5]

MEDICAL MANAGEMENT OF ACUTE RENAL COLIC

Management of acute renal colic depends on the patient's clinical status and results of imaging studies. Three imaging modalities are available to assess stone burden and location: plain radiography, unenhanced helical computed tomography scan, and ultrasonography.

Plain Radiography

Plain radiography may reveal radiopaque calcium and struvite stones, and possibly cystine stones, but will not reveal nonopaque uric acid stones. Overlying stool and bowel gas may interfere with visualization. Precise stone localization is not possible.

Unenhanced Helical Computed Tomography Scan

Precise localization of stones and visualization of other pathologies make unenhanced helical computed tomography scan the preferred test. However, radiation risk and cost are concerns.

Ultrasound

Ultrasound is the initial imaging modality in pregnancy, but concern over radiation with computed tomography has prompted interest in using ultrasound as the initial

Table 4
Presenting patterns of pain differ according to the site of obstruction from a stone, and diagnoses that can mimic renal colic also differ in these respective locations

Site of Obstruction	Pattern of Pain	Differential Diagnosis
Ureteropelvic junction Proximal ureter	Flank pain; no radiation to groin Flank pain radiating to lumbar area	Right side: acute cholecystitis Left side: acute pancreatitis, peptic ulcer, gastritis
Mid to distal ureter	Flank pain radiating to groin and genitalia	Right side: acute appendicitis Left side: acute diverticulitis
Ureterovesical junction	Urinary frequency, urgency, dysuria, suprapubic pain, with or without diarrhea or tenesmus	Both sexes: acute cystitis/ urethritis Males: acute prostatitis, testicular torsion, incarcerated hernia Females: pelvic inflammatory disease, ovarian cyst rupture

diagnostic test for a suspected symptomatic stone. A recent study produced favorable outcomes with this approach, although the results need to be confirmed.[53] Yearly follow-up ultrasound should be done for a few years after an initial stone and indefinitely in those at high risk of recurrence.[54]

Most ureteral stones 5 mm or smaller pass spontaneously, whereas those 10 mm or greater usually require surgical intervention. Proximal stones are less likely to pass than distal ones. For stones intermediate in size, medical expulsive therapy (MET) may facilitate stone passage in patients whose symptoms do not demand immediate intervention. The selective alpha blocker tamsulosin (0.4 mg/d) is the best studied medication, followed by the calcium channel blocker nifedipine (30 mg XR daily), with or without steroids.[55,56] However, results with MET have been inconsistent. A recent large, well-designed, randomized trial (SUSPEND) failed to show any benefit from either tamsulosin or nifedipine.[57] In contrast, 3 other recent randomized controlled trials comparing either tamsulosin or alfuzosin (another alpha blocker) with standard care showed benefit from MET in terms of increased expulsion rate and shortening of expulsion time for distal ureteral stones.[58–60] A possible explanation for the different results may be related to stone size and location. In the SUSPEND trial, only 25% of stones were greater than 5 mm, only about 65% were in the distal third of the ureter, and the authors did not report the relative effect of MET on stones less than 5 mm versus 5 mm or larger. In the other 3 trials, all stones were in the distal ureter and benefit from MET versus standard care was seen only with stones 5 mm or larger.[58–60] Thus, the benefit from MET may be limited to patients with distal stones 5 mm or larger.

Another intriguing therapy to facilitate stone passage in men may be sexual intercourse. A small randomized controlled study showed that sexual intercourse 3 to 4 times a week for up to 4 weeks increased the probability of earlier passage of stones 6 mm and smaller compared with either tamsulosin or standard care.[61] The postulated mechanism is release of nitric oxide (the main neurotransmitter involved in erection during sexual intercourse) from nitrergic nerve endings in the distal ureter, which results in ureteral muscle relaxation.

Treatment also includes analgesics and antiemetics as needed. Stones that do not pass within 4 weeks should be surgically removed to prevent infection, renal deterioration, and ureteral stricture.[62] **Fig. 7** provides an algorithm for the management of acute renal colic.

Evaluation and treatment should not end with the passage or removal of a kidney stone. To prevent recurrences, further diagnostic evaluation and interventions are necessary, but are often neglected.

DIAGNOSTIC EVALUATION

There are 3 steps in the diagnostic evaluation of kidney stones directed at preventing recurrences:

- History and physical examination to uncover risk factors: family history, systemic disease, and dietary and environmental risk factors.
- Laboratory testing (blood and urine) to further identify systemic disease and risk factors:
  - *Blood tests:* **Table 5** lists diagnostically useful tests and their purpose.
  - *Urinalysis:* Specific gravity provides information on fluid intake.
    pH and morphology of crystals, if present, provide clues as to stone type.
    Presence of white blood cells suggests accompanying infection.
    Proteinuria or sediment abnormalities indicate kidney disease.

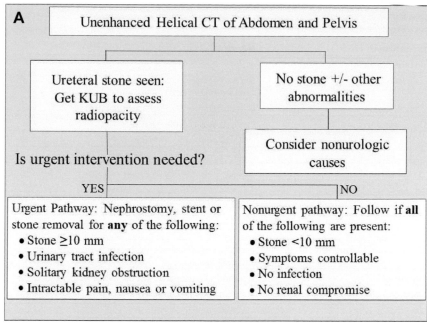

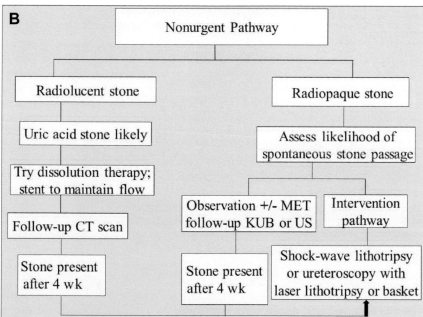

Fig. 7. Medical management of acute renal colic. (*A*) Initial path directed from computed tomography (CT) scan diagnosis to urgent intervention. (*B*) Path directed at nonurgent intervention. KUB, plain X-ray of the kidney, ureter and bladder; MET, medical expulsive therapy; US, ultrasonography. (*Adapted from* Teichman JMH. Acute renal colic from ureteral calculus. N Engl J Med 2004;350:687.)

Table 5 Blood tests useful in the evaluation of nephrolithiasis	
Measurement	**Purpose**
All stone formers	
Calcium	Detect primary hyperparathyroidism, sarcoidosis or vitamin D excess
Phosphorus	Detect primary hyperparathyroidism
Bicarbonate	Detect renal tubular acidosis
Chloride	Detect renal tubular acidosis
Potassium	Detect renal tubular acidosis or gastrointestinal disease
Glucose/HbA1c	Detect diabetes (associated with low urine pH and uric acid stones)
Uric acid	Detect hyperuricemia
Creatinine	Detect chronic kidney disease
Special tests	
Parathyroid hormone	If calcium is elevated or primary hyperparathyroidism is suspected
Calcitriol	If vitamin D excess or sarcoidosis is suspected
Angiotensin converting enzyme	If sarcoidosis is suspected

Abbreviation: HbA1c, hemoglobin A1c.

- *24-Hour urine:* Metabolic profiling of lithogenic constituents and supersaturation indices.
  Reserve this for recurrent stone formers or high-risk first-time stone formers (**Box 3**).
  Collections should be done on the patient's usual diet and fluid intake and not before at least 1 month after the passage or removal of a stone. At least 2 collections should be done to confirm results.[54]
- Analysis of stone composition: This should always be done, preferably by laboratories that specialize in stone analysis. Stone composition has diagnostic value in identifying metabolic causes of nephrolithiasis.[63] Because stone type can change over time, recurrent stones should also be analyzed in patients failing therapy.

Box 3 Indications for 24-hour urine profiling of lithogenic constituents
Recurrent stone formers

First-time stone formers at high risk for recurrence
  Solitary kidney
  Residual stones in kidney
  Systemic diseases that predispose to recurrent stones
  Uric acid, struvite, or cystine stone formers
  High risk score on Recurrence of Kidney Stone nomogram

Because of spontaneous variation, it is recommended that at least 2 collections be obtained before targeting therapy based on results. Also, the profile should be repeated 4 to 6 weeks after therapy is started to see if the desired effect has been obtained.
Data from Goldfarb DS, Arowojolu O. Metabolic evaluation of first-time and recurrent stone formers. Urol Clin North Am 2013;40:13–20.

- Bone mineral density testing: Hypercalciuric stone formers experience increased bone resorption. In 1 study, their vertebral fracture rate was 4-fold greater than in the general population.[64] Therefore, hypercalciuric patients should be tested for osteoporosis.

PREVENTION OF RECURRENT STONES

Being able to predict which first-time stone formers will have symptomatic recurrences would help clinicians to determine the intensity of initial evaluation and preventive treatment. Recently, a prediction tool designed to address this issue was developed at the Mayo Clinic.[65] Known as the Recurrence of Kidney Stone (ROKS) Nomogram, it is available on-line at http://www.qxmd.com/calculate-online/nephrology/recurrence-of-kidney-stone-roks and as a downloadable app for iOS or Android devices. It is not intended for rare stone types or genetic disorders, and it needs to be validated in other geographic climates and in more ethnically diverse populations. However, it offers clinicians some guidance for preventive therapy.

Medical prophylaxis works.[51,52] It also results in a better quality of life than repeated ureteroscopic procedures.[66] Yet, a survey of stone patients and urologists revealed sharply different responses to questions regarding chronic medical prophylaxis versus tolerance of stone recurrence and surgical intervention. Whereas 80% to 90% of patients preferred medical prophylaxis over passing another stone or requiring surgery, most urologists thought the opposite.[67] Thus, the reluctance of clinicians to promote prophylactic measures, along with inconsistent patient adherence, conspires to limit the effectiveness of these interventions. There are 3 types of prophylactic interventions: fluid intake, dietary management, and pharmacologic management.

Fluid Intake

The 2014 guidelines from the American Urologic Association and the American College of Physicians recommend sufficient fluid intake to generate at least 2 to 2.5 L of urine per day.[68,69] By decreasing the concentration of lithogenic urinary constituents, liberal fluid intake has been shown to benefit all stone formers, regardless of stone type.[52,70,71] However, not all fluids are created equal. Some types of fluids, such as those containing fructose or sucrose, or sodas acidified with phosphoric acid, can promote stones.[72,73] Among 194,000 participants in the NHS I and II and HPFS cohorts followed for more than 8 years, significant differences in stone risk were found between various beverages[73] (**Fig. 8**).

Dietary Management

Two dietary approaches can be used: empirical versus targeted. For first-time calcium stone formers who are not at high risk for recurrence (see **Box 3**), empirical treatment with a diet of normal calcium content, and low content of animal protein, sodium, and fructose, coupled with liberal fluid intake should suffice. The DASH diet (Dietary Approach to Stop Hypertension), which is high in potassium, fruits, and vegetables and relatively low in animal protein, conforms very well to these recommendations and has been shown to reduce stone recurrences.[74] Dietary management should also address obesity and the metabolic syndrome if present.

For high-risk first-time calcium stone formers and recurrent stone formers, a targeted approach based on stone composition and 24-hour urine metabolic profiling may produce better outcomes.[75] Although, evidence from randomized clinical trials is insufficient to conclude that such testing reduces stone recurrence, there is support for this approach among experts.[52,54,68,69,76]

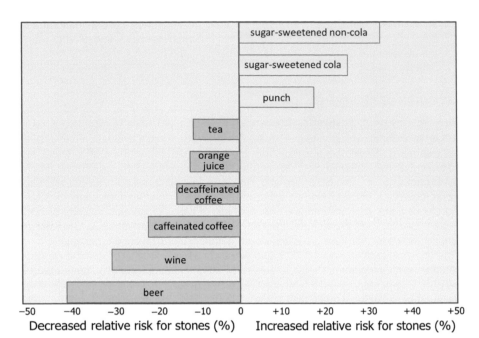

Fig. 8. Effect of various beverages on risk for kidney stones. The graph compares the relative risk of consuming 1 or more drinks per day of each beverage versus less than 1 drink per week (the zero point). Data are derived from the NHS I and II and HPFS cohorts reported in Ref.[73]

Patients with hyperoxaluria should limit foods high in oxalate content, the most common of which are spinach, nuts, and chocolate. A complete listing of oxalate-containing foods can be found online at regepi.bwh.harvard.edu/health/nutrition. html. **Table 6** summarizes the dietary recommendations for calcium stone prevention.

There are no studies regarding dietary intervention for hyperuricosuria, but reduced intake of nondairy animal protein (ie, purines) and increased dietary alkali (fruits and vegetables) are recommended in the current guidelines.[68] Referral to a dietitian to initiate and monitor therapy is advisable.[76]

Table 6
Dietary recommendations for calcium stone prevention

Diet Constituent	Dose	Patient Selection
Calcium	1000–1200 mg/d dietary (not as supplements)	All calcium stones
Sodium	2300 mg/d (100 mmol/d)	Hypercalciuria Hyperuricosuria
Animal protein	<0.8–1.0 g/kg/d	Hypercalciuria Hyperuricosuria
Oxalate	<100 mg/d	Hyperoxaluria

Data from Borghi L, Schanchi T, Meschi T, et al. Comparison of two diets for the prevention of recurrent stones in idiopathic hypercalciuria. N Engl J Med 2002;346:77–84.

Table 7 Medications for prevention of recurrent nephrolithiasis		
Drug	**Dose**	**Patient Selection**
Thiazide diuretics	Hydrochlorothiazide: 50 mg/d Chlorthalidone: 25 mg/d Indapamide: 2.5 mg/d	Hypercalciuria and normocalciuria with calcium stones
Potassium alkali	Potassium citrate: 10–20 mEq 2–3 times daily	Hypocitraturia with calcium stones; normocitraturia with low urine pH; uric acid stones
Allopurinol	100–300 mg/d	Hyperuricemia or hyperuricosuria with calcium stones

Pharmacologic Management

For recurrent stone formers, especially those not responsive to nonpharmacologic measures, and for high-risk first-time stone formers, directed pharmacologic therapy is indicated. **Table 7** summarizes medications that randomized clinical trials have shown to reduce stone recurrence risk, although the strength of evidence for efficacy is only moderate.[52]

Thiazide diuretics
Thiazides increase renal tubular calcium reabsorption and are indicated for patients with calcium stones, with or without hypercalciuruia. Composite results from 5 randomized clinical trials show a relative risk reduction of 48%.[52]

Potassium citrate
Potassium citrate increases the urinary excretion of citrate, a calcium stone inhibitor, and also increases urine pH. It is indicated for calcium stones associated with hypocitraturia and/or low urine pH. In 4 randomized clinical trials, citrate therapy reduced recurrence rates by 75%. However, withdrawals owing to adverse events were high.[52] Because low urine pH is the major determinant of uric acid stone formation, citrate is also the primary treatment for the prevention and dissolution of uric acid stones. Most patients with uric acid stones do not have hyperuricosuria, but all have low urine pH.[77] Urine alkalinization also protects against cystine stones.

Allopurinol
Allopurinol inhibits uric acid production and is indicated for calcium stone formers with hyperuricemia and/or hyperuricosuria. In 2 randomized clinical trials, allopurinol reduced stone recurrence by 41%.[52] There are no randomized clinical trials for uric acid stone prevention, but allopurinol is used as second-line therapy if urinary alkalinization with citrate fails.

Acetohydroxamic acid
This urease inhibitor has been used for recurrent struvite stones, which are due to chronic infection with urease-producing bacteria, and tend to be very large, forming staghorn calculi that fill the renal pelvis. Three randomized clinical trials showed reduction in stone growth but not recurrence, and major adverse events were frequent.[52]

Antibiotics
Surgical removal with antibiotics before and after surgery is the treatment of choice for struvite stones. Antibiotics, of course, are also indicated whenever an obstructing stone is accompanied by infection.

SUMMARY

Kidney stones extract a high price in terms of suffering as well as a financial burden. Recognizing which patients are at high risk and practicing preventive medicine is key. The ROKS calculator allows the PA to predict who has the highest chance for reoccurrence. Taking steps to prevent further damage in the high risk patient decreases the incidence of morbidity for the kidney patient

REFERENCES

1. Eknoyan G. History of urolithiasis. Clin Rev Bone Miner Metab 2004;2:177–85.
2. Shah J, Whitfield HN. Urolithiasis through the ages. BJU Int 2002;89:801–10.
3. Edvardsson VO, Goldfarb DS, Lieske JC, et al. Hereditary causes of kidney stones and chronic kidney disease. Pediatr Nephrol 2013;28:1923–42.
4. Bird VG, Canales BK, Shields JM. Stratifying surgical therapy. In: Monga M, Penniston KL, Goldfarb DS, editors. Pocket guide to kidney stone prevention. Heidelberg (Germany): Springer; 2015. p. 149–59.
5. Krambeck AE, Lieske JC, Li X, et al. Effect of age on the clinical presentation of incident symptomatic urolithiasis in the general population. J Urol 2013;189:158–64.
6. Scales CD, Smith AC, Hanley JM, et al. Prevalence of kidney stones in the United States. Eur Urol 2012;62:160–5.
7. Borghi L, Schanchi T, Meschi T, et al. Comparison of two diets for the prevention of recurrent stones in idiopathic hypercalciuria. N Engl J Med 2002;346:77–84.
8. Ghani KR, Sammon JD, Karakiewicz PI, et al. Trends in surgery for upper urinary tract calculi in the USA using the Nationwide Inpatient sample: 1999-2009. BJU Int 2013;112:224–30.
9. Romero V, Akpinar H, Assimos DG. Kidney stones: a global picture of prevalence, incidence, and associated risk factors. Rev Urol 2010;12:e86–96.
10. Worcester EM, Coe FL. Calcium kidney stones. N Engl J Med 2010;363:954–63.
11. Fwu C-W, Eggers PW, Kimmel PL, et al. Emergency department visits, use of imaging, and drugs for urolithiasis have increased in the United States. Kidney Int 2013;83:479–86.
12. Pearle MS, Calhoun EA, Curhan GC, et al. Urologic diseases in America project: urolithiasis. J Urol 2005;173:848–57.
13. Litwin MS, Saigal CS. Urinary tract stones. In: Urologic Diseases in America, editor. US Department of Health and Human Services, Public Health Service, National Institutes of Health, National Institute of Diabetes and Digestive and Kidney Diseases. Washington, DC: US Government Printing Office; 2012. p. 316–20. NIH Publication No. 12-7865.
14. Coe FL, Parks JH, Asplin JR. The pathogenesis and treatment of kidneys stones. N Engl J Med 1992;327:1141–52.
15. Bushinsky DA, Coe FL, Moe OW. Nephrolithiasis. In: Taal MW, Chertow GM, Marsden PA, et al, editors. Brenner & Rector's the kidney. 9th edition. Philadelphia: Elsevier; 2012. p. 1455.
16. Fakheri RJ, Goldfarb DS. Ambient temperature as a contributor to kidney stone formation: implications of global warming. Kidney Int 2011;79:1178–85.
17. Soucie JM, Coates RJ, McClellan W, et al. Relation between geographic variability in kidney stones prevalence and risk factors for stones. Am J Epidemiol 1996;143:487–95.
18. Fakheri RJ, Goldfarb DS. Association of nephrolithiasis prevalence rates with ambient temperature in the United States: a re-analysis. Kidney Int 2009;76:798.

19. Chen Y-K, Lin H-C, Chen C-S, et al. Seasonal variations in urinary calculi attacks and their association with climate: a population based study. J Urol 2008;179: 564–9.

20. Breyer BN, Sen S, Aaronson DS, et al. Use of Google Insights for search to track seasonal and geographic kidney stone incidence in the United States. Urology 2011;78:267–71.

21. Brikowski TH, Lotan Y, Pearle MS. Climate-related increase in the prevalence of urolithiasis in the United States. Proc Natl Acad Sci U S A 2008;105: 9841–6.

22. Evans K, Costabile RA. Time to development of symptomatic calculi in a high risk environment. J Urol 2005;173:858–61.

23. Curhan GC, Willett WC, Rimm EB, et al. Family history and risk of kidney stones. J Am Soc Nephrol 1997;8:1568–73.

24. Taylor EN, Curhan GC. Differences in 24-hour urine composition between black and white women. J Am Soc Nephrol 2007;18:654–9.

25. Mente A, Honey RJ, McLaughlin JR, et al. Ethnic differences in relative risk of idiopathic calcium nephrolithiasis in North America. J Urol 2007;178:1992–7.

26. Goldfarb DS, Fischer ME, Keich Y, et al. A twin study of genetic and dietary influences on nephrolithiasis: a report from the Vietnam Era Twin (VET) Registry. Kidney Int 2005;67:1053–61.

27. Curhan GC, Willett WC, Rimm EB, et al. A prospective study of dietary calcium and other nutrients and the risk of symptomatic kidney stones. N Engl J Med 1993;328:833–8.

28. Curhan GC, Willett WC, Speizer FE, et al. Comparison of dietary calcium with supplemental calcium and other nutrients as factors affecting the risk for kidney stones in women. Ann Intern Med 1997;126:497–504.

29. Curhan GC, Willett WC, Knight EL, et al. Dietary factors and the risk of incident kidney stones in younger women. Arch Intern Med 2004;164:885–91.

30. Taylor EN, Curhan GC. Determinants of 24-hour urinary oxalate excretion. Clin J Am Soc Nephrol 2008;3:1453–60.

31. Holmes RP, Assimos DG. The impact of dietary oxalate on kidney stone formation. Urol Res 2004;32:311–6.

32. Heilberg IP, Goldfarb DS. Optimal nutrition for kidney stone disease. Adv Chronic Kidney Dis 2013;20:165–74.

33. Taylor EN, Curhan GC. Oxalate intake and the risk for nephrolithiasis. J Am Soc Nephrol 2007;18:2198–204.

34. Holmes RP, Ambrosius WT, Assimos DG. Dietary oxalate loads and renal oxalate handling. J Urol 2005;174:943–7.

35. Taylor EN, Curhan GC. Fructose consumption and the risk of kidney stones. Kidney Int 2008;73:207–12.

36. Knight J, Assimos DG, Easter L, et al. Metabolism of fructose to oxalate and glycolate. Horm Metab Res 2010;42:868–73.

37. Muldowney FP, Freaney R, Moloney MF. Importance of dietary sodium in the hypercalciuria syndrome. Kidney Int 1982;22:292–6.

38. Taylor EN, Stampfer MJ, Curhan GC. Dietary factors and the risk of incident kidney stones in men: new insights after 14 years of follow-up. J Am Soc Nephrol 2004;15:3225–32.

39. Kok DJ, Lestra JA, Doorenbos CJ, et al. The effects of dietary excesses in animal protein and in sodium on the composition and the crystallization kinetics of calcium oxalate monohydrate in urines of healthy men. J Clin Endocrinol Metab 1990;71:861–7.

40. Krieger NS, Asplin JR, Frick KK, et al. Effect of potassium citrate on calcium phosphate stones in a model of hypercalciuria. J Am Soc Nephrol 2015. [Epub ahead of print].
41. Baxmann AC, Mendonca CD, Heilberg IP. Effect of vitamin C supplements on urinary oxalate and pH in calcium stone-forming patients. Kidney Int 2003;63:1066–71.
42. Nguyen S, Baggerly L, French C, et al. 25-hydroxyvitamin D in the range of 20 to 100 ng/ml and incidence of kidney stones. Am J Public Health 2014;104:1783–7.
43. Clayman RV, Williams RD. Oxalate urolithiasis following jejunoileal bypass. Surg Clin North Am 1979;59:1071–7.
44. Matlaga BR, Shore AD, Magnuson T, et al. Effect of gastric bypass surgery on kidney stone disease. J Urol 2009;181:2673–7.
45. Wu JN, Craig J, Chamie K, et al. Urolithiasis risk factors in the bariatric population undergoing gastric bypass surgery. Surg Obes Relat Dis 2013;9:83–7.
46. Taylor EN, Stampfer MJ, Curhan CG. Obesity, weight gain, and the risk of kidney stones. J Am Med Assoc 2005;293:455–62.
47. West B, Luke A, Durazo-Arvisu RA, et al. Metabolic syndrome and self-reported history of kidney stones: the National Health and Nutrition Examination Survey (NHANES III) 1988-1994. Am J Kidney Dis 2008;51:741–7.
48. Weinberg AE, Patel CJ, Chertow GM, et al. Diabetic severity and risk of kidney stone disease. Eur Urol 2014;65:242–7.
49. Daudon M, Traxer O, Conort P, et al. Type 2 diabetes increases the risk for uric acid stones. J Am Soc Nephrol 2006;17:2026–33.
50. Curhan GC, Willett WC, Speizer FE, et al. Twenty-four-hour chemistries and the risk of kidney stones among women and men. Kidney Int 2001;59:2290–8.
51. Lee YH, Huang WC, Tsai JY, et al. The efficacy of potassium citrate based medical prophylaxis for preventing upper urinary tract calculi: a midterm follow-up study. J Urol 1999;161:1453–7.
52. Fink HA, Wilt TJ, Eidman KE, et al. Medical management to prevent recurrent nephrolithiasis in adults: a systematic review for an American College of Physicians clinical guideline. Ann Intern Med 2013;158:535–43.
53. Smith-Bindman R, Aubin C, Bailitz AJ, et al. Ultrasonography versus computed tomography for suspected nephrolithiasis. N Engl J Med 2014;371:1100–10.
54. Goldfarb DS, Arowojolu O. Metabolic evaluation of first-time and recurrent stone formers. Urol Clin North Am 2013;40:13–20.
55. Coll DM, Varanelli MJ, Smith RC. Relationship of spontaneous passage of ureteral calculi to stone size and location as revealed by unenhanced helical CT. Am J Roentgenol 2002;178:101–9.
56. Campschroer T, Zhu Y, Duijvesz D, et al. Alpha-blockers as medical expulsive therapy for ureteral stones. Cochrane Database Syst Rev 2014;(4):CD008509.
57. Pickard R, Starr K, Maclennan G, et al. Medical expulsive therapy in adults with ureteric colic: a multicenter, randomized, placebo-controlled trial. Lancet 2015; 386(9991):341–9.
58. El Said NO, El Wakeel L, Kamal KM, et al. Alfuzosin treatment improves the rate and time for stone expulsion in patients with distal ureteral stones: a prospective randomized controlled study. Pharmacotherapy 2015;35(5):470–6.
59. Ahmed A, Al-sayed A. Tamsulosin versus Alfuzosin in the treatment of patients with distal ureteral stones: prospective, randomized, comparative study. Korean J Urol 2010;51:193–7.
60. Furyk JS, Chu K, Banks C, et al. Distal ureteric stones and tamsulosin: a double-blind, placebo-controlled, randomized, multicenter trial. Ann Emerg Med 2015. [Epub ahead of print].

61. Doluoglu OG, Demirbas A, Killnc MF, et al. Can sexual intercourse be an alternative therapy for distal ureteral stones? A prospective, randomized, controlled study. Urol 2015;86:19–24.

62. Teichman JMH. Acute renal colic from ureteral calculus. N Engl J Med 2004;350: 684–93.

63. Pak CYC, Poindexter JR, Adams-Huet B, et al. Predictive value of kidney stone composition in the detection of metabolic abnormalities. Am J Med 2003;115: 26–32.

64. Heilberg IP, Weisinger JR. Bone disease in idiopathic hypercalciuria. Curr Opin Nephrol Hypertens 2006;15:394–402.

65. Rule AD, Lieske JC, Li X, et al. The ROKS nomogram for predicting a second symptomatic stone episode. J Am Soc Nephrol 2014;25:2878–86.

66. Bensalah K, Tuncel A, Gupta A, et al. Determinants of quality of life for patients with kidney stones. J Urol 2008;179:2238–43.

67. Bensalah K, Tuncel A, Raman JD, et al. How physician and patient perceptions differ regarding medical management of stone disease. J Urol 2009;182: 998–1004.

68. Pearle MS, Goldfarb DS, Assimos DG, et al. Medical management of kidney stones: AUA guideline. J Urol 2014;192:316–24.

69. Qaseem A, Dallas P, Forciea MA, et al. Dietary and pharmacologic management to prevent recurrent nephrolithiasis in adults: A clinical practice guideline from the American College of Physicians. Ann Intern Med 2014;161:659–67.

70. Fink HA, Akornor JW, Garimella PS, et al. Diet, fluid, or supplements for secondary prevention of nephrolithiasis: a systematic review and meta-analysis of randomized trials. Eur Urol 2009;56:72–80.

71. Borghi L, Meschi T, Amato F, et al. Urinary volume, water and recurrences in idiopathic calcium nephrolithiasis: a 5-year randomized prospective study. J Urol 1996;155:839–43.

72. Shuster J, Jenkins A, Logan C, et al. Soft drink consumption and urinary stone recurrence: a randomized prevention trial. J Clin Epidemiol 1992;45:911–6.

73. Ferraro PM, Taylor EN, Gambaro G, et al. Soda and other beverages and the risk of kidney stones. Clin J Am Soc Nephrol 2013;8:1389–95.

74. Taylor EN, Fung TT, Curhan GC. DASH-style diet associates with reduced risk for kidney stones. J Am Soc Nephrol 2009;20:2253–9.

75. Kocvara R, Plasgura P, Petrik A, et al. A prospective study of nonmedical prophylaxis after a first kidney stone. BJU Int 1999;84:393–8.

76. Penniston KL, Nakada SY. Diet and alternative therapies in the management of stone disease. Urol Clin North Am 2013;40:31–46.

77. Shekarriz B, Stoller ML. Uric acid nephrolithiasis: current concepts and controversies. J Urol 2002;168:1307–14.

Acute Kidney Injury
The Ugly Truth

Erica N. Davis, MHS, PA-C*

KEYWORDS

- Acute kidney injury • KDIGO • Continuous renal replacement therapy • AKIN
- RIFLE

KEY POINTS

- Acute kidney injury (AKI) is a common cause of morbidity and mortality in hospitalized patients.
- The Kidney Disease Improving Global Outcomes (KDIGO) guidelines are the most recent guidelines for the definition and staging of AKI. These were preceded by the risk, injury, failure, loss, and end-stage renal disease (RIFLE) and Acute Kidney Injury Network (AKIN) criteria.
- Acute tubular necrosis is the most common cause of AKI in hospitalized patients, accounting for 45% of all in-hospital AKI.
- The mainstay of treatment of AKI is the prompt identification of the underlying cause and aggressive hemodynamic support.

ACUTE KIDNEY INJURY: THE UGLY TRUTH

Acute kidney injury (AKI) is a common and complex problem. The incidence of AKI severe enough to warrant renal replacement therapy (RRT) has an occurance of 2 to 300 per million population per year; while AKI without the need for RRT occurs in 2 to 3000 per million population per year.[1] Close to two-thirds of all patients in the critical care setting will develop AKI and approximately 5% of intensive care unit (ICU) patients will develop AKI severe enough to warrant RRT.[1] AKI is typically caused by renal ischemia and is characterized by the abrupt decline in urine production and rise in serum creatinine.

AKI was without a consensus definition until 2002 when the Acute Dialysis Quality Initiative (ADQI), an expert panel, developed the risk, injury, failure, loss, and end-stage renal disease (RIFLE) criteria classification of acute renal failure. It includes 3 classes of increasing severity of renal failure (risk, injury, and failure) and 2 outcome

Disclosure Statement: The author has nothing to disclose.
Metropolitan Nephrology Associates, 2616 Sherwood Hall Lane, Suite 209, Alexandria, VA 22306, USA
* 401 13th Street Northeast #102, Washington, DC 20002.
E-mail address: endavis@hotmail.com

Physician Assist Clin 1 (2016) 149–159
http://dx.doi.org/10.1016/j.cpha.2015.09.006
2405-7991/16/$ – see front matter © 2016 Elsevier Inc. All rights reserved.

variables (loss, and end-stage renal disease [ESRD]). The classes of severity of kidney failure are based on increase in serum creatinine, decrease in glomerular filtration rate (GFR) and reduction in urine output (UOP). The outcome variables establish time frames for determination of prolonged loss of function (>4 weeks) and the development of ESRD.[2]

Following the development of the RIFLE criteria, the Acute Kidney Injury Network (AKIN), which recommended the term AKI be used to represent the entire spectrum of acute renal failure, was formed in 2004. It also set forth a staging system for AKI reflecting quantitative changes in serum creatinine and UOP. AKIN varies from RIFLE by defining AKI as reduced function over a 48-hour period versus the 7 days suggested by RIFLE. AKIN also includes less severe injury in its diagnostic criteria and removes GFR, which is unpredictable during AKI. The AKIN criteria are predicated on 2 factors: that volume status has been optimized and the presence of urinary tract obstructions has been excluded. The need for RRT was not included in the AKIN criteria because this was thought to be an outcome of AKI.[2,3] To further complicate the picture, a third criteria was proposed in 2012 when the Kidney Disease Improving Global Outcomes (KDIGO) released Clinical Practice Guidelines for AKI. These guidelines, developed by the world's kidney experts and agreed to by all participating countries, sought to provide comprehensive evidenced-based recommendations and improve patient care in the setting of AKI. The KDIGO guidelines simplified the definition of AKI down to any 1 of the following 3 criteria:

1. An increase in serum creatinine by 0.3 mg/dL or more within 48 hours
2. An increase in serum creatinine to 1.5 times the baseline or more within the last 7 days
3. A UOP of less than 0.5 mL/kg/h for 6 hours.

AKI can then be further staged for severity according to additional severity criteria[4] **(Table 1)**.

Table 1
The 3 acute kidney injury classification systems

Stage	UOP	RIFLE	AKIN	KDIGO
1	<0.5 mL/kg/h for 6 h	*Risk:* Increase in SCr of 1.5× or decrease in GFR >25%	Increase in SCr 1.5× baseline or ≥3.0 mg/dL	Increase in SCr of 1.5–1.9× baseline or ≥0.3 mg/dL increase in SCr
2	<0.5 mL/kg/h for 12 h	*Injury:* Increase in SCr 2× or decrease in GFR >50%	Increase in SCr 2× baseline	Increase in SCr of 2–2.9× baseline
3	<0.3 mL/kg/h for 24 h or anuria for 12 h	*Failure:* Increase in SCr 3× or decrease in GFR >75%	Increase in SCr 3× baseline or ≥4 mg/dL (with acute rise of >0.5 mg/dl)	Increase in SCr of >3× baseline or increase in SCr ≥4.0 mg/dL or initiation of RRT

Loss and ESRD of the RIFLE criteria are not included in this staging chart because they are considered outcome variables.
Abbreviation: SCr, serum creatinine.
Adapted from Kristensen SD, Knuuti J, Saraste A, et al. 2014 ESC/ESA Guidelines on non-cardiac surgery: cardiovascular assessment and management: The Joint Task Force on non-cardiac surgery: cardiovascular assessment and management of the European Society of Cardiology (ESC) and the European Society of Anaesthesiology (ESA). Eur Heart J 2014;35:2383–431; with permission.

MORBIDITY AND MORTALITY OF ACUTE KIDNEY INJURY

AKI results in significant increases in mortality and morbidity of affected patients. AKI is more likely to occur in older men and those with diabetes and pre-existing chronic kidney disease (CKD). Blacks are at much higher risk of developing AKI than whites or other races. In 2012, the incidence rate of AKI in blacks was 68.8 per 1000 patient years compared with 40.1 in whites. Since 2003, there has been a significant racial disparity with black patients twice as likely to have an episode of AKI, even when controlling for other factors.[5] Patients with 1 episode of AKI are much more likely to suffer recurrent episodes, develop CKD, or have progression of their pre-existing CKD. Thus, with the addition of these known risk factors, the patient most likely to have an episode of AKI is the hospitalized black, diabetic, CKD patient. The most likely diagnoses contributing to AKI include cardiovascular disease, sepsis and other infections, iatrogenic and neoplasms.[6]

In the year following a hospital admission with AKI, 30% of patients without CKD before their episode of AKI will be reclassified as having some degree of CKD (**Fig. 1**). There are a small number (<1%) who will develop ESRD after a hospitalization with AKI.[5] A 2012 study found that AKI occurred in 1 of 5 hospital admissions and was associated with a fourfold increase in mortality.[6] They also found that this mortality association is independent of other factors, such as the severity of other comorbid conditions, and is an independent effect for AKI itself. The odds ratio for death was also higher among those patients with prolonged hospitalizations and serum creatinine values that did not peak until after hospital day 7 (**Fig. 2**).[6]

CAUSE OF ACUTE KIDNEY INJURY

The causes of AKI are varied but fall into 3 main categories:

- Prerenal
- Intrarenal
- Postrenal

The most common cause of AKI in an outpatient setting is prerenal azotemia characterized by decreased renal blood flow or perfusion. This can often be seen in the

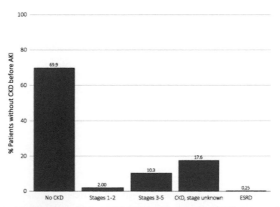

Fig. 1. Renal status 1 year after first AKI hospitalization in Medicare patients (2010–2011). (*From* U.S. Renal Data System. USRDS 2014 annual data report: atlas of end-stage renal disease in the United States. Bethesda (MD): National Institutes of Health, National Institute of Diabetes and Digestive and Kidney Diseases; 2014.)

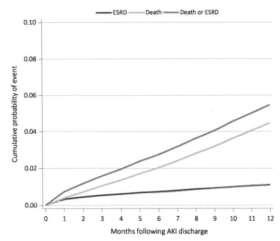

Fig. 2. Probability of death or ESRD 1 year after AKI hospitalization in Medicare patients (2010–2011). (*From* U.S. Renal Data System. USRDS 2014 annual data report: atlas of end-stage renal disease in the United States. Bethesda (MD); National Institutes of Health, National Institute of Diabetes and Digestive and Kidney Diseases; 2014.)

volume depletion associated with gastrointestinal losses such as vomiting or diarrhea. It also occurs as a result of heart failure (cardiorenal syndrome) when pump failure results in poor perfusion of the kidneys. Diuretics, vasoactive medication such as angiotensin converting enzyme inhibitor (ACEi), and nonsteroidal anti-inflammatory drugs (NSAIDs) are also common factors in the development of AKI in the outpatient setting as well as the inpatient setting:

- Diuretics reduce glomerular blood flow through intravascular volume depletion
- ACEi cause vasodilatation of the efferent arteriole, causing a decrease in the filtration rate across the glomerulus
- NSAIDs inhibit prostaglandins, which cause vasodilation of the afferent arteriole, thereby causing unopposed constriction of the afferent arteriole resulting in decreased renal flow[7]

The concomitant use of 2 or 3 of these classes of mediations is often enough to result in significant prerenal AKI. Intrarenal AKI is caused by damage to the structures within the kidney and can be vascular, tubular, glomerular, or interstitial. The most common cause of intrarenal failure, and by far the most common cause of AKI in the hospitalized patient, is acute tubular necrosis (ATN), which occurs in close to half of all cases.[8] Of all cases of AKI in the hospital, 65% to 75% occur due to either ATN or prerenal causes.

ATN is the death of the tubular epithelial cells. ATN occurs for 3 major reasons:

- Renal ischemia
- Sepsis
- Nephrotoxins

All causes of prerenal AKI, with the exception of heart failure, can cause ischemic ATN, especially if there is concomitant sepsis or hypotension. It is not well understood why patients with cardiorenal syndrome are not likely to develop ATN.[9] Patients with sepsis are likely to have hypotension and a subsequent decrease in renal perfusion, exposure to endotoxins, the release of cytokines (eg, tumor necrosis factor, certain interleukins), and the release of oxidants from neutrophils. All of these factors are contributors to the development of ATN.[10,11] In addition to reduction in renal perfusion and the endogenous release of toxins, there are many drugs that can lead to ATN. Some of the most common are platinum containing chemotherapeutics (eg, cisplatin), radiocontrast dye, aminoglycosides (eg, gentamycin), and antiretrovirals (eg, tenofovir).[9]

To aid in determining if ATN is present, a fractional excretion of sodium (FENa) can be obtained (**Fig. 3**). If the result is greater than 2%, it is considered ATN. There may or may not be granular casts in the urine; though, when seen, they are pathognomonic for ATN and are referred to as muddy brown casts.

Postrenal failure occurs due to the obstruction of urine outflow via

- Prostatic hypertrophy
- Calculi
- Tumors
- Strictures

Urinary tract obstructions account for 1 in 10 AKI cases in hospitalized patients. Hydronephrosis is often the sequelae of severe or prolonged cases of obstruction. Postobstructive diuresis (POD) is defined as UOP greater than 200 mL/h for 2 consecutive hours or greater than 3L of urine in 24 hours. Patients with pathologic POD are at risk for severe volume depletion, electrolyte imbalances, and even hypovolemic shock; all of which can serve to further worsen the initial AKI.[12] However, if POD lasts less than 24 hours, it is classified as physiologic and is self-limiting.

DIAGNOSIS OF ACUTE KIDNEY INJURY

The diagnostic approach to AKI starts with a complete and detailed history. The history must include recent drug history, radiocontrast exposure, and the presence of urinary symptoms. Vitally important is the presence of recent or current hypotension. During the physical examination, it is important to evaluate the patient's fluid status. Look for peripheral edema, orthopnea, jugular venous distention, and, if possible, orthostasis. If AKI is suspected, look for suspicious history: sepsis, heart failure or signs of a systemic illness (eg, lupus or vasculitis). Treating the underlying cause of the AKI is 1 of the most important steps in management of AKI.

Determining the baseline serum creatinine helps to determine if the elevated creatinine is chronic or has occurred acutely or subacutely over the course of days to weeks to months. Urinalysis is a vital step as it can help establish a differential diagnosis. The presence or absence of casts, such as granular or white blood cell casts, can narrow the differential to ATN or acute interstitial nephritis. The presence of hyaline casts can signify volume depletion. Urine electrolytes, such as those used to calculate the FENa, can help differentiate the cause of AKI. A FENa of less than 1% indicates a prerenal cause of AKI, with the caveat that a FENa less than 1% is not 100% diagnostic of prerenal causes. A low FENa can be seen in rhabdomyolysis and contrast-induced nephropathy giving the false impression of a prerenal cause. A FENa greater than 2% indicates an intrinsic cause such as ATN. A value between 1% and 2% can be seen in either prerenal or intrarenal. Diuretic therapy and diseases of sodium wasting can falsely elevate the FENa above 1% and careful consideration must be given to this.

$$FENa\ \% = (U_{Na} \times S_{Cr}) / (S_{Na} \times U_{Cr}) \times 100$$

Fig. 3. Calculation of FENa. SCr, serum creatinine; S_{Na}, serum sodium concentration; U_{cr}, urine creatinine concentration; UNa, urinary sodium concentration.

KIDNEY IMAGING AND BIOPSY

The performance of a kidney ultrasound can be important in the workup of AKI. It is noninvasive and typically readily available. It can help to determine if a patient has evidence of CKD, such as a thinned kidney cortex or increased parenchymal echogenicity. Small shrunken kidneys or asymmetric kidneys may be an indicator that renovascular disease is a factor in the AKI. The presence of hydronephrosis often indicates an obstruction of some type. Ultrasonography of the bladder should also be performed to evaluate for bladder outlet obstruction. Kidney biopsy is a much more invasive procedure and often reserved for use in the following instances:

1. When there is the absence of an obvious cause of the AKI
2. Extrarenal manifestations suggestive of a systemic disease are present
3. There is the presence of proteinuria, hematuria, or casts in the urine
4. There is suspicion of parenchymal disease other than ATN
5. There is AKI lasting longer than 3 weeks or prolonged anuria[13]

TREATMENT OF ACUTE KIDNEY INJURY

First and foremost in the treatment of AKI is the discontinuation of all nephrotoxic agents such as NSAIDs or aminoglycosides. Once offending medications are stopped, all other medications should be evaluated for dosing changes. As the kidney function declines, GFR becomes less reliable; often the pharmacist is the best resource for evaluating the doses of medications.[14] GFR calculations for medication dosing require that the GFR be stable. In the rapidly changing AKI patient, this is rarely true. These changes should be made quickly and occur concurrently with a rapid assessment of volume status. Volume resuscitation can be achieved by the use of either crystalloid or colloid solutions. Colloid solutions are considerably more expensive and recent studies have shown the use of hydroxyethyl starch (6% HES) to be associated with increased mortality and AKI resulting in the increased need for RRT.[15,16] Early goal-directed therapy (EGDT) as defined by Rivers and colleagues[17] in 2001 was aimed at the treatment of severe sepsis and shock and involves adjustments of cardiac preload, afterload, and contractility to balance oxygen delivery to decrease severe organ dysfunction. The Rivers and colleagues[17] study, however, did not evaluate AKI as an endpoint. More recent studies have shown that, in the setting of ATN, the most common cause of AKI in the hospitalized patient, aggressive fluid resuscitation aimed at reversing renal ischemia and diluting nephrotoxins may compromise kidney recovery secondary to volume overload.[18] Despite the conventional view that EGDT improves end-organ perfusion, the liberal administration of intravenous fluids in the attempt to reach a target central venous pressure often leads to positive fluid balance and volume overload. In the critically ill patient, a positive fluid balance of 5% to 10% of total body weight is associated with worsening organ dysfunction without any beneficial effect on kidney function and, in fact, is associated with increased mortality.[19] These new data have led to the common use of vasopressors to improve kidney perfusion in the critically ill patient without significantly contributing to volume overload.

Vasopressors, such as norepinephrine and vasopressin, are often used to help maintain kidney perfusion after intravascular volume depletion has been restored with fluid resuscitation. Dopamine has been found to increase UOP through a diuretic effect; however, it does not significantly reduce the risk of kidney dysfunction.[20] In addition, it should not be used for prophylaxis against AKI because it has several adverse effects, including a decrease in T-cell function, a proarrhythmic effect, and depression of the respiratory drive.[4,20] Norepinephrine, the drug of choice for systemic vasodilation, constricts both the afferent and efferent arterioles, which does not have a favorable effect on glomerular filtration. Vasopressin, on the other hand, increases resistance in the efferent arterioles with little effect on the afferent arterioles, leading to increased kidney blood flow and enhanced diuresis. Despite this seemingly favorable physiologic profile, there was no significant reduction in mortality rates in critically ill patients when vasopressin was used.[21]

Loop diuretics, such as furosemide, are commonly used in patients with AKI to improve UOP. The rationale is that active sodium transport would decrease oxygen demand, debris from the tubules may be washed out and there may be increased renal blood flow and renal vasodilation. Despite this seemingly favorable profile, loop diuretics have proven to have no significant effect on mortality or the need for RRT.[22] Diuretics are not recommended for the prevention or treatment of AKI but are recommended for the management of fluid overload and electrolyte disturbances, which typically occur during AKI.[4]

Vasodilator therapy, such as fenoldopam, has been used to improve renal blood in an effort to prevent AKI; however, further randomized clinical trials are necessary for further confirmation of benefit and its use is not currently recommended by the KDIGO guidelines. The use of natriuretic peptides, such as atrial natriuretic peptide and nesiritide, are theorized to increase GFR via afferent vasodilation and efferent vasoconstriction. However, neither is currently recommended for use by the KDIGO guidelines.

Most treatment during AKI is supportive and often includes nutritional support. There are little data on nutritional clinical endpoints. The current KDIGO guidelines recommend that nutrition be given via the enteral route (when possible) for a total intake of 20 to 30 kcal/kg/d. Protein restriction should be avoided in the AKI patient with this recommendation based on the degree of catabolism and whether the patient is on RRT.[4] Patients on RRT or who are hypercatabolic are recommended to receive up to 1.7 g/kg/d of protein compared with non-RRT, noncatabolic patients who are recommended to receive 0.8 to 1.0 g/kg/d.[4] In addition, stress hyperglycemia is common in critically ill patients and, given that diabetic patients are much more likely to develop AKI, glycemic control is imperative. The most recent KDIGO guidelines recommend the use of insulin therapy to maintain a target glucose of 110 to 149 mg/dl.[4]

RENAL REPLACEMENT THERAPY

The optimal timing for the initiation of dialysis in AKI is not defined and is a subject of much debate. The decision to start dialysis is often based on clinical features such as volume overload, uremic complications, hyperkalemia, and severe acidosis. Often the initiation of RRT is delayed due to concerns about the risks associated with RRT and the lingering hope that the patient may recover on her or his own. Risks of starting RRT include

- Hypotension
- Arrhythmias
- Vascular access complications (infection, bleeding, anesthesia)

There are various forms of RRT that can be used in AKI, including

- Intermittent hemodialysis (IHD)
- Continuous RRT (CRRT)
- Peritoneal dialysis (PD)

An important concept to understand in RRT is the difference between hemodialysis and hemofiltration. In hemodialysis, blood runs countercurrent to a dialysis solution, or dialysate, and solutes are cleared by diffusion across a semipermeable membrane. In hemofiltration, fluid is removed via a hydrostatic pressure gradient and solutes are cleared by convection across a semipermeable membrane. There is no dialysate; instead, an isotonic replacement fluid is added to the blood to replace electrolytes and volume. There are large amounts of fluid removed during hemofiltration and normal blood volume must be maintained.[23] The 2 modalities can be combined in hemodiafiltration in which both a dialysate and replacement fluid are used.

In IHD the removal of solutes is rapid and efficient, making it an ideal choice for the removal of toxins. The downside to IHD is the potential for hypotension related to rapid fluid removal, particularly in patients who may have hemodynamic instability. IHD typically occurs through a dual venous access, via a Quinton (nontunneled) catheter or permcath (tunneled) catheter. Each dialysis session typically lasts anywhere from 3 to 5 hours and usually occurs 3 to 7 times per week, depending on the patient. Having a shorter dialysis time period allows for patients to be more readily available for other diagnostic procedures or therapies necessary for their care. It also decreases the patient's exposure to anticoagulation, reducing the risk for significant bleeding. Isolated ultrafiltration (UF), which removes fluid only, can also be used in an intermittent format in patients requiring more aggressive fluid removal but who do not need more frequent solute removal. In UF, hydrostatic pressure is the driving force for fluid removal and small solutes are removed due to the semipermeable membrane. The small solutes are removed at the same rate as water and their overall concentration does not change.[23]

In CRRT, the removal of solutes occurs through convection across a semipermeable membrane over a 24-hour period. Although convection is less efficient than the diffusion used in IHD, the continuous nature of the therapy compensates for this difference.[24] Venous access for CRRT can occur through dual venous access as in IHD or through arterial and venous access. All types of CRRT afford better hemodynamic stability through slower fluid removal, more effective control of acid-base balance and electrolyte status, and the improved removal of uremic toxins and inflammatory mediators, specifically in patients with sepsis.[24] There is also great flexibility in the various types of CRRT. The newer, user-friendly machines make offering CRRT more feasible. Despite the benefits to CRRT, there are significant disadvantages. These are mainly related to the need for prolonged exposure to anticoagulants thus increasing the risk of bleeding and the requirement and cost of additional nursing staff, dialysis machines, and solutions.[23] As can be surmised, this adds significantly to the cost of treating the patient; although a decrease in the number of days in the ICU can outweigh the cost in some instances.

There are various types of CRRT and each can be performed using either arteriovenous (AV) access or venovenous access (VV). For simplicity, the VV designation will be used here. Types of CRRT include

- Continuous VV hemodialysis (CVVHD), in which diffusion is the primary means of solute removal; the amount of fluid that can be ultrafiltered is low and typically ranges between 3 to 6 L per day
- Continuous VV hemofiltration (CVVHF) without dialysate and without diffusion; the amount of fluid ultrafiltered is large and replacement fluid is used to restore electrolyte balance and maintain normal blood volumes
- CVVHDF: a combination of both CVVHD and CVVHF

- Slow continuous UF (SCUF); similar to that of isolated UF but carried out over a longer time period.
- Sustained low-efficiency dialysis (SLED); an extended form of IHD with reduced blood flow and dialysate flow rates, occurring over a 6 to 10 hour timeframe

SLED can achieve similar benefits of CRRT in institutions where CRRT equipment or personnel are unavailable.[25] SLED is often performed overnight, allowing the patient to be available during the day for other treatment modalities and diagnostics.

PD is a nonvascular alternative to provide dialysis in the acute setting. It is often used in low-resource settings or for children. PD is technically much simpler than IHD or CRRT and there is no need for vascular access or anticoagulation. This contributes to a more stable hemodynamic profile. That said, the development of CRRT modalities has resulted in a decline in both the use of and expertise in PD as a treatment of AKI.[26]

A Cochrane Review of 15 randomized controlled trails with a total of 1550 AKI subjects found similar outcomes in subjects treated with CRRT versus IHD in hospital mortality, ICU mortality, length of hospitalization, and kidney recovery.[24] Often, there is a high rate of crossover between modalities and patients are often treated via both CRRT and IDH during the course of their hospitalization. The choice of modality of RRT should be dictated by local expertise and the availability of equipment and personnel.

THE FUTURE OF ACUTE KIDNEY INJURY

All 3 AKI classification systems are based on serum creatinine concentrations, which can be an unreliable surrogate for GFR due to nonkidney factors such as age, gender, race, and body size. In the setting of acute changes in GFR, creatinine is insensitive to small decreases and its increase can lag behind actual kidney function. Cystatin-C is a low molecular weight cysteine proteinase inhibitor synthesized by all nucleated cells, is freely filtered by the glomerulus, nearly completely reabsorbed, and not secreted by the tubules. It performs better than creatinine in the early detection of AKI in various settings, including the emergency department, ICU, and postoperatively.[27–29] Changes in cystatin C early in the course of AKI are also more strongly associated with the eventual need for RRT and with mortality.[30] Adoption of the routine use of cystatin C as a measure of kidney function will likely lead to the earlier diagnosis of AKI and, thus, earlier interventions with the potential to limit the devastating effects of AKI.

SUMMARY

AKI is a condition with a poor short-term prognosis and high rates of mortality. The rates of mortality vary across studies and range anywhere from 40% to 70%. Clear concomitant features that portend a worse outcome include advanced age, the presence of sepsis or respiratory failure, liver failure, or thrombocytopenia. Even when AKI is mild and resolves, there are both negative short-term and long-term impacts. Almost 30% of patients without CKD before their AKI hospitalization will be reclassified as having some degree of CKD or change in their stage of CKD in the subsequent year. These patients are at substantially higher risk of developing subsequent episodes of AKI, which further compounds their morbidity and mortality. Unfortunately, there are currently no pharmacologic agents that have been clinically validated for the treatment of established AKI. There are insufficient data to recommend a particular approach to RRT in the patient with AKI. The major goals in the treatment of AKI are the prompt identification and treatment of the underlying cause along with aggressive hemodynamic support. Despite the advances in medical care and RRT, mortality and morbidity in AKI remain high.

REFERENCES

1. Hoste EA, Schurgers M. Epidemiology of AKI: how big is the problem. Crit Care Med 2008;36:S146–51.
2. Bisen WV, Vanholder R, Lamrire N, et al. RIFLE and beyond. Clin J Am Soc Nephrol 2006;1:1314–9.
3. Mehta RL, Kellum JA, Shah SV. Acute Kidney Injury Network: a report of an initiative to improve outcomes in acute kidney injury. Crit Care 2007;11:R31.
4. Kidney Disease: Improving Global Outcomes (KDIGO) Acute Kidney Injury Work Group. KDIGO clinical practice guideline for acute kidney injury. Kidney Int Suppl 2012;2:1–138.
5. U.S. Renal Data System. USRDS 2014 annual data report: atlas of end-stage renal disease in the United States. Bethesda (MD): National Institutes of Health, National Institute of Diabetes and Digestive and Kidney Diseases; 2014.
6. Wang HE, Muntner P, Chertow GM, et al. Acute kidney injury and mortality in hospitalized patients. Am J Nephrol 2012;35:349–55.
7. PL Detail-Document, the "Triple Whammy". Pharmacist's Letter/Prescriber's Letter 2013.
8. Liano F, Pascual J. Epidemiology of acute renal failure: a prospective, multicenter, community based study. Madrid Acute Renal Failure Study Group. Kidney Int 1996;50:811.
9. Erdburegger U, Okusa MD. Etiology and diagnosis of prerenal disease and acute tubular necrosis in acute kidney injury. UptoDate 2014;7216:26.
10. Linas SL, Whittenburg D, Repine JE. Role of neutrophil derived oxidants and elastase in lipopolysaccharide-mediated injury. Kidney Int 1991;39(4):618.
11. Khan RZ, Badr KF. Endotoxin and renal function: perspectives to the understanding of septic acute renal failure and toxic shock. Nephrol Dial Transplant 1999; 14(4):814.
12. Halbegwachs C. Postobstructive diuresis: pay close attention to urinary retention. Can Fam Physician 2015;61(2):137–42.
13. Lopez-Gomez JM, Rivera F. Renal biopsy findings in ARF in the cohort of patients in the Spanish Registry of Glomerulonephritis. Clin J Am Soc Nephrol 2008;3: 674–81.
14. Matzke G, Aronoff GR, Atkinson AJ, et al. Drug dosing consideration in patients with acute and chronic kidney disease-a clinical update from kidney disease: improving global outcomes (KDIGO). Kidney Int 2011;80(11):1122–37.
15. Shaw AD, Kellum JA. The risk of AKI in patients treated with intravenous solutions containing hydroxyethyl starch. Clin J AM Soc Nephorl 2013;8:497–503.
16. Myburg JA, Finfer S, Bellomo R. Hydroxyethyl starch or saline for fluid resuscitation in intensive care. N Engl J Med 2012;367(20):1901–11.
17. Rivers E, Nguyen B, Havstad S, et al. Early goal-directed therapy in the treatment of severe sepsis and septic shock. N Engl J Med 2001;345(19):1369–77.
18. Prowle JR, Echcverri JE, Ligabo EV, et al. Fluid balance and acute kidney injury. Nat Rev Nephrol 2010;6:107–15.
19. Ahmed W, Memon JI, Rehmain R, et al. Outcome of patients with acute kidney injury in severe sepsis and septic shock with early goal-directed therapy in an intensive care unit. Saudi J Kidney Dis Transpl 2014;25(3):544–51.

20. Bellomo R, Chapman M, Finfer S, et al. Low-dose dopamine in patients with early renal dysfunction: a placebo-controlled randomised trial. Australian and New Zealand Intensive Care Society (ANZICS) clinical trials group. Lancet 2000; 356:2139–43.

21. Russell JA, Walley KR, Singer J, et al. Vasopressin versus norepinephrine infusion in patients with septic shock. N Engl J Med 2008;358:877–84.

22. Bagshaw SM, Delaney A, Haase M, et al. Loop diuretics in the management of acute renal failure: a systematic review and meta-analysis. Crit Care Resusc 2007;9(1):60–8.

23. Sam R. Hemodialysis: diffusion and ultrafiltration. Austin J Nephrol Hypertens 2014;1(2):1010.

24. Rabindranath K, Adans J, Mcleod AU, et al. Intermittent versus continuous renal replacement therapy for acute renal failure in adults. Cochrane Database Syst Rev 2007;(3):CD003773.

25. Daugirdas JT, Blake PG, Ing TS, editors. Handbook of dialysis. 4th edition. Philadelphia: Lippinoctt Williams & Wilkins; 2007.

26. Chionh CY, Soni SS, Finkelstein FO, et al. Use of peritoneal dialysis in acute kidney injury: a systematic review. Clin J Am Nephorl 2013;8:1649–60.

27. Soto K, Coelho S, Rodrigues B, et al. Cystatin C as a marker of acute kidney injury in the emergency department. Clin J Am Soc Nephrol 2010;5(10):1745–54.

28. Nejat M, Pickering JW, Walker RJ, et al. Rapid detection of acute kidney injury by plasma cystatin C in the intensive care unit. Nephrol Dial Transplant 2010;25(10): 3283–9.

29. Zappitelli M, Krawczeski CD, Devarajan P, et al. Early post-operative serum cystatin C predicts severe acute kidney injury following pediatric cardiac surgery. Kidney Int 2011;80(6):655–62.

30. Belcher JM, Sanyal AJ, Garcia-Tsao G, et al. Early trends in cystatin C and outcomes with cirrhosis in acute kidney injury. Int J Nephrol 2014;2014:708585, 8.

ABCs of the Intensive Care Unit

Catherine Clark Wells, DNP, ACNP-BC, CNN-NP, FNKF

KEYWORDS

- Continuous renal replacement therapy (CRRT) • Hemofiltration • Hemodialysis
- Acute kidney injury (AKI)

KEY POINTS

- Acute kidney injury (AKI) is the most common cause for nephrology referrals in the intensive care unit and is often treatable and preventable.
- Treatment of AKI should be individualized for the recovery of kidney function through conservative management of the AKI, prevention of secondary AKI, and either intermittent or continuous renal replacement therapies, as indicated.
- There is no clear evidence to prove superiority of intermittent versus continuous therapies or any specific renal replacement modality.
- All renal replacement therapies should be delivered in accordance with individualized goals of therapy and with utmost safety goals.

INTRODUCTION

Modern nephrology practice merges care across the spectrum of both acute and chronic kidney disease (CKD): inpatient, outpatient, critical care, as well as stable patient management. Whereas, historically, the nephrology team was often viewed as the dialysis management team, nephrology specialists now additionally provide critical care support for prevention and treatment of acute kidney injury (AKI), fluid management expertise via diuresis and ultrafiltration (UF), hemodynamic support, electrolyte and acid-base management, and support for CKD. Dialysis or renal replacement therapy (RRT) is one of many ways the nephrology team can support the intensive care unit (ICU). However, as with most medical therapies, RRT is continuously changing in an effort to improve the quality, safety, and efficacy of patient care.

In the ICU, there are primarily 2 categories of patients with kidney-related issues: (1) patients with AKI and (2) patients with a primary critical illness and a secondary kidney

Disclosures: Sanofi (education support).
Division of Nephrology, University of Mississippi, 2500 North State Street, Jackson, MS 39216, USA
E-mail address: cwells@umc.edu

Physician Assist Clin 1 (2016) 161–174
http://dx.doi.org/10.1016/j.cpha.2015.09.004
2405-7991/16/$ – see front matter Published by Elsevier Inc.

physicianassistant.theclinics.com

comorbidity such as CKD, end-stage renal disease or dialysis patients, kidney transplant, and so forth. Most hospital consults are for AKI.[1] Because AKI is treatable and often preventable, it is commonly the focus of nephrology in the ICU. In fact, this is a growing subspecialty within nephrology with associated research and, recently, the first set of guidelines published.[2] However, evidence on AKI and acute kidney disease (AKD) is still lacking for optimal and complete management.

ACUTE KIDNEY INJURY

There is little evidence guiding a formal definition of AKI. Guidelines recommend diagnosing AKI based on changes in serum creatinine over time ($\geq$0.3 mg/dL within 48 hours or $\geq$1.5 times baseline within the past 7 days) or a persistent decline in urine output (<0.5 mL/kg/h for 6 hours) (**Table 1**).[2] Additionally, current guidelines recommend staging the severity of AKI according to the rise of the serum creatinine over time and/or the decline in urine output over time. There is currently no evidence for use of staging in treatment of AKI but severity of AKI via staging does correlate with outcomes.[2] In addition to staging, providers are encouraged to diligently determine the cause of AKI, thoroughly assess risks and exposures associated with AKI, monitor creatinine and urine output throughout treatment, and assess patients 3 months after AKI for presence of CKD.[2] The Kidney Disease Improving Global Outcomes (KDIGO) guidelines defined the 3-month period of decreased glomerular filtration rate (GFR) after AKI as AKD; these patients should not be misdiagnosed with CKD because the pathophysiology is often different and many patients continue to recover.[2]

Most commonly, AKI is initially caused by prerenal physiologic changes, such as hypovolemia, decreased cardiac output, and severe peripheral vasodilation. If these changes are addressed quickly, AKI is usually easily reversible. However, in many patients, prerenal changes can lead to critical illness. Sepsis is the most common cause of AKI. It is associated first with only prerenal changes (eg, peripheral vasodilation, hypotension) and only intrarenal cellular changes when renal perfusion cannot be restored.[3] If renal perfusion is not promptly restored in any patient with prerenal AKI, cellular damage can result.[4] Intrarenal causes of AKI are conditions that affect the cellular structures within the kidney, most often the tubules, vasculature, and/or interstitial space. Intrarenal AKI is most often characterized as acute tubular necrosis,

Table 1
KDIGO guidelines for diagnosis and staging of acute kidney injury (stage based on creatinine or urine output criteria)

AKI	Creatinine Changes	Urine Output
—	↑ by $\geq$0.3 mg/dL (26.5 μmol/L) within 48 h ↑ by 1.5 times within 7 d	<0.5 mL/kg/h for 6 h —
Stage 1	↑ by 1.5–1.9 times baseline ↑ by $\geq$0.3 mg/dL (26.5 μmol/L)	<0.5 mL/kg/h for 6–12 h —
Stage 2	↑ by 2.0–2.9 times baseline	<0.5 mL/kg/h for $\geq$12 h
Stage 3	↑ by 3.0 times baseline ↑ to 4.0 mg/dl Initiation of RRT ↓ GFR to 35 mL/min1.73 m^2 (if >18 y old)	<0.3 mL/kg/h for $\geq$24 h Anuria for $\geq$12 h — —

Adapted from Palevsky PM, Liu KD, Brophy PD, et al. KDOQI US Commentary on the 2012 KDIGO clinical practice guideline for acute kidney injury. Am J Kidney Dis 2013;61(5):649–72.

which is most often caused by persistent poor perfusion, drugs (eg, nonsteroidal anti-inflammatory drugs, contrast dye, antibiotics), maladaptive immune responses, and vasculitis.[4] Postrenal causes of AKI are much less common and result from complete or partial obstruction of the structures that drain urine away from the kidneys (ureters, bladder, and urethra). This can be caused by overgrowth of internal structures, malignant growths, foreign objects, and so forth.[4]

The medical consequences of AKI are related to the loss of the normal functions of the kidneys. Healthy kidneys should maintain a normal range of balance of electrolytes, balance acid-base, help manage blood pressure (BP) and fluid removal (via renin, angiotensin, aldosterone, and sodium management), contribute to erythropoiesis (via erythropoietin), support vitamin D hydroxylation, support gluconeogenesis, and so forth. During AKI, the damaged portions of the kidney temporarily fail and, at times, require RRT to ensure patient safety and survival. Most often, ICU personnel note imbalance in electrolytes, acidosis, and/or hemodynamic instability in association with AKI. However, patients may also have bleeding disorders, decreased immune response, or neurologic and/or muscular consequences of kidney failure.[4] **Table 2** further defines these complications of AKI.

ACUTE KIDNEY INJURY RISK AND OUTCOMES

According to most recent reports, 1.9% of hospital admissions included the diagnoses of acute renal diseases[5] and incidence has been increasing approximately 11% per year.[3] AKI increases mortality and hospital length of stay. In addition, it leads to complications such as respiratory, hematologic, hepatic, neurologic, and cardiovascular acute organ dysfunctions.[5] AKI is increasingly common in the ICU and patients are 3 times more likely to experience AKI if they require an ICU stay.[3] Up to 30% of ICU patients have AKI versus 11% of total hospitalized patients.[6] The disparity between the ICU and floor is likely to be directly related to patient risk but the cause of the overall rise in AKI cases has not been clearly defined. There are 2 possible reasons: either more circumstances in the ICU are causing AKI or there are now more of the types of ICU patients who experience AKI (ie, sicker patients staying longer in the hospitals).

AKI is an independent predictor of mortality and associated with a higher mortality when patients require ICU care. First-year mortality for AKI has been previously reported as 52.8% to 60.7%, with variation between individual centers providing treatment.[7–13] More recent data in larger populations of AKI patients requiring RRT (n = 1,108,017) reports a general decline from 49.9% in 1996–2000 to 45% in 2006–2010 (adjusted HR 0.83 [95% CI, 0.79–0.87]), and a decline in 1 year mortality from 57.2% in 1996 to 2000, to 52.8% in 2006 to 2010 (adjusted HR 0.84, 95% CI 0.80–0.88).[7]

Mortality is higher for patients with more severe episodes of AKI.[8] However, mortality is not likely directly related to use of RRT.[9] However, RRT and non-RRT AKI patient groups are difficult to compare. Elseviers and colleagues[10] found AKI subjects receiving RRT versus conservative management had higher acuity and associated higher mortality. They also observed large but linear intercenter differences in both patient acuity and mortality between 4 study centers. The Beginning and Ending Supportive Therapy (BEST) investigators also found a higher acuity among AKI patients requiring RRT (n = 1250 per 1584). This RRT group experienced hemodynamic instability, higher central venous pressures, higher potassium values, lower pH, and lower bicarbonate values.[11] Crude RRT mortality was 62.4% versus 37.4% in the non-RRT group (P<.001) but there was no difference in mortality once adjusted (propensity and multivariable) to accommodate patient acuity and conditions.[11] There are many

Table 2
Consequences and complications of acute kidney injury requiring management in the intensive care unit

Complication		Common Timing of Finding	Common Signs	Treatment Options
Electrolyte Changes	Hyperkalemia	AKI or anuria	Arrhythmias	Diuretics
	Hypokalemia	Diuretics AKI recovery or polyuric phase	Hemodynamic changes	Replace
	Hypocalcemia	CRRT		Replace
	Hyponatremia	Hypervolemia or decreased clearance of free water	Tissue (ie, cerebral) edema	Diuresis vs UF with close monitoring
	Hyperphosphatemia	AKI or anuria	Hypocalcemia	Bind or CRRT
	Hypophosphatemia	CRRT	Weakness	Replace
Acid-Base	Acidosis	AKI or anuria AKI recovery or polyuric phase	Decreased cardiac output Vasodilation Low BP Cellular dysfunction	Replace bicarbonate RRT
	Alkalosis	CRRT Diuretics	Respiratory dysfunction	RRT Dosing correction

Inability to Regulate Sodium and Water	AKI or anuria	Organ dysfunction	Diuretics
Volume overload	AKI or anuria	Respiratory dysfunction	UF
Pleural effusion			Site-specific drainage
Dehydration	AKI recovery or polyuric phase	Prerenal AKI	Replace fluid
		Hypoperfusion	
		Hypotension	
		Tachycardia	
Anemia	Severe AKI or CKD	—	Transfuse
			ESA management
Decreased immune response	Severe AKI or CKD	Infection	Prevention strategies
			Treat as needed
Bleeding	Severe AKI or CKD	Bleeding or bruising	Prevention
	Platelet dysfunction		
Decreased muscle mass	Severe AKI or CKD	Low creatinine compared with GFR	Nutrition support
		Malnutrition	
Neurologic	Severe AKI or CKD	Mental status changes	RRT
		Seizures	
Inflammation	Throughout AKI	Organ crosstalk and related dysfunction	Unknown
		Respiratory dysfunction	

Abbreviation: ESA, erythropoietin stimulating agent.
Data from Refs. [2,4,30,42]

reasons for not initiating RRT in patients with AKI. Some AKI patients have adequate urinary output and can be observed closely without RRT. Others avoid RRT because of plans to withdraw care or they are not willing to risk chronic RRT requirements.[11] For AKI patients, RRT is supportive care and the patient and family must agree with the overall plan of care.

The risk for AKI is highest in patients with advanced age, female gender, hypoalbuminuria, dehydration or volume depletion, black race, and previous AKI episode.[4] Comorbidities associated with AKI include CKD, heart disease, liver disease, pulmonary disease, and diabetes mellitus.[9,11–14] Additional risks and correlatives can include nephrotoxic agents, lactate greater than 4 mmol/L, higher blood urea nitrogen to creatinine ratio at initiation of RRT, multiple organ dysfunction, sepsis, and shock, as well as increased ventilator and vasopressor requirements.[4,14] Patients at highest risk of the worse outcomes are those with persistent (vs transient) AKI or worse AKI defined as a higher creatinine at onset of injury.[15] Patients with persistent or worse AKI episodes are also more likely to require chronic dialysis therapy.[15] Among AKI survivors requiring RRT, 25.1% depend on RRT after the AKI episode.[7]

Despite initial improvement, there is a trend toward progressively worsening kidney function during long-term follow-up. Recent studies have revealed that AKI survivors have a better estimated GFR at hospital discharge than at 50 to 60 month follow-up.[16,17] Further research is needed to clearly define this correlation; however, kidney function may decline in some patients in the years following (besides the expected age-related loss of function) AKI. The goal for follow-up is still to maximize kidney recovery and provide long-term follow-up for patients after severe AKI.[2]

To overcome risk and manage this high-mortality AKI, treatment in the ICU is multifaceted. Despite this, Ali and colleagues[8] discovered that a consulting nephrologist only treated 25% of AKI patients.

For nephrology, the goal of treatment is to maintain end-organ perfusion and maximize kidney recovery after AKD while ensuring patient safety (due to failed kidney functions) and supporting general critical care patient management. This includes managing recovery as well as preventing secondary AKI.[2] Use of renal replacement therapies must comply with these principles as well.

TREATMENT OF ACUTE KIDNEY INJURY IN CRITICAL CARE PATIENTS

AKI patients can be treated conservatively or with RRT based on patient condition and comorbidities as well as the capabilities of the hospital system. Conservative management of AKI rarely requires prescribing medication. Management most often centers on removing all sources of harm to the recovering kidneys (eg, pharmaceutical, dietary).[2] When the kidneys fail to provide their usual functions and maintain patient safety (ie, electrolyte and acid-base balance), renal replacement, or support must be considered. Before choosing RRT, choose a goal of therapy for the patient. RRTs are not always interchangeable and it is rare for centers to provide all available choices for RRT.

The RRT delivery system is critical to patient safety and quality.[2] System dynamics can change patient outcomes. During AKI, complications of RRT can vary widely depending on the type of RRT chosen to treat the patient but, generally, the primary complications of RRT are hemodynamic changes; electrolyte imbalances; blood loss due to circuit clotting or heparin anticoagulation; infection; and loss of water-soluble vitamins, and trace elements, as well as, potentially, amino acids or proteins.[2,20–22]

In the ICU, there are options for RRT. RRT can be provided by peritoneal dialysis (PD), hemodialysis (HD), or hemofiltration (HF), and patients can be treated continuously or intermittently. Intermittent can refer to treatments that last any number of hours but most commonly 2 to 4 hours. There are numerous therapies, acronyms, and anacronyms in RRT literature. However, individualized patient plans are created based on patient condition and the risks and benefits of each RRT category.

Peritoneal Dialysis

Acute PD is rare in the ICU but, when chosen, is used for patients with the most severe hemodynamic instability. PD uses active diffusion across the peritoneal membrane (**Fig. 1**) using the peritoneal capillaries and standardized fluid instilled into the peritoneal space via a peritoneal catheter. Blood is directly filtered and does not have to be removed from the capillaries. No anticoagulation is required.

The Achilles heel of acute or ICU use of PD is the catheter. Acutely placed PD catheters tend to leak, especially if large volumes are used for therapy. Currently, there is insufficient evidence either in favor or against PD for AKI.[18] There is disparity among studies reporting both mortality outcomes and adverse events (such as peritonitis); therefore, further research is needed.[18]

Hemotherapies

When PD is not a viable option, RRT is delivered by filtering blood directly on an extracorporeal circuit. Blood is removed from the blood with a pump and filtered through a semipermeable membrane. There are several different commercial machines available to provide these hemotherapies. All machines include a blood pump, fluid pumps, and safety sensors with clamps to prevent air embolus and damage from high pressures on blood cells. There are 3 different hemotherapies, which can also be provided in combination. They are HD, HF, and UF.

HD is the most commonly used RRT. HD uses simple diffusion to remove unwanted waste products and balance electrolytes in the blood. HD filters have a collection of straw-like, semipermeable membranes that are designed to allow removal of small to medium-size molecules.

HF is used less often in the United States; it is currently only available during continuous therapies. HF is based on the concept of convection. Convection is removal of large volumes of plasma water across a similar semipermeable membrane. However, this hemofilter is different. It is designed to allow removal of larger molecules than the filter used for HD. Practically, HF is removal of plasma water (called effluent). Plasma water contains the uremic toxins, electrolytes, and so forth that need to be removed. However, sufficient therapy requires removing 20 to 35 mL/kg of plasma water per hour.[2] It is not safe to remove this much volume from a patient without replacing the volume. Volume is replaced by fluid that resembles ideal plasma water (equivalent amount), called replacement fluid.

Many investigators think that HF or convection removes more harmful middle molecules than HD.[19–21] However, there is no clear evidence for the use of HF versus HD or using hemodiafiltration (HDF) versus simple HF.[21] The molecular clearance of HF has also led some investigators to propose high-volume HF (HVHF) for septic patients with AKI. This requires high volumes of fluid removed or replaced per hour. HVHF is defined as high as 50 to 70 mL/kg/h and intermittent very HVHF as 100 to 120 mL/kg/h.[22] However, after multiple studies, there is no clear evidence that HVHF improves patient outcomes but it does increase the risk for adverse events such as hypophosphatemia, hypokalemia, and drug dosing errors.[23] HVHF is generally not recommended.[2]

UF is removal of plasma water using hydrostatic pressure against the semipermeable membrane. RRT machines can control the volume removed (accuracy depends

PERITONEAL DIALYSIS

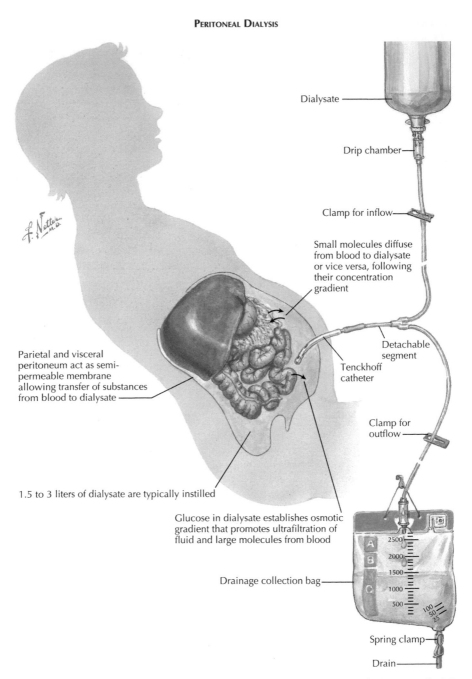

Dialysate

Drip chamber

Clamp for inflow

Small molecules diffuse from blood to dialysate or vice versa, following their concentration gradient

Detachable segment

Parietal and visceral peritoneum act as semi-permeable membrane allowing transfer of substances from blood to dialysate

Tenckhoff catheter

Clamp for outflow

1.5 to 3 liters of dialysate are typically instilled

Glucose in dialysate establishes osmotic gradient that promotes ultrafiltration of fluid and large molecules from blood

Drainage collection bag

2500
2000
1500
1000
500
100
50
25

Spring clamp

Drain

Fig. 1. Peritoneal dialysis. Copyright © 2016. Used with permission of Elsevier. All rights reserved. www.netterimages.com.

Concepts

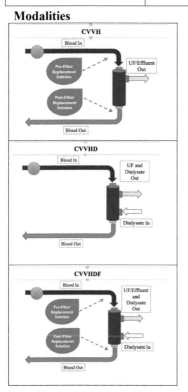

Modalities

Fig. 2. CRRT modalities. CVVH, continuous venovenous hemofiltration; CVVHD, continuous venovenous hemodialysis; CVVHDF, continuous venovenous hemodiafiltration.

on the machine and should be monitored). This is plasma water; therefore, UF does have the same toxins and electrolytes as HF effluent. Therefore, UF and HF are equivalent therapies conceptually but used at remarkably different rates. UF is used for removing volume due to fluid overload and, most often, fluid is removed slowly. **Fig. 2** shows circuit diagrams of different modalities.

Continuous Versus Intermittent

Continuous and intermittent therapies are complementary in the ICU. Both have risks and benefits. Unfortunately, available evidence does not clearly guide the choice between continuous and intermittent therapy.[2,24] There have been multiple studies attempting to clearly define benefits in patient survival with either therapy but, when inclusive AKI populations are studied, there is no clear role for one therapy versus the other. However, comparing these therapies in a clinical trial has had issues and limitations. One struggle of randomized controlled trials is the interplay between subject acuity and provider preference. This either interferes with randomization or produces modality crossover during the trial. A significant number of subjects are often treated with both modalities as a result of crossover. Also, intermittent therapies have more clear guidelines for practice than continuous therapies. This leads to more consistency among subjects treated with intermittent therapies and great variation in the continuous therapies groups.[2] Thus, direct comparisons must be put aside and these therapies individually assessed.

Continuous RRT (CRRT) refers to HD, HF, and the combination of these therapies prescribed with a goal of running 24 hours a day. This requires a large diameter central venous dialysis catheter, not a tunneled dialysis catheter.[2] The most common CRRTs are continuous venovenous HD (CVVHD); continuous venovenous HF (CVVH); and continuous venovenous HDF (CVVHDF), which combines HD and HF. All 3 modalities of CRRT can additionally remove fluid (ultrafiltrate or effluent). There is not sufficient evidence to claim superiority of one versus another CRRT modality.[2] However, use of CRRT as the initial RRT modality has risen from 23.2% to 40% from 1996 to 2010.[7]

Intermittent dialysis (IHD) refers to HD treatments that are typically 2 to 4 hours, most often 3 to 5 days per week in hospitalized patients. Due to the equipment available in the United States, most intermittent dialysis treatments are HD or slow low-efficiency HD, now called prolonged intermittent RRT.

Because continuous therapies are designed for 24 hours of therapy, they run more slowly than intermittent treatments. Solute exchange is slower, as is fluid removal. Therefore, patients often tolerate treatments of CRRT better than IHD.[25] There is no clear evidence of survival benefit with one specific modality or continuous versus intermittent therapies but there is evidence that CRRT is beneficial in a few specific patient populations. Because it is slow and continuous, CRRT avoids the consequences of abrupt solute and osmolyte shifts.[25] Thus, it provides more stable hemodynamics, stable osmolality, and intracranial pressure (ICP) with improved cumulative volume removal. Patients are more hemodynamically stable on CRRT than IHD; systolic and mean BP is far worse during IHD treatments than CRRT.[11,26] Slow, consistent removal of solutes (particularly sodium and larger osmolytes) makes CRRT safer for patients who require a stable ICP. ICP remains stable during CRRT but spikes dangerously high during IHD treatments.[27] Fluid removal also benefits from CRRT. ICU patients are at risk for decompensating during RRT; higher acuity patients generally tolerate CRRT better than IHD.

However, CRRT is not the ideal therapy for all patients. CRRT requires a catheter; existing arteriovenous fistulas (AVFs) and arteriovenous grafts (AVGs) are not safe to use for continuous therapies.[2] AVFs and AVGs require needle cannulation and they can become dislodged easily, causing bleeding and exsanguination. Also, because of slow solute removal, CRRT does not remove electrolytes quickly; therefore, in the event of hyperkalemia or other electrolyte emergency, IHD may be the more appropriate initial therapy.[25,28]

Issues of CRRT versus intermittent dialysis will never resolve with one dialysis therapy standing as best for all patients. These are complementary therapies. The patient condition and the system competency to provide that therapy must be assessed before initiating any treatment.

Complications

Complications and adverse events are often preventable but still require diligent monitoring from a trained nursing staff. The most common adverse events common to CRRT and IHD are hypotension or hemodynamic alterations, arrhythmias, clotting of the extracorporeal circuit, catheter-associated complications (infection or dysfunction), and bleeding (related to heparin anticoagulation).[2,29–31] To prevent adverse events, an educated and experienced staff with opportunities for ongoing competency via simulations is vital.[32,33]

When CRRT is effective, it will deplete both good and bad solutes from a patient's blood. Electrolyte and acid-base abnormalities are common with CRRT, especially depletion of calcium, phosphorous, potassium, and magnesium.[30,31] These electrolytes should be continuously monitored and replaced as indicated. CRRT complications are most commonly related to hypocalcemia followed by hypophosphotemia.[30,31] CRRT will also clear certain drugs very effectively. It is wise to consult with pharmacy daily regarding drug dosing because kidney function is commonly unstable for AKI patients.[30,34] Nutrition should be carefully monitored because both CRRT and IHD will deplete minerals and water-soluble vitamins, and CRRT will also deplete amino acids.[35] CRRT will cause hypothermia as well. Most modern machines have blood warmers available but patient temperature should still be carefully monitored.[30,31]

Fluid Management in Critical Care Patients

Fluid management plans must be individualized, based on comorbidities, and readdressed often because overcorrection can be harmful. Fluid overload greater than 10% at initiation of dialysis is independently associated with a 2-fold increase in mortality.[36] Additionally, fluid volume overload is associated with underestimation of serum creatinine, increased ventilator days, increased ICU days, cardiovascular failure, end-organ failure, poor wound healing, poor tissue perfusion, and infection.[37,38] When possible, fluid is removed via diuresis through the kidneys. However, when this fails, UF can be achieved either through intermittent or continuous dialysis. When diuresis fails, UF is available via intermittent HD or CRRT.

Intermittent dialysis sessions are typically 3 to 4 hours (rarely 2 or 5 hours), every other day. Fluid is removed in short bursts; as much fluid as possible without compromising patient condition. Alternately, fluid removal with CRRT is continuous and slow because the machines are running up to 24 hours a day. CRRT results in larger fluid volume removed due to persistent and sustained fluid removal.[36] One subset of the Program to Improve Care in Acute Renal Disease (PICARD) AKI trial evaluated 396 subjects treated with CRRT versus IHD. CRRT was more likely to reduce the percentage of total fluid volume overload. IHD subjects actually accumulated fluid over time because of postdialysis fluid boluses due to hemodynamic instability. There was a higher mortality associated with fluid overload at dialysis cessation (OR 2.52 95% CI 1.55–4.08).[36] Thus, it is prudent to consider the strategy for removal rather than solely the volume of fluid to be removed with critically ill patients. However, this strategy only works if it is actively removing fluid. If CRRT machines are constantly interrupted for procedures, testing or clotting, volume removal and other CRRT goals will not be met.

Anticoagulation

Extracorporeal circuits and filters function better with anticoagulation that is included in the dialysis prescription. All RRT modalities are equally ineffective if the goals of treatment cannot be met, which can occur if the system clots and the treatment is interrupted or terminated. Thus, pharmaceutical anticoagulants are often used to improve success. Choice of anticoagulation depends on the type of circuit, length of the treatment, and available evidence for safety and efficacy.

The most prevalent choice of anticoagulation for IHD is unfractionated heparin used for almost all patients who do not have a heparin allergy, a history of heparin-induced thrombocytopenia, or other relative contraindications.[39] However, IHD can, at times, be accomplished without anticoagulation.

CRRT is generally more difficult without anticoagulation than IHD. However, there are centers that perform CRRT without anticoagulation as well. Without anticoagulation, the CRRT circuit and filter will need to be exchanged more frequently due to clotting and clogging of the lines and the filter. At times, clotting or clogging occurs so frequently that effective CRRT is not possible without anticoagulation.

There are options for anticoagulation during CRRT but the most commonly used anticoagulation during CRRT is regional citrate. Regional citrate anticoagulation (RCA) is used throughout the world, including the United States. However, it is not approved by the US Food and Drug Administration for use during CRRT. Because of this, RCA is recommended for use by the KDIGO worldwide guidelines for AKI and CRRT but the US KDOQI workgroup could not recommend RCA for use within the United States.[2] Yet there are at least 6 randomized controlled trials showing RCA is effective as a circuit anticoagulant and safer than heparin (decreased risk of bleeding).[4,40,41] There are also multiple published protocols for using RCA during CRRT.

SUMMARY

The nephrology team is now a large part of the critical care environment, primarily caring for patients with AKI. Despite evidence that nephrology is not always consulted, nephrology teams are seeing increasingly greater numbers of AKI patients for conservative management, prevention strategies, and RRT. There remains the need for all available types of RRT in the ICU when used wisely, monitored correctly, and when proper patient follow-up is established. Nevertheless, RRT does have significant adverse events that require a knowledgeable user and ongoing education of the ICU staff.

The nephrologist should be integral to the ICU team. Patients at risk for AKI can often be managed conservatively and disease progression slowed or prevented. RRT, when individualized to the patient's condition and outcome goals, can shorten ICU stays, prevent further kidney damage, and improve outcomes. However, the care and management of the AKI patient is dynamic and continuous education is essential for all staff.

REFERENCES

1. Koyner JL, Cerdá J, Goldstein SL, et al. The daily burden of acute kidney injury: a survey of U.S. nephrologists on World Kidney Day. Am J Kidney Dis 2014;64(3): 394–401.
2. Palevsky PM, Liu KD, Brophy PD, et al. KDOQI US commentary on the 2012 KDIGO clinical practice guideline for acute kidney injury. Am J Kidney Dis 2013;61(5):649–72.
3. Xue JL, Daniels F, Star RA, et al. Incidence and mortality of acute renal failure in Medicare beneficiaries, 1992 to 2001. J Am Soc Nephrol 2006;17(4):1135–42.
4. Freidrich JO, Wald R, Bagshaw, et al. Hemofiltration compared to hemodialysis for acute kidney injury: systematic review and met analysis. Crit Care 2012; 16(4):1–16.
5. Liangos O, Wald R, O'Bell JW, et al. Epidemiology and outcomes of acute renal failure in hospitalized patients: a national survey. Clin J Am Soc Nephrol 2006; 1(1):43–51.
6. Joannidis M, Metnitz PGH. Epidemiology and natural history of acute renal failure in the ICU. Crit Care Clin 2005;21(2):239–49.

7. Wald R, McArthur E, Adhikari NK, et al. Changing incidence and outcomes following dialysis-requiring acute kidney injury among critically ill adults: a population-based cohort study. Am J Kidney Dis 2015;65(6):870–7.
8. Ali T, Khan I, Simpson W, et al. Incidence and outcomes in acute kidney injury: a comprehensive population-based study. J Am Soc Nephrol 2007;18(4): 1292–8.
9. Van Berendoncks AM, Elseviers MM, Lins RL, et al. Outcome of acute kidney injury with different treatment options: long-term follow-up. Clin J Am Soc Nephrol 2010;5(10):1755–62.
10. Elseviers MM, Lins RL, Van der Niepen P, et al. Renal replacement therapy is an independent risk factor for mortality in critically ill patients with acute kidney injury. Crit Care 2010;14(6):R221.
11. Bagshaw SM, Uchino S, Kellum JA, et al. Association between renal replacement therapy in critically ill patients with severe acute kidney injury and mortality. J Crit Care 2013;28(6):1011–8.
12. Ponte B, Felipe C, Muriel A, et al. Long-term functional evolution after an acute kidney injury: a 10-year study. Nephrol Dial Transplant 2008;23(12):3859–66.
13. Allegretti AS, Steele DJ, David-Kasdan JA, et al. Continuous renal replacement therapy outcomes in acute kidney injury and end-stage renal disease: a cohort study. Crit Care 2013;17(3):R109.
14. Perinel SMD, Vincent F, Lautrette A, et al. Transient and persistent acute kidney injury and the risk of hospital mortality in critically ill patients: results of a multi-center cohort study. Crit Care Med 2015;43(8):e269–75.
15. Chawla LS, Amdur RL, Amodeo S, et al. The severity of acute kidney injury predicts progression to chronic kidney disease. Kidney Int 2011;79(12):1361–9.
16. Macedo E, Zanetta DMT, Abdulkader RCRM. Long-term follow-up of patients after acute kidney injury: patterns of renal functional recovery. PLoS One 2012;7(5): e36388.
17. Duran PA, Concepcion LA. Survival after acute kidney injury requiring dialysis: long-term follow up. Hemodial Int 2014;18:S1–6.
18. Chionh CY, Soni SS, Finkelstein FO, et al. Use of peritoneal dialysis in AKI: a systematic review. Clin J Am Soc Nephrol 2013;8(10):1649–60.
19. Morgera S, Slowinski T, Melzer C, et al. Renal replacement therapy with high-cutoff hemofilters: impact of convection and diffusion on cytokine clearances and protein status. Am J Kidney Dis 2004;43(3):444–53.
20. Clark WR, Hamburger RJ, Lysaght MJ. Effect of membrane composition and structure on solute removal and biocompatibility in hemodialysis. Kidney Int 1999;56(6):2005–15.
21. Friedrich JO, Wald R, Bagshaw SM, et al. Hemofiltration compared to hemodialysis for acute kidney injury: systematic review and meta-analysis. Crit Care 2012; 16(4):R146.
22. Honoré PM, Jacobs R, Boer W, et al. New insights regarding rationale, therapeutic target and dose of hemofiltration and hybrid therapies in septic acute kidney injury. Blood Purif 2012;33(1–3):44–51.
23. Clark E, Molnar AO, Joannes-Boyau O, et al. High-volume hemofiltration for septic acute kidney injury: a systematic review and meta-analysis. Crit Care 2014; 18(1):R7.
24. Schefold JC, von Haehling S, Pschowski R, et al. The effect of continuous versus intermittent renal replacement therapy on the outcome of critically ill patients with acute renal failure (CONVINT): a prospective randomized controlled trial. Crit Care 2014;18(1):R11.

25. Liao Z, Zhang W, Hardy PA, et al. Kinetic comparison of different acute dialysis therapies. Artif Organs 2003;27(9):802.
26. Augustine JJ, Sandy D, Seifert TH, et al. A randomized controlled trial comparing intermittent with continuous dialysis in patients with ARF. Am J Kidney Dis 2004; 44(6):1000–7.
27. Davenport A. Continuous renal replacement therapies in patients with acute neurological injury. Semin Dial 2009;22(2):165–8.
28. Agar BU, Culleton BF, Fluck R, et al. Potassium kinetics during hemodialysis. Hemodial Int 2015;19(1):23–32.
29. Shingarev R, Wille K, Tolwani A. Management of complications in renal replacement therapy. Semin Dial 2011;24(2):164–8.
30. Moliner MJ, Honore PM, Sánchez-Izquierdo Riera JA, et al. Handling continuous renal replacement therapy-related adverse effects in intensive care unit patients: the dialytrauma concept. Blood Purif 2012;34(2):177–85.
31. Akhoundi A, Singh B, Vela M, et al. Incidence of adverse events during continuous renal replacement therapy. Blood Purif 2015;39(4):333–9.
32. Graham P, Lischer E. Nursing issues in renal replacement therapy: organization, manpower assessment, competency evaluation and quality improvement processes. Semin Dial 2011;24(2):183–7.
33. Mottes T, Owens T, Niedner M, et al. Improving delivery of continuous renal replacement therapy: impact of a simulation-based educational intervention. Pediatr Crit Care Med 2013;14(8):747–54.
34. Jiang S-P, Xu YY, Ping-Yang, et al. Improving antimicrobial dosing in critically ill patients receiving continuous venovenous hemofiltration and the effect of pharmacist dosing adjustment. Eur J Intern Med 2014;25(10):930–5.
35. Maursetter L, Kight CE, Mennig J, et al. Review of the mechanism and nutrition recommendations for patients undergoing continuous renal replacement therapy. Nutr Clin Pract 2011;26(4):382–90.
36. Bouchard J, Soroko SB, Chertow GM, et al. Fluid accumulation, survival and recovery of kidney function in critically ill patients with acute kidney injury. Kidney Int 2009;76(4):422–7.
37. Cerda J, Sheinfeld G, Ronco C. Fluid overload in critically ill patients with acute kidney injury. Blood Purif 2010;29(4):331–8.
38. Macedo E, Bouchard J, Soroko SH, et al. Fluid accumulation, recognition and staging of acute kidney injury in critically-ill patients. Crit Care 2010;14(3):R82.
39. Foundation NK. KDOQI clinical practice guidelines and clinical practice recommendations for 2006 updates: hemodialysis adequacy, peritoneal dialysis adequacy, and vascular access. Am J Kidney Dis 2006;48(Suppl 1):S1–322.
40. Schilder L, Nurmohamed SA, Bosch FH, et al. Citrate anticoagulation versus systemic heparinisation in continuous venovenous hemofiltration in critically ill patients with acute kidney injury: a multi-center randomized clinical trial. Crit Care 2014;18(4):472.
41. Oudemans-van Straaten HM, Bosman RJ, Koopman M, et al. Citrate anticoagulation for continuous venovenous hemofiltration. Crit Care Med 2009;37(2): 545–52.
42. Hoste E, De Corte W. Clinical consequences of acute kidney injury. Contrib Nephrol 2011;174:56–64.

Pediatrics
The Forgotten Stepchild of Nephrology

Molly E. Band, MHS, PA-C*, Cynthia D'Alessandri-Silva, MD

KEYWORDS

- Pediatrics • Chronic kidney disease
- Congenital anomalies of the kidney and urinary tract (CAKUT) • Growth and nutrition

KEY POINTS

- The causes of chronic kidney disease in the pediatric population vary significantly from that of the adult population.
- In addition to the medical complications of chronic kidney disease in the pediatric population, special attention should be paid to psychosocial and developmental issues that arise.
- The period of transition of a pediatric patient with chronic kidney disease from Pediatric Nephrology to Adult Nephrology is a difficult time for both parents and patients.

INTRODUCTION

Chronic kidney disease (CKD) is a devastating disease that can occur at any age. There are particular challenges that arise in the pediatric population requiring the expertise of a pediatric nephrologist in the management of CKD. Specific complications that are prevalent in children with CKD include impaired growth, psychosocial adjustments of the children and their families, and other issues that are age-specific, including immunizations. There is much more knowledge available regarding the epidemiology of adult-onset CKD versus childhood-onset CKD. More research is required in pediatric CKD because this can aid in the early identification and diagnosis of CKD, aggressive treatment of the complications, as well as identification of (this keeps parallel structure) preventable risk factors in the progression of CKD.[1,2]

DEFINITION

In 2002, the National Kidney Foundation's Kidney Disease Outcomes Quality Initiative (NKF K/DOQI) established guidelines on CKD, divided into 5 categories

Disclosure: The authors have nothing to disclose.
Pediatric Nephrology, Connecticut Children's Medical Center, 282 Washington Street, Hartford, CT 06106, USA
* Corresponding author.
E-mail address: mband@connecticutchildrens.org

2405-7991/16/$ – see front matter © 2016 Elsevier Inc. All rights reserved.

(**Table 1**).[3] This classification system is applicable to children over 2 years of age, because the glomerular filtration rate (GFR) does not reach normal adult values until after 2 years of age. The criteria for CKD include the presence of kidney damage for greater than or equal to 3 months or a GFR of less than 60 mL/min/1.73 m^2 for greater than or equal to 3 months. Kidney damage is defined by structural or functional abnormalities of the kidney, including abnormalities in the composition of the blood or urine, abnormalities seen on radiographic imaging studies, or abnormalities revealed on kidney biopsy testing. This definition is regardless of the pathologic cause of CKD.[1,3]

EPIDEMIOLOGY

Although extensive epidemiologic data are available for the adult population with CKD, little epidemiologic data are available for the pediatric population. This is possibly due in part to the historical absence of a standardized definition of CKD. In addition, estimating GFR becomes challenging in a child, as it varies based on age, gender, and body size.[1,3]

Most epidemiologic data that are available in pediatric patients come from end-stage renal disease (ESRD) registries. In 2008, the prevalence of renal replacement therapy was estimated to be between 18 and 100 per million of children, aged 0 to 19 years.[1] According to the 2014 US Renal Data System, there were 1161 children in 2012 that began ESRD care. The incidence of ESRD in the United States peaked in 2003 and has been slowly decreasing since 2008.[4] There is a reported 10-year survival rate of 80% for adolescent-onset ESRD.[5]

The prevalence of CKD among pediatric patients is not known.[5] There is a reported prevalence of CKD of 1.5 to 3.0 per 1,000,000 among children younger than 16 years of age.[6]

CAUSE

The cause of CKD in children is vastly different than those in adults. Congenital disorders are the primary cause of CKD in children, accounting for nearly half of all causes, including congenital anomalies of the kidney and urinary tract (CAKUT), such as vesicoureteral reflux (VUR), genitourinary tract obstruction, urinary tract infections, and hereditary nephropathies. Another prevalent cause of CKD in children is glomerulonephritis.[1]

The causes of CKD in children vary by age and race.[1,5] CAKUT and hereditary nephropathies are more common in younger children, compared with glomerulonephritis, which is more common in children over the age of 12 years. African Americans and

Table 1		
Definition and classification of chronic kidney disease		
Stage	**GFR (mL/min/1.73 m^2)**	**Definition**
1	≥90	Kidney damage with normal or increased GFR
2	60–89	Mild reduction in GFR
3	30–59	Moderate reduction in GFR
4	15–29	Severe reduction in GFR
5	<15	Kidney failure

Data from Hogg RJ, Furth S, Portman R, et al. National Kidney Foundation's Kidney Disease Outcomes Quality Initiative clinical practice guidelines for chronic kidney disease in children and adolescents: evaluation, classification, and stratification. Pediatrics 2003;111:1416–21.

Latinos have a higher incidence of CKD.[5] Focal segmental glomerulosclerosis is 3 times more common in black patients than in Caucasian patients[1] (**Fig. 1**).

COMPLICATIONS
Hematologic

Anemia is a known complication of CKD and is defined as hemoglobin (Hgb) levels less than 12.1 to 13.5 g/dL for boys and less than 11.4 to 11.5 g/dL for girls, for children ages 1 to 19 years.[5,7] The most common cause of anemia in CKD is erythropoietin deficiency as a result of insufficient production by the diseased kidney, but other causes can include blood loss, iron deficiency, bone marrow suppression, and malnutrition, among others.[5,6] The prevalence of anemia in children with CKD increases with the progression of CKD.[5] The prevalence of anemia in children with stage 1 CKD is 31.2%, compared with 93.3% in stages 4 and 5 CKD.[7]

Anemia in children with CKD is managed with recombinant human erythropoiesis-stimulating agents and iron supplementation. Iron supplementation can be given orally or parenterally. Oral iron therapy is dosed at 2 to 3 mg/kg/d of elemental iron, divided into 2 or 3 doses. Erythropoietin is administered subcutaneously at a dose of 30 to 300 units/kg/wk for an initial dose, and up to 60 to 600 units/kg/wk. The injection is given in 1, 2, or 3 doses per week.[6]

Many of the recommendations regarding erythropoietin use in children are extrapolated from adult data, as pediatric data are limited. There are risks and benefits to normalizing Hgb with recombinant human erythropoiesis-stimulating agents. Reported benefits include improvement in cognitive function and scholastic performance, improvement in growth and nutrition, cardiovascular (CV) benefits, and decreased mortality.[6,7] The risks include hypertension, thrombosis, and atherosclerosis. To minimize the risks of epoetin (Epogen, Procrit), the NKF K/DOQI has suggested target Hgb levels of 11 to 12 g/dL.[7]

Cardiovascular

Cardiovascular disease (CVD) mortality is very low in the general pediatric population.[8] CKD in children, particularly children on dialysis, is a major risk factor for CV-related

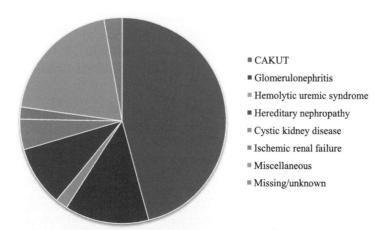

- CAKUT
- Glomerulonephritis
- Hemolytic uremic syndrome
- Hereditary nephropathy
- Cystic kidney disease
- Ischemic renal failure
- Miscellaneous
- Missing/unknown

Fig. 1. Causes of pediatric CKD. (*Data from* Harambat J, van Stralen KJ, Kim JJ, et al. Epidemiology of chronic kidney disease in children. Pediatr Nephrol 2012;27:363–73.)

morbidity and mortality. Studies have shown that CVD begins developing in early stages of CKD and increases promptly after initiation of dialysis. CVD is the most common cause of mortality in children with ESRD, and in adults with childhood onset of CKD.[5,8,9] CV death rates are comparable in children receiving peritoneal dialysis and hemodialysis. In contrast, the risk of CV death is lower in transplant recipients.[8]

The cause of CV-related mortality varies greatly between adults with ESRD compared with children with CKD. Although coronary artery disease and congestive heart failure are the leading causes of CV-related mortality in adults, cardiac arrest is the most common cause of CV death in children with CKD. Additional causes of CV death in children with CKD include arrhythmia, cardiomyopathy, and cerebrovascular disease.[8]

The risk factors for development of CVD in children can be divided into 2 groups, including traditional risk factors and uremia-related risk factors.[8,9] Traditional risk factors include hypertension, dyslipidemia, obesity, and hyperglycemia. Hypertension is the most common traditional risk factor for the development of CVD. Uncontrolled hypertension is more common in children with ESRD compared with earlier stages of CKD.[10] Hypertension in a child is defined by an elevated blood pressure recording on at least 3 separate occasions, at least 1 week apart. Hypertension is determined by the child's age, sex, and height percentiles. Hypertension is graded as prehypertension, stage I hypertension, stage II hypertension, and hypertensive urgency and emergency (**Table 2**).[6] Obesity, dyslipidemia, and abnormal insulin and glucose metabolism increase after kidney transplantation.[10] Although data are scarce, dyslipidemia is a known risk factor for atherosclerotic disease in children with CKD. Saland and colleagues[11] described risk factors for dyslipidemia, which include reduced GFR, nephrotic range proteinuria, older age, and obesity.[11]

Uremia-related risk factors include volume overload, anemia, hyperparathyroidism, abnormalities in calcium-phosphorus metabolism, and hypoalbuminemia.[8,10] These risk factors are more pertinent in patients with advanced CKD on maintenance dialysis, apart from anemia, which can be present in early CKD.[10] Volume overload is commonly related to interdialytic weight gain and inability to achieve dry weight after dialysis.[10] Volume overload is associated with increased rate of hypertension and structural and functional cardiac abnormalities, including left ventricular hypertrophy (LVH).[10] Anemia is prevalent and poorly controlled in pediatric patients with CKD despite the use of erythropoiesis-stimulating agents and iron supplementation.[8,10] Derangements in calcium-phosphorus metabolism, including hyperparathyroidism, are strong risk factors for progression of CVD. Hyperparathyroidism is common in pediatric patients with CKD and can contribute to the progression of LVH.[8]

Table 2 Grades of hypertension	
Grade	**Definition**
Prehypertension	Average systolic or diastolic pressure between the 90th and 95th percentile for age, sex, and height
Stage I hypertension	Average systolic or diastolic pressure greater than or equal to the 95th percentile for age, sex, and height
Stage II hypertension	Average systolic or diastolic pressure more than 5 mm Hg greater than the 95th percentile for age, sex, and height
Hypertensive urgency and emergency	Average systolic or diastolic pressure more than 5 mm Hg greater than the 95th percentile for age, sex, and height AND clinical symptoms of headache, vomiting, seizures, or encephalopathy

Data from Whyte DA, Fine RN. Chronic kidney disease in children. Pediatr Rev 2008;29:335–41.

LVH is the most common cardiac abnormality found in pediatric patients with CKD.[8] LVH can develop in early stages of CKD and becomes more prevalent and severe as kidney function declines.[8,10] Mitsnefes and colleagues[12] revealed that eccentric LVH is the most common geometric pattern among children with CKD, over concentric LVH. Risk factors for progression of LVH include older age, higher baseline intact parathyroid hormone (PTH), and lower Hgb.[12]

The above-mentioned risks for CVD should be managed with prevention strategies and aggressive medical therapy. Management of CV risk in children with CKD includes avoidance of long-term dialysis. Avoidance of dialysis with pre-emptive kidney transplantation has been shown to reduce the risk for CVD in children.[10] Other management techniques include aggressive management of hypertension, including treatment and avoidance of volume overload, treatment of anemia with iron therapy and erythropoiesis stimulating agents, and treatment of hyperparathyroidism.[10,12]

Growth and Nutrition

Reduced dietary intake, malnutrition, and impediment of growth are known complications of CKD in pediatric patients. Nutritional status is of such high importance in children because of the effects it has on growth, sexual and neurocognitive development. There are many differences between the nutritional requirements of children versus adults.[13,14] Factors that affect nutrition in children with CKD include birth weight and gestational age, additional comorbidities, residual kidney function, presence of sodium wasting, acidosis, and anemia, among others.[13] As discussed previously, one of the most common causes of CKD in children is kidney dysplasia associated with congenital abnormalities. With this, there are increased urinary sodium and water losses, which can cause failure to gain weight.[13,15]

Because of the complexities that surround nutritional management and requirements in children, nutritional status should be followed closely by the pediatrician, pediatric nephrologist, and a pediatric renal dietitian.[13–15] There is not a consensus of the appropriate interval of nutritional assessment for children with CKD. The factors that should be taken into account when determining nutritional assessment and follow-up include the child's age, stage of CKD, and presence or absence of growth failure. As part of a child's nutritional assessment, recumbent length for children less than 2 years old, or standing height for children older than 2 years old, and weight should be obtained. These parameters will be used to plot and track along growth charts and can be used to calculate body mass index.[13–15] Head circumference is another growth parameter that is important in children under 3 years of age. Children with CKD have been shown to have poor head growth, which can correlate to brain growth.[14]

Development and progression of oral and gross motor skills occur during the infancy period. However, acute and chronic illnesses can disrupt this normal development. Infants require close monitoring and follow-up because anorexia, vomiting, and altered taste sensation are common during this developmental stage.[13,15] Additional challenges for infants with CKD include decreased appetite, early satiety, and delayed gastric emptying.[15] In addition, growth and developmental deficits during infancy may not fully improve with intervention. Thus, prevention and early intervention are prudent.[14] Such interventions include enteral feeding with a nasogastric tube or gastrostomy tube which can help maintain normal growth in children with CKD and have the potential to allow for catch-up growth.[13]

On the other end of the spectrum, obesity is an emerging problem in children with CKD, particularly after kidney transplantation. Several factors influence this, including treatment with steroids. As the use of steroid-sparing protocols begin to increase, it will be interesting to see if the rates of obesity are affected.[13]

Bone and Mineral Disorders

As CKD progresses, mineral metabolism is significantly affected, termed chronic kidney disease mineral and bone disorder (CKD-MBD). This term encompasses secondary hyperparathyroidism, renal osteodystrophy, disorders of vitamin D metabolism, hyperphosphatemia, and disorders of calcium.[16,17]

CKD poses several risk factors for vitamin deficiency, which include increased urinary losses of vitamin D–binding protein and albumin and decreased intake seen with dietary restrictions.[18] In early stages of CKD, there is a decrease in circulating levels of 1,25-dihydroxycholecalciferol (1,25[OH]$_2$D). In turn, this leads to impaired intestinal absorption of calcium and subsequent hypocalcemia. Hypocalcemia is a powerful stimulant for the release of PTH, causing an increase in serum PTH and secondary hyperparathyroidism. The elevated level of PTH helps to maintain normocalcemia by releasing calcium from bone. With this resorption of bone, there is an increase in the amount of phosphate that needs to be excreted. However, as CKD progresses, there is a decrease in functional nephrons, causing hyperphosphatemia. Hyperphosphatemia is another stimulator for PTH release, causing worsening of secondary hyperparathyroidism.[16,17] The consequences of CKD-MBD include poor growth, bony deformities, and fractures.[16]

Targeted therapy for CKD-MBD includes treatment and prevention of vitamin D deficiency, hypocalcemia, and hyperphosphatemia. Treatment and prevention of vitamin D deficiency become paramount in CKD-MBD. K/DOQI has set guidelines for the repletion of vitamin D in patients with CKD (**Table 3**).[19]

Important notice should also be taken for phosphorus control. Various mechanisms for treatment and prevention of hyperphosphatemia exist and include dietary restrictions and the use of phosphate binders. Patients and parents should receive individualized dietary counseling on phosphorus restrictions. Phosphorus binders work by binding dietary phosphorus in the gastrointestinal tract allowing for elimination via fecal material. There are several formulations of phosphorus binders, including aluminum-containing, magnesium-containing, calcium-based, and non-calcium-based binders. Aluminum-containing phosphorus binders are used sparingly because of the known side effects, including encephalopathy that can be seen with decreased GFR. Magnesium-containing phosphorus binders are used infrequently, because they are not as effective. Calcium-containing phosphorus binders are used commonly and include calcium carbonate and calcium acetate. If hypercalcemia becomes a concern, sevelamer hydrochloride (Renagel) and sevelamer carbonate (Renvela) can be used for phosphorus binding. These agents do not contain calcium, magnesium, or aluminum.[17]

PATHOGENESIS/PROGRESSION

The progression of CKD is influenced by multiple factors, including underlying disease and severity of injury present on presentation, among others.[1,5] Specifically for children

Table 3 Vitamin D repletion	
Serum 25 (OH)D Level (ng/mL)	Vitamin D Dose (IU)
<5	8000 daily for 4 wk, followed by 4000 daily for 8 wk
5–15	4000 daily for 12 wk
16–30	2000 daily for 12 wk

Data from KDOQI Work Group. KDIGO Clinical practice guideline for nutrition in children with CKD: 2008 update. Am J Kidney Dis 2009;53:S1–123.

with CKD, time periods of rapid growth increase the filtration demands of the kidneys. Thus, large increases in body mass during infancy and puberty can result in deterioration of kidney function. In addition to periods of rapid growth, acute kidney injury can also affect the progression of CKD. Injuries include infections or episodes of pyelonephritis, periods of dehydration, and nephrotoxic drugs. Other influences include the duration of disease, initiation of therapy, hypertension, and proteinuria.[5] Data from the North American Pediatric Renal Trials and Collaborative Studies Registry (NAPRTCS) revealed that the rate of progression of CKD to ESRD was inversely proportional to baseline GFR. In addition, NAPRTCS revealed that pediatric patients with CKD stages 2 to 3 progressed to ESRD at a rate of 17% at 1 year, and 39% at 3 years.[2]

Interventions such as the judicious use of an angiotensin-converting enzyme inhibitor for hypertension and proteinuria have been shown to decrease the rate of progression of disease in children, specifically with primary glomerulopathies or renal hypoplasia.[5]

Children with a primary congenital kidney disorder as the cause of their CKD show a slower progression of CKD when compared with children with glomerulonephritis.[1,2] Novak and colleagues[2] studied the rate of progression of kidney disease to ESRD in children with VUR to children with other causes of CKD. Patients were divided into 3 cohorts: those with VUR as a cause of CKD, those with congenital kidney aplasia, hypoplasia, or dysplasia as a cause of CKD, and those with CKD due to all other causes. This retrospective cohort study using data from NAPRTCS revealed that children with VUR as a cause for their CKD had a slower rate of progression to ESRD when compared with patients with renal aplasia and all other causes of CKD. This study also revealed that children with older age, more advanced stages of CKD, and a history of urinary tract infections were at risk for progression of CKD to ESRD.[2]

IMMUNIZATIONS

Immunizations are vital in decreasing the risk of vaccine-preventable diseases in children. Children with CKD on conservative therapy, those requiring dialysis (both hemodialysis and peritoneal dialysis), and those who have received kidney transplantation are at a higher risk for infection compared with healthy children.[20,21] In the aforementioned patient population, infections have significant consequences, including increased morbidity and mortality, increased hospitalization rates, and increased medical, social, and economic costs.[21]

There are several factors that contribute to the greater infection risk in children with CKD. For patients who carry a diagnosis of nephrotic syndrome, urinary losses of complement pathway factors contribute to an increased infection risk. In addition to nephrotic syndrome, other additional kidney diseases are treated with immunosuppressive agents, adding to this risk. Multiple other co-morbidities influence the infection risk profile of patients with CKD such as malnutrition and uremia. Dialysis catheters, both hemodialysis and peritoneal dialysis, are associated with increased risk for bacteremia, exit-site infections, or peritonitis.[21] In addition, children undergoing dialysis require frequent hepatitis B antibody titers, as hepatitis B antibodies are removed with dialysis.[5,6]

When children with CKD are preparing for kidney transplantation, important notice must be taken to the child's immunization status. If possible, immunizations should be completed before kidney transplantation because live vaccines are contraindicated after transplant. Common live vaccinations include LAIV (live, attenuated influenza vaccine), MMR (measles, mumps, rubella) vaccine, and VAR (varicella) vaccine. Children who have not completed their live vaccine schedule before transplantation, they are susceptible to contracting measles, mumps, rubella, and varicella. Some transplant centers will accelerate the immunization schedule before transplantation for optimal protection. Discussion among the primary pediatrician, pediatric nephrologist, and transplant team is crucial.[5,6]

It is important for pediatric primary care providers and subspecialists to be knowledgeable on the guidelines for vaccinating both healthy children and those children with specific medical conditions. The Center for Disease Control and Prevention (CDC) Advisory Committee on Immunization Practices (ACIP) and the Committee on Infectious Diseases of the American Academy of Pediatrics provide the recommended immunization schedule for healthy children, which is updated annually, most recently in 2015. Available at: http://www.cdc.gov/vaccines/schedules/hcp/imz/child-adolescent.html.[20] In addition, the CDC provides vaccination guidelines for patients with CKD and those on dialysis.[21] The most recent recommendations from the CDC ACIP were published in 2012.[22,23]

QUALITY OF LIFE

Caregivers of children with chronic illnesses, including CKD, often have many roles and responsibilities. There are significant burdens, including time, financial, and emotional struggles that families and caregivers experience. Overall, more research is needed to identify caregiver struggles for children with chronic illnesses.

Tong and colleagues[24] performed 20 interviews of caregivers for children with CKD. This group highlighted 4 main themes when interviewing caregivers of children with CKD, including absorbing the clinical environment, medicalizing parenting, disruption of family norms, and coping strategies. Although this study was small, the findings were in line with other reviews. This study revealed that caregivers had difficulty understanding the diagnosis, including the lifelong nature of CKD. Caregivers often had the responsibility of performing medical interventions, such as injections and dialysis. There was often a disruption in normal family dynamics, affecting employment, finances, and social life. There also tended to be tension between spouses revolving around guilt and blame. Some families experienced difficulty giving appropriate attention to siblings of children with CKD. This study also identified that families of children with CKD sought coping through both internal and external avenues.[24]

Gerson and colleagues[25] compared the health-related quality of life (HRQoL) of children with CKD with their healthy cohorts. This study comprised 402 patients, aged 2 to 16, with mild to moderate CKD. This study provided evidence that children with mild to moderate CKD had poorer HRQoL when compared with healthy children, including poorer physical, social, emotional, and school functioning. The authors of this study hypothesized that poorer school function was related to school days missed for medical visits or cognitive functioning, as it relates to worsening kidney function. The results of this study did not reveal an association with the severity of CKD and HRQoL impairment. Surprisingly, patients who have been diagnosed with CKD for a longer period of time were reported via parent feedback to have better physical and emotional functioning, when compared with patients who had CKD for less time. This study also revealed that both youth with mild to moderate CKD and their parents reported that short stature was associated with a negative impact on overall quality of life. Last, this study revealed that advanced maternal education with greater than 16 years of education was associated with higher HRQoL scores, when compared with children whose mother had less than a high school education.[25]

TRANSITION

Transition and transfer of care from pediatric to adult care for patients with CKD and those who have received kidney transplantation pose unique challenges. This time period requires seamless and continuous care with appropriate communication between pediatric and adult teams. This process has recently been examined more closely for several reasons, including the increased rate of young adult patient survival with CKD. Adolescence is an age group that is at risk for noncompliance during the time of transition from pediatric to adult care, for reasons including physical, psychological, and sexual changes during this period.[26] Adolescents can exhibit rebellious behavior and experimentation as they develop more independence. When compared with younger children, adolescents have lower 5-year survival rates of kidney transplants.[27] Another challenge is that the adult nephrologist may be less familiar with the common causes of CKD in pediatric patients, including hereditary conditions and congenital abnormalities.[26]

The International Society of Nephrology and the International Pediatric Nephrology Association have developed a consensus statement outlining recommendations on how providers should help patients achieve transfer of care from pediatrics to adult nephrology.[26] This consensus statement recommends that the transition process be personalized, begin early in adolescence, and happen in a gradual manner. The transition plan should be developmentally and intellectually appropriate for each patient. The timing of transition should be done when the patient is in a stable period without crises, and after completion of school. The consensus statement also recommends that the patient and family be seen together by pediatric and adult teams before completion of transfer of care.[26]

Harden and colleagues[27] developed an integrated transition clinic for young adults with CKD for the many reasons discussed above. In this transition clinic, patients aged 15 to 18 years are seen jointly by both pediatric and adult teams until transfer of care is deemed appropriate as it relates to educational, employment, and social development. The outcomes of this transition clinic showed decreased rate of transplant failure and decreased rate of late acute rejection.[27]

An optimal transition period and transfer of care should provide uninterrupted care and be developmentally appropriate.[28]

SUMMARY

Children with CKD require the expertise of a pediatric nephrology team, including providers, nursing staff, social work, dietitians, and transplant team. It is also important for the pediatric nephrology team to work closely with the child's pediatrician to ensure the needs of the child are met. This multidisciplinary team should work closely together to manage not only the child's CKD but also the comorbidities that accompany CKD. As these children transition into adulthood, it is also important for adult nephrologists to be aware of the various causes of pediatric CKD, including congenital and hereditary disorders.

REFERENCES

1. Harambat J, van Stralen KJ, Kim JJ, et al. Epidemiology of chronic kidney disease in children. Pediatr Nephrol 2012;27:363–73.
2. Novak TE, Mathews R, Martz K, et al. Progression of chronic kidney disease in children with vesicoureteral reflux: the North American Pediatric Renal Trials Collaborative Studies Database. J Urol 2009;182:1678–82.

3. Hogg RJ, Furth S, Portman R, et al. National Kidney Foundation's Kidney Disease Outcomes Quality Initiative clinical practice guidelines for chronic kidney disease in children and adolescents: evaluation, classification, and stratification. Pediatrics 2003;111:1416–21.
4. United States Renal Data System (USRDS). Pediatric ESRD. Chapter 7. 2014.
5. Massengill SF, Ferris M. Chronic kidney disease in children and adolescents. Pediatr Rev 2014;35:16–29.
6. Whyte DA, Fine RN. Chronic kidney disease in children. Pediatr Rev 2008;29: 335–41.
7. Keithi-Reddy SR, Singh AK. Hemoglobin target in chronic kidney disease: a pediatric perspective. Pediatr Nephrol 2009;24:431–4.
8. Mitsnefes MM. Cardiovascular disease in children with chronic kidney disease. J Am Soc Nephrol 2012;23:578–85.
9. Shroff R, Degi A, Kerti A, et al. Cardiovascular risk assessment in children with chronic kidney disease. Pediatr Nephrol 2013;28:875–84.
10. Wilson AC, Mitsnefes MM. Cardiovascular disease in CKD in children: update on risk factors, risk assessment, and management. Am J Kidney Dis 2009;54(2): 345–60.
11. Saland JM, Pierce CB, Mifsnefes MM, et al. Dyslipidemia in children with chronic kidney disease. Kidney Int 2010;78:1154–63.
12. Mitsnefes MM, Kimball TR, Kartal J, et al. Progression of left ventricular hypertrophy in children with early chronic kidney disease: 2-year follow-up study. J Pediatr 2006;149:671–5.
13. Rees L, Jones H. Nutritional management and growth in children with chronic kidney disease. Pediatr Nephrol 2013;28:527–36.
14. Foster BJ, Leonard MB. Measuring nutritional status in children with chronic kidney disease. Am J Clin Nutr 2004;80:801–14.
15. Secker D. Nutrition management of chronic kidney disease in the pediatric patient. In: Byham-Gray L, Stover J, Wisen K, editors. A clinical guide to nutrition care in kidney disease. 2nd edition. 2013. p. 157–88.
16. Wesseling-Perry K. Bone disease in pediatric chronic kidney disease. Pediatr Nephrol 2013;28:569–76.
17. Norwood K. Chronic kidney disease: mineral and bone disorders. In: Byham-Gray L, Stover J, Wisen K, editors. A clinical guide to nutrition care in kidney disease. 2nd edition. Chicago, IL: Academy of Nutrition and Dietetics; 2013. p. 239–61.
18. Kalkwarf HJ, Denburg MR, Strife CF, et al. Vitamin D deficiency is common in children and adolescents with chronic kidney disease. Kidney Int 2012;81:690–7.
19. KDOQI Work Group. KDIGO Clinical practice guideline for nutrition in children with CKD: 2008 update. Am J Kidney Dis 2009;53:S1–123.
20. Center for Disease Control Recommended immunization schedule for persons aged 0-18. Chicago, IL: Academy of Nutrition and Dietetics; 2015.
21. Neu AM. Immunizations in children with chronic kidney disease. Pediatr Nephrol 2012;27:1257–63.
22. Esposito S, Mastrolia MV, Prada E, et al. Vaccine administration in children with chronic kidney disease. Vaccine 2014;13:6601–6.
23. Guidelines for vaccinating kidney dialysis patients and patients with chronic kidney disease. Summarized from Recommendations of the Advisory Committee on Immunization Practices (ACIP). December 2012.
24. Tong A, Lowe A, Sainsbury P, et al. Parental perspectives on caring for a child with chronic kidney disease: an in-depth interview study. Child Care Health Dev 2010;36:549–57.

25. Gerson AC, Wentz A, Abraham AG, et al. Health-related quality of life of children with mild to moderate chronic kidney disease. Pediatrics 2010;125:e349–57.
26. Watson AR, Harden PN, Ferris ME, et al. Transition from pediatric to adult renal services: a consensus statement by the International Society of Nephrology (ISN) and the International Pediatric Nephrology Association (IPNA). Kidney Int 2011;80:704–7.
27. Harden PN, Walsh G, Bandler N, et al. Bridging the gap: an integrated paediatric to adult clinical service for young adults with kidney failure. BMJ 2012;344:1–8.
28. American Academy of Pediatrics, American Academy of Family Practitioners, American College of Physicians-American Society of Internal Medicine. A consensus statement on health care transition for young adults with special health care needs. Pediatrics 2002;110:1304–6.

Health Disparities in Chronic Kidney Disease
The Role of Social Factors

Jenna Norton, MPH

KEYWORDS

- Chronic kidney disease • Health disparities • Social determinants of health
- African Americans • Blacks • Hispanics • Race • Ethnicity

KEY POINTS

- Black and Hispanic Americans bear a disproportionate burden of chronic kidney disease (CKD) and end-stage renal disease in the United States.
- Racial/ethnic differences in the social determinants of health may contribute significantly to CKD disparities.
- Clinicians can counteract CKD disparities by understanding how social determinants of health may affect their patients, promoting integrated collaborative CKD care, and acknowledging and counteracting implicit biases.

INTRODUCTION

Chronic kidney disease (CKD) is progressive, often leading to kidney failure, and is associated with increased hospitalizations, cardiovascular events, and mortality.[1] In the United States, the burden of CKD is born disproportionately by racial/ethnic minority populations, especially black and Hispanic Americans.[2] A complex and interacting set of issues, including genetics and social factors, likely contribute to racial/ethnic disparities in CKD. This article reviews the burden of CKD on black and Hispanic Americans, considers sources of disparity with emphasis on underacknowledged but potentially modifiable social factors, and suggests opportunities for clinicians to counteract CKD disparities.

CHRONIC KIDNEY DISEASE IN BLACK AMERICANS

Black individuals may have lower prevalence of CKD than white individuals based on estimated glomerular filtration rate (eGFR) alone[3]; however, their CKD rates are higher

Disclosures: Ms J. Norton reports no biomedical financial interests or potential conflicts of interest.
Kidney and Urologic Science Translation, National Kidney Disease Education Program, Department of Kidney, Urologic and Hematologic Diseases, National Institute of Diabetes and Digestive and Kidney Diseases, National Institutes of Health, 6707 Democracy Blvd, 6th floor, Bethesda, MD 20817, USA
E-mail address: Jenna.norton@nih.gov

Physician Assist Clin 1 (2016) 187–204
http://dx.doi.org/10.1016/j.cpha.2015.09.009
2405-7991/16/$ – see front matter © 2016 Elsevier Inc. All rights reserved.

physicianassistant.theclinics.com

than in white individuals (**Fig. 1**) when assessing CKD based on both eGFR and albuminuria.[2,4] Additionally, risk for progression to end-stage renal disease (ESRD) appears to differ by race (**Fig. 2**).[5,6] Black individuals are 3.5 times more likely to progress to ESRD than white individuals.[4] Despite making up only 13% of the US population,[7] black individuals account for more than 30% of Americans with ESRD.[2] Further, black individuals start dialysis at younger average ages than white individuals, leading to a greater proportion of life spent on dialysis.[4] Of note, black individuals appear to survive longer on dialysis than white individuals[8]. However, this survival advantage disappears in younger black individuals; higher mortality has been shown in black individuals younger than 30 when adjusting for Hispanic ethnicity[9] and black individuals younger than 50 when accounting for kidney transplantation as a competing risk.[10]

CHRONIC KIDNEY DISEASE IN HISPANIC AMERICANS

Data on early CKD among Hispanic individuals is limited. National Health and Nutrition Examination Survey (NHANES) data suggest nearly 19% of Mexican Americans may have CKD compared with approximately 15% of non-Hispanic white individuals (NHW) (see **Fig. 1**)[4]. However, it is unlikely that CKD rates among Mexican American individuals accurately reflect rates across the heterogeneous Hispanic American population. More robust data on ESRD suggest the prevalence in Hispanic individuals is increasing. Since 2000, the number of Hispanic individuals with ESRD has more than doubled.[2] Additionally, Hispanic individuals are 1.5 times more likely to progress to ESRD than non-Hispanic individuals (**Fig. 3**).[2] However, as with black individuals, Hispanic individuals tend to survive longer on dialysis than their non-Hispanic counterparts.[11]

SOURCES OF DISPARITIES IN CHRONIC KIDNEY DISEASE

Racial/ethnic CKD disparities are likely due to a complex and interacting set of biologic and social issues. Recent studies have considered the role of these factors in black[12–14] and Hispanic individuals.[14–16] In black individuals, controlling for social, lifestyle/behavior, and biologic factors accounted for 44%[13] to 82%[17] of increased risk of kidney function decline, leaving some of the increased risk unexplained.

Genetics

Heritable traits play a role in CKD disparities, especially those seen between black and white individuals. Variants of the apolipoprotein L1 (APOL1) gene common to people of African but not European descent may account for much of the increased risk for nondiabetic CKD in black individuals.[18–20] Estimates suggest APOL1 risk variants

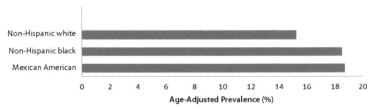

Fig. 1. Age-Adjusted Prevalence of CKD Among US Adults Aged 20 Years and Older by Race Ethnicity, 1999–2010. The prevalence of CKD, based on eGFR and urine albumin, is higher among both Mexican American and non-Hispanic black individuals compared with NHWs. (*From* Centers for Disease Control and Prevention. National chronic kidney disease fact sheet. Atlanta (GA): US Department of Health and Human Services; 2014.)

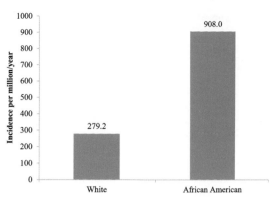

Fig. 2. Adjusted ESRD Incidence per Million/Year by Race in the United States, 2012. The incidence of ESRD is 3.3 times higher in African American than white individuals. (*From* US Renal Data System. USRDS 2014 annual data report. Bethesda (MD): National Institute of Diabetes and Digestive and Kidney Diseases; 2014.)

may account for more than 50% of the increased ESRD risk seen among black individuals compared with white individuals.[21]

Disparities in Chronic Kidney Disease Risk Factors

Prevalence of diabetes and hypertension, the 2 leading ESRD causes in the United States (**Fig. 4**),[2] are disproportionately high among black and Hispanic individuals compared with white individuals. A study by Tarver-Carr and colleagues[13] found the age-adjusted incidence of CKD attributable to diabetes or hypertension was almost 12 times higher in black individuals than in white individuals.

Diabetes
Both black and Hispanic individuals have significantly elevated prevalence of diabetes at 13.2% and 12.8%, respectively, nearly double the rate of 7.6% among NHWs (**Fig. 5**).[22]

Hypertension
Rates of hypertension are higher in black individuals than both NHWs and Hispanic individuals (**Fig. 6**)[23] and black individuals tend to develop hypertension at younger

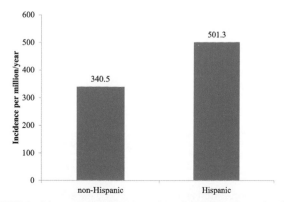

Fig. 3. Adjusted ESRD Incidence per million/year by Ethnicity in the United States, 2012. The incidence of ESRD is 1.5 times higher in Hispanic than non-Hispanic individuals. (*From* US Renal Data System. USRDS 2014 annual data report. Bethesda (MD): National Institute of Diabetes and Digestive and Kidney Diseases; 2014.)

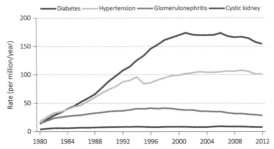

Fig. 4. Trends in Adjusted ESRD Incidence Rate by Primary Cause in the US, 1980–2012. Diabetes remains the primary cause of ESRD, followed by hypertension. (*From* US Renal Data System. USRDS 2014 annual data report. Bethesda (MD): National Institute of Diabetes and Digestive and Kidney Diseases; 2014.)

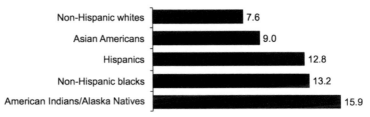

Fig. 5. Age-Adjusted Prevalence of Diagnosed Diabetes Among US Adults Aged 20 Years and Older by Race/Ethnicity, 2010–2012. The prevalence of diabetes is higher among both Hispanic and non-Hispanic black individuals compared with NHWs. (*From* Centers for Disease Control and Prevention. National diabetes statistics report. Atlanta (GA): US Department of Health and Human Services; 2014.)

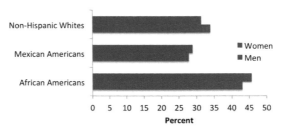

Fig. 6. Prevalence of Hypertension among US Adults by Race/Ethnicity. The prevalence of hypertension is higher among non-Hispanic black individuals compared with NHWs. (*From* Centers for Disease Control and Prevention. High blood pressure facts. Washington, DC: US Department of Health and Human Services; 2015. Available from: http://www.cdc.gov/bloodpressure/facts.htm. Accessed June 30, 2015.)

ages than other populations.[24] Although hypertension is less prevalent in Hispanic individuals, Mexican American individuals may have higher rates of uncontrolled hypertension[25] and incidence of ESRD due to hypertension[26] compared with NHWs.

Social Determinants of Health

Because racial/ethnic groups are constructed to a large degree by belief systems rather than inherent biologic categories, much of the racial/ethnic disparity in CKD (and other conditions) may be due to nonbiologic factors, such as social determinants of health (SDOHs). SDOHs include a variety of social and economic factors that differentially influence health across racial/ethnic groups. SDOHs may affect health outcomes by reducing access to resources (eg, healthy food, quality care, safe places for physical activity), increasing risk of exposure to work-based and neighborhood-based toxins, exacerbating stress and stress-related health outcomes, and creating competing demands that reduce capacity to self-manage health. Additionally, SDOHs are known to influence prenatal development, which is increasingly recognized as important to kidney function later in life; a growing body of evidence links in utero insults, such as maternal diabetes, preeclampsia, and fetal drug exposure, to abnormal nephrogenesis and increased risk for hypertension and CKD.[27]

As noted by Crews and colleagues,[12] the "downstream" SDOHs, including lifestyle and constitutional factors, are most cited as potential sources of CKD disparity, whereas more causal, "upstream" determinants, such as environmental and living conditions, remain understudied. Healthy People 2020 (HP2020)[28] organizes SDOH into 5 key areas (economic stability, education, social and community context, health and health care, and neighborhood and built environment; **Fig. 7**), which provide a helpful framework for reviewing the effect of SDOHs on CKD disparities.

Economic stability

Both black and Hispanic individuals experience disproportionate rates of poverty, unemployment, food insecurity, and housing instability, which are key HP2020 indicators

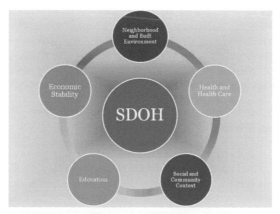

Fig. 7. A Framework of SDOH from Healthy People 2020. HP2020 organizes SDOH into 5 key areas: neighborhood and built environment, health and health care, social and community context, education, and economic stability. These areas provide a helpful framework for considering the role of SDOHs in racial/ethnic CKD disparity. (*From* Healthy People 2020. Social determinants of health. Washington, DC: Department of Health and Human Services; 2015. Available at: http://www.healthypeople.gov/2020/topics-objectives/topic/social-determinants-health. Accessed May 13, 2015.)

of *economic stability*. Each of these indicators is associated with increased incidence or complications of CKD.

Poverty Nearly 26% of black individuals and 23% of Hispanic individuals live below the poverty line in the United States compared with fewer than 12% of white individuals.[29] Poverty associates strongly with CKD,[30] and recent research by Garrity and colleagues[31] suggests poverty among adults initiating dialysis may be increasing over time. Additionally, numerous studies have shown poverty relates more strongly to CKD in black individuals than white individuals,[32,33] suggesting poverty is a driver of CKD disparities.

Unemployment In 2013, 13.1% of black individuals and 9.1% of Hispanic individuals were unemployed compared with 6.5% of white individuals.[34] Among those employed, only 29% of black individuals and 20% of Hispanic individuals worked in the highest paying occupational category compared with 39% of white individuals.[34] Both unemployment[35] and employment in lower paying or working class occupations[36,37] are associated with increased CKD rates. However, this association may be bidirectional, as ESRD has been shown to negatively impact employment.[38] Among those with CKD, unemployment and working class employment are linked to depression[39] and hyperphosphatemia,[40] which may exacerbate disease progression, as well as reduced access to transplantation.[41]

Food insecurity Food insecurity (lack of "access at all times to enough food for an active, healthy life"[42]) is experienced by 24.6% of non-Hispanic black and 23.3% of Hispanic households compared with 11.2% of NHW households.[43] Food insecurity is associated with higher CKD prevalence[44] and conditions that may contribute to CKD, including obesity,[45] cardiovascular disease,[45] hypertension,[46] and diabetes.[45,47]

Housing instability Data on housing instability and homelessness are limited, especially relating to CKD. Available data suggest black individuals are overrepresented among the homeless population.[48] Homelessness is directly associated with CKD-related mortality,[49,50] emergency room use,[50] late nephrology referral,[49] and progression to ESRD.[50,51]

Neighborhood and built environment
Racial/ethnic segregation persists to an alarming degree within the United States and is associated with higher risk of CKD-related conditions, including cardiovascular disease[52,53] and hypertension[54] among black individuals and obesity among black and Hispanic women.[55] Of the HP2020 *neighborhood and built environment* areas, all but crime and violence appear to associate with CKD disparities.

Access to healthy foods Compared with NHW communities, predominantly black communities have fewer healthy food sources (eg, supermarkets)[55] and higher density of fast food restaurants and convenience stores.[56] Although evidence is less robust, food deserts also appear to be more common in Hispanic than non-Hispanic communities.[57,58] As a central strategy for managing blood pressure, diabetes, dyslipidemia, anemia, hypoalbuminemia, hyperkalemia, metabolic acidosis, and bone disease,[59] nutrition, and therefore access to healthy foods, is important for both prevention and management of CKD. Lacking access to healthy foods may be a barrier to nutrition management in CKD. The processed foods available in food deserts are often high in sodium and of low nutritional quality. Additionally, these foods may have high (and undisclosed) amounts of phosphorus,[60] and high serum phosphorus levels are associated with mortality in CKD.[61] Additionally, increased dietary acid load, resulting from diets low in fruits and vegetables and high in meats, may reduce kidney function and is associated with poverty and African American race.[62]

Quality of housing and environmental conditions Extensive environmental justice literature shows racial/ethnic minorities experience unequal exposure to environmental hazards. Predominantly black and Hispanic communities have more toxic waste sites[63] and poorer air quality[64,65] compared with white communities. Additionally, black individuals and Hispanic individuals are more likely than white individuals to live in overcrowded[66] housing. These poor housing and environmental conditions may disproportionately expose racial/ethnic minorities to nephrotoxic agents. For example, low-level lead exposure, which can result from lead-based paint in homes, is more common among black children[67] and is associated with CKD incidence and progression.[68] Further, disparities in built environment, such as neighborhood walkability and safe places for physical activity, exist across race/ethnicity[69,70] and may contribute to CKD risk factors such as diabetes and hypertension.

Health and health care
Racial and ethnic differences in all HP2020 *health and health care* aspects, including access to health care, access to primary care, and health literacy, may have a role in CKD disparities.

Access to health care/primary care Reduced access to health care, including primary care, for Hispanic and black individuals has been demonstrated repeatedly.[71–73] In an Agency for Healthcare Research and Quality study,[73] black and Hispanic individuals fared worse than white individuals on approximately half and two-thirds of access to care measures, respectively. Compared with white individuals, a greater proportion of Hispanic and black individuals lack health insurance, a significant mediator of care access.[72–74] The Affordable Care Act may help equalize access to insurance, and in turn, health care; however, poverty-associated barriers, such as limited transportation options and lack of paid sick leave, may continue to limit the ability of disadvantaged populations to access care.[74] Reduced health care access is associated with ESRD,[75] and lack of insurance correlates with ESRD onset[76] and reduced GFR at dialysis initiation.[77]

Health literacy Limited health literacy affects black and Hispanic individuals more than white individuals; 24% of black individuals and 41% of Hispanic individuals have below basic health literacy compared with 9% of white individuals.[78] Low health literacy is associated with lower CKD knowledge,[79] reduced kidney function,[80,81] and lower kidney transplant rates.[82,83] Additionally, dialysis patients with low health literacy missed more dialysis appointments, had reduced blood pressure control,[84] increased mortality,[85] and poorer self-management[86], and experienced greater kidney-related hospitalization.[87]

Social and community context
Of the 4 aspects (social cohesion, civic participation, perceptions of discrimination, and incarceration) included under the HP2020 *social and community context* area, the following 3 associate with CKD.

Social cohesion There is conflicting literature around levels of social cohesion and social support and how they associate with health outcomes across racial/ethnic groups. Some studies suggest black individuals may have smaller social networks and lower social engagement than white individuals,[88,89] whereas others have found no difference in level of social support.[90] For Hispanic individuals, studies have suggested larger familial but smaller friend-based social support systems compared with non-Hispanic individuals.[16,91] Several studies have suggested that social support may counteract negative health effects of stress,[92,93] which may be particularly relevant to minority groups that experience increased stress related to acculturation[94] and perceived discrimination.[94] In patients with CKD, reduced social support is linked with disease progression in Hispanic individuals[16] and is associated with reduced mental and physical health in black individuals.[95] Further, low levels of social support are associated with increased mortality[96,97] and lower adherence to treatment[98] in ESRD patients.

Perceptions of discrimination Stress-related health issues resulting from perceived discrimination are well documented among both black[99,100] and Hispanic individuals,[100,101] particularly relating to hypertension[102] and diabetes.[103,104] Additionally, medical mistrust is more prevalent among racial/ethnic minorities,[105] and may affect patient decisions about care. For example, mistrust about how donated kidneys are allocated to patients may reduce interest in transplantation among black patients.[106] More research is needed to understand how perceived discrimination and medical mistrust may be associated with CKD.

Incarceration Black and Hispanic individuals account for 13% and 17% of the US population[7] but 38% and 34% of the inmate population, respectively.[107] The effect of incarceration on CKD has not been studied; however, incarceration is associated with weight gain[108] and hypertension,[109,110] which may exacerbate CKD. Additionally, incarceration is associated with increased poverty,[111] which feeds back into numerous SDOH.

Education

Educational attainment is an independent predictor of worse outcomes in CKD.[112] Black and Hispanic individuals fair worse than white individuals across all *education* aspects outlined by HP2020: early childhood education, high school graduation, higher education, and language/literacy.

Early childhood education and development Several studies indicate racial/ethnic disparities exist in early childhood education and development.[113–115] Hispanic children attend preschool at lower rates than white children.[115,116] Whereas black and white children attend preschool at similar rates, black children may receive lower-quality care.[114,116] No studies have assessed the relationship between early childhood education/development and CKD; however, as discussed previously, environmental exposures (eg, lead) disproportionately affect racial/ethnic minority groups, including youth and pregnant women. Exposure to such toxins during fetal development and early childhood negatively affects childhood development.[116] Yet, Shoham and colleagues[37] found no evidence to support a connection between childhood socioeconomic status and CKD later in life. Additional research is needed to understand associations between childhood education/development and CKD.

High school graduation/higher education Freshman graduation rates are 76% among Hispanic individuals and 68% among black individuals compared with 85% among white individuals.[117] Of those who graduate high school, US Census Bureau data suggest a roughly equal number of black and white students, approximately 70%, enroll in college, compared with only 59% of Hispanic students[118]; however, low sample size may bias these data. Individuals who do not graduate high school are more likely to have albuminuria[119] and disability with CKD[120] compared with those who graduate. Additionally, obtaining a college degree is associated with higher kidney function,[121,122] reduced albuminuria,[122] and lower risk of CKD-related conditions (hypertension, diabetes, and cardiovascular disease).[122]

Language and literacy

Language barriers are a particular issue among Hispanic individuals, whereas low literacy affects both black and Hispanic individuals. Among the 12.9% of Americans who spoke Spanish in 2011, nearly half spoke English less than very well.[123] Among Hispanic individuals with diabetes, low English proficiency is associated with suboptimal clinician interactions[124] and reduced glycemic control[125] which may increase CKD risk. Compared with 12% of the general population, 39% of Hispanic and 20% of black adults read at below basic levels.[126] There is little or no research on associations between overall literacy and CKD, but associations between health literacy and CKD were discussed previously.

Implicit Bias Among Clinicians

CKD care delivery varies by race/ethnicity. For example, black and Hispanic patients with CKD may be more likely than white patients to have delayed[127] or no[128] referral to nephrology. Additionally, referral to and use of kidney transplantation, generally considered a superior treatment, is lower for black than white patients.[129–131] However, disparity in care delivery does not exist in all settings. Consistency in CKD care across race seen within the Department of Defense[132] suggests universal access to care may mitigate disparity in care delivery.

Although differences in access to care, patient preference, and health status may contribute to differences in care, explicit or implicit biases within the health care system also may play a role. Some physicians[133] and nurses[134] have implicit biases in favor of white patients compared with other groups, with mixed effect on treatment decisions.[134,135] van Ryn and Fu[136] describe several pathways (eg, influencing patient self-perceptions, differences in content or manner of communication, providing variable access to treatments) by which clinician attitudes may influence patient outcomes. Specific to CKD, nephrologists who believed that patient-physician communication and trust were not reasons for racial disparities in health-care were also less to give their black patients information about kidney transplant.[137]

Interaction of Social and Biologic Factors

Social and genetic factors may interact in complex ways to drive racial/ethnic disparities in CKD. For example, as previously discussed, carrying 2 APOL1 risk variants dramatically increases CKD risk. Yet, not all individuals with 2 APOL1 risk variants develop CKD, which may suggest gene-environment interactions.[138] As suggested by Crews and colleagues,[12] SDOHs may provide the "second hit" that causes some but not all individuals with 2 APOL1 risk variants to develop ESRD. Additionally, SDOHs may account for some of the increased rates of diabetes and hypertension among racial/ethnic minorities, which in turn increases risk for CKD.

ADDRESSING DISPARITIES IN THE CLINICAL SETTING

With the contribution of complex social and institutional issues to CKD disparities, addressing these disparities may seem beyond the scope of the individual clinician. Although eradicating these disparities will likely require concerted effort from a variety of stakeholders, practicing clinicians may be able to help reduce CKD disparities by the following.

Understanding That Social Determinants of Health May Affect Individual Patient Ability to Self-Manage

It is important to understand how social issues affect patients and their ability to manage CKD and related conditions. For example, Gutierrez[139] contends that nutrition management efforts in CKD must consider individual patient access to healthy foods. As part of self-management support, ask whether your patient has access to safe places for physical activity, transportation to various health care settings, and paid sick time to attend health appointments. For patients who need additional support, engage social workers, who are trained to help individuals facing social barriers to health. Provide patients with culturally appropriate, low health literacy materials, such as those available from the National Kidney Disease Education Program (http://nkdep.nih.gov).

Promoting an Integrated, Collaborative Approach to Chronic Kidney Disease Care

A review of disparities in CKD suggests integrated, collaborative approaches to CKD care may reduce disparities.[30] For example, application of the Chronic Care Model, a framework for improving chronic disease care that integrates the patient, community, organization, practice, and health system, to diabetes and CKD care within the Indian Health Service is associated with significantly reduced ESRD rates among Native Americans and may provide a model for reducing disparities in other communities.[140]

Being Aware of and Countering Implicit Biases

Even those who consciously eschew racism may be susceptible to implicit biases that they do not consciously recognize. Harvard University's Project Implicit (https://implicit.harvard.edu/implicit/research/) allows individuals to test their own implicit biases. Simply being aware of implicit biases may reduce differences in care delivery.[141] Additionally, several studies suggest providers may be able to reduce biases by being trained on communicating about race,[142] consciously focusing on individual patient aspects and perspectives,[134] and participating in targeted experiences with minorities.[143]

SUMMARY

CKD imposes a greater burden on racial/ethnic minority groups in the United States. At least in African American individuals, a significant portion of this disparity likely results from genetic factors; however, the effects of social factors on CKD outcomes are often underappreciated and may be more amenable to intervention. Despite the complex nature of these disparities, clinicians may be able to counteract disparities by understanding how SDOHs may affect their patients, promoting integrated collaborative CKD care, and acknowledging and countering implicit biases.

ACKNOWLEDGMENTS

Thanks to Andrew S. Narva, MD, FACP, FASN; Kevin Abbott, MD, MPH; and Nilka Ríos Burrows, MPH, for review and guidance on the development of this article.

REFERENCES

1. Go AS, Chertow GM, Fan D, et al. Chronic kidney disease and the risks of death, cardiovascular events, and hospitalization. N Engl J Med 2004;351(13):1296–305.
2. US Renal Data System. USRDS 2014 annual data report. Bethesda (MD): National Institute of Diabetes and Digestive and Kidney Diseases; 2014.

3. Grams ME, Chow EK, Segev DL, et al. Lifetime incidence of CKD stages 3-5 in the United States. Am J Kidney Dis 2013;62(2):245–52.
4. Centers for Disease Control and Prevention. National chronic kidney disease fact sheet. Atlanta (GA): US Department of Health and Human Services; 2014.
5. Hsu CY, Lin F, Vittinghoff E, et al. Racial differences in the progression from chronic renal insufficiency to end-stage renal disease in the United States. J Am Soc Nephrol 2003;14(11):2902–7.
6. McClellan W, Warnock DG, McClure L, et al. Racial differences in the prevalence of chronic kidney disease among participants in the Reasons for Geographic and Racial Differences in Stroke Cohort Study. J Am Soc Nephrol 2006;17(6):1710–5.
7. US Census Bureau. State and county quickfacts. Washington, DC: US Department of Commerce; 2015. Available at: http://quickfacts.census.gov/qfd/states/00000.html. Accessed June 30, 2015.
8. Kovesdy CP, Anderson JE, Derose SF, et al. Outcomes associated with race in males with nondialysis-dependent chronic kidney disease. Clin J Am Soc Nephrol 2009;4(5):973–8.
9. Yan G, Norris KC, Yu AJ, et al. The relationship of age, race, and ethnicity with survival in dialysis patients. Clin J Am Soc Nephrol 2013;8(6):953–61.
10. Kucirka LM, Grams ME, Lessler J, et al. Age and racial disparities in dialysis survival. JAMA 2011;306(6):620–6.
11. Jolly SE, Burrows NR, Chen SC, et al. Racial and ethnic differences in mortality among individuals with chronic kidney disease: results from the Kidney Early Evaluation Program (KEEP). Clin J Am Soc Nephrol 2011;6(8):1858–65.
12. Crews DC, Pfaff T, Powe NR. Socioeconomic factors and racial disparities in kidney disease outcomes. Semin Nephrol 2013;33(5):468–75.
13. Tarver-Carr ME, Powe NR, Eberhardt MS, et al. Excess risk of chronic kidney disease among African-American versus white subjects in the United States: a population-based study of potential explanatory factors. J Am Soc Nephrol 2002;13(9):2363–70.
14. Nicholas SB, Kalantar-Zadeh K, Norris KC. Racial disparities in kidney disease outcomes. Semin Nephrol 2013;33(5):409–15.
15. Lora CM, Daviglus ML, Kusek JW, et al. Chronic kidney disease in United States Hispanics: a growing public health problem. Ethn Dis 2009;19(4):466–72.
16. Lora CM, Gordon EJ, Sharp LK, et al. Progression of CKD in Hispanics: potential roles of health literacy, acculturation, and social support. Am J Kidney Dis 2011; 58(2):282–90.
17. Krop JS, Coresh J, Chambless LE, et al. A community-based study of explanatory factors for the excess risk for early renal function decline in blacks vs whites with diabetes: the Atherosclerosis Risk in Communities study. Arch Intern Med 1999;159(15):1777–83.
18. Genovese G, Friedman DJ, Ross MD, et al. Association of trypanolytic ApoL1 variants with kidney disease in African Americans. Science 2010;329(5993): 841–5.
19. Freedman BI, Kopp JB, Langefeld CD, et al. The apolipoprotein L1 (APOL1) gene and nondiabetic nephropathy in African Americans. J Am Soc Nephrol 2010;21(9):1422–6.
20. Kopp JB, Nelson GW, Sampath K, et al. APOL1 genetic variants in focal segmental glomerulosclerosis and HIV-associated nephropathy. J Am Soc Nephrol 2011;22(11):2129–37.
21. Williams SF, Nicholas SB, Vaziri ND, et al. African Americans, hypertension and the renin angiotensin system. World J Cardiol 2014;6(9):878–89.

22. Centers for Disease Control and Prevention. National diabetes statistics report. Atlanta (GA): US Department of Health and Human Services; 2014.
23. Centers for Disease Control and Prevention. High blood pressure facts. Atlanta, GA: US Department of Health and Human Services; 2015. Available at: http://www.cdc.gov/bloodpressure/facts.htm. Accessed June 30, 2015.
24. Mozzafarian D, Benjamin EJ, Go AS, et al. Heart Disease and Stroke Statistics-2015 Update: a report from the American Heart Association. Circulation 2015;e29–322.
25. Hajjar I, Kotchen JM, Kotchen TA. Hypertension: trends in prevalence, incidence, and control. Annu Rev Public Health 2006;27:465–90.
26. Pugh JA, Stern MP, Haffner SM, et al. Excess incidence of treatment of end-stage renal disease in Mexican Americans. Am J Epidemiol 1988;127(1):135–44.
27. Luyckx VA, Brenner BM. Birth weight, malnutrition and kidney-associated outcomes–a global concern. Nat Rev Nephrol 2015;11(3):135–49.
28. Healthy People 2020. Social determinants of health. Washington, DC: Department of Health and Human Services; 2015. Available at: http://www.healthypeople.gov/2020/topics-objectives/topic/social-determinants-health. Accessed May 13, 2015.
29. US Census Bureau. Poverty rates for selected detailed race and Hispanic Groups by state and place: 2007–2011. Washington, DC: US Department of Commerce; 2013. Available from: https://www.census.gov/prod/2013pubs/acsbr11-17.pdf. Accessed June 30, 2015.
30. Nicholas SB, Kalantar-Zadeh K, Norris KC. Socioeconomic disparities in chronic kidney disease. Adv Chronic Kidney Dis 2015;22(1):6–15.
31. Garrity BH, Kramer H, Vellanki K, et al. Time trends in the association of ESRD incidence with area-level poverty in the US population. Hemodial Int 2015. [Epub ahead of print].
32. Crews DC, McClellan WM, Shoham DA, et al. Low income and albuminuria among REGARDS (Reasons for Geographic and Racial Differences in Stroke) study participants. Am J Kidney Dis 2012;60(5):779–86.
33. Crews DC, Charles RF, Evans MK, et al. Poverty, race, and CKD in a racially and socioeconomically diverse urban population. Am J Kidney Dis 2010;55(6):992–1000.
34. US Bureau of Labor Statistics. Labor force characteristics by race and ethnicity, 2013. Washington, DC: US Department of Labor; 2014. Available at: http://www.bls.gov/cps/cpsrace2013.pdf. Accessed June 30, 2015.
35. White SL, McGeechan K, Jones M, et al. Socioeconomic disadvantage and kidney disease in the United States, Australia, and Thailand. Am J Public Health 2008;98(7):1306–13.
36. Shoham DA, Vupputuri S, Diez Roux AV, et al. Kidney disease in life-course socioeconomic context: the Atherosclerosis Risk in Communities (ARIC) Study. Am J Kidney Dis 2007;49(2):217–26.
37. Shoham DA, Vupputuri S, Kaufman JS, et al. Kidney disease and the cumulative burden of life course socioeconomic conditions: the Atherosclerosis Risk in Communities (ARIC) study. Soc Sci Med 2008;67(8):1311–20.
38. Murray PD, Dobbels F, Lonsdale DC, et al. Impact of end-stage kidney disease on academic achievement and employment in young adults: a mixed methods study. J Adolesc Health 2014;55(4):505–12.
39. Fischer MJ, Kimmel PL, Greene T, et al. Sociodemographic factors contribute to the depressive affect among African Americans with chronic kidney disease. Kidney Int 2010;77(11):1010–9.

40. Gutiérrez OM, Anderson C, Isakova T, et al. Low socioeconomic status associates with higher serum phosphate irrespective of race. J Am Soc Nephrol 2010; 21(11):1953–60.
41. Sandhu GS, Khattak M, Pavlakis M, et al. Recipient's unemployment restricts access to renal transplantation. Clin Transplant 2013;27(4):598–606.
42. Economic Research Service. Food security in the U.S. Washington, DC: U. S. Department of Agriculture; 2015. Available at: http://www.ers.usda.gov/topics/food-nutrition-assistance/food-security-in-the-us/key-statistics-graphics.aspx. Accessed June 30, 2015.
43. Coleman-Jensen A, Nord M, Singh A. Household food security in the United States in 2012. Washington, DC: US Department of Agriculture; 2013.
44. Crews DC, Kuczmarski MF, Grubbs V, et al. Effect of food insecurity on chronic kidney disease in lower-income Americans. Am J Nephrol 2014;39(1):27–35.
45. Castillo DC, Ramsey NL, Yu SS, et al. Inconsistent access to food and cardiometabolic disease: the effect of food insecurity. Curr Cardiovasc Risk Rep 2012;6(3):245–50.
46. Seligman HK, Laraia BA, Kushel MB. Food insecurity is associated with chronic disease among low-income NHANES participants. J Nutr 2010; 140(2):304–10.
47. Seligman HK, Jacobs EA, López A, et al. Food insecurity and glycemic control among low-income patients with type 2 diabetes. Diabetes Care 2012;35(2): 233–8.
48. Substance Abuse and Mental Health Services Administration. Current statistics on the prevalence and characteristics of people experiencing homelessness in the United States. Rockville (MD): SAMHSA; 2011.
49. Obialo CI, Ofili EO, Quarshie A, et al. Ultralate referral and presentation for renal replacement therapy: socioeconomic implications. Am J Kidney Dis 2005;46(5): 881–6.
50. Hall YN, Choi AI, Himmelfarb J, et al. Homelessness and CKD: a cohort study. Clin J Am Soc Nephrol 2012;7(7):1094–102.
51. Maziarz M, Chertow GM, Himmelfarb J, et al. Homelessness and risk of end-stage renal disease. J Health Care Poor Underserved 2014;25(3):1231–44.
52. Kershaw KN, Osypuk TL, Do DP, et al. Neighborhood-level racial/ethnic residential segregation and incident cardiovascular disease: the multi-ethnic study of atherosclerosis. Circulation 2015;131(2):141–8.
53. Kershaw KN, Albrecht SS. Racial/ethnic residential segregation and cardiovascular disease risk. Curr Cardiovasc Risk Rep 2015;9(3):10.
54. Kershaw KN, Diez Roux AV, Burgard SA, et al. Metropolitan-level racial residential segregation and black-white disparities in hypertension. Am J Epidemiol 2011;174(5):537–45.
55. Walker RE, Keane CR, Burke JG. Disparities and access to healthy food in the United States: a review of food deserts literature. Health Place 2010;16(5): 876–84.
56. Hilmers A, Hilmers DC, Dave J. Neighborhood disparities in access to healthy foods and their effects on environmental justice. Am J Public Health 2012; 102(9):1644–54.
57. Bower KM, Thorpe RJ Jr, Rohde C, et al. The intersection of neighborhood racial segregation, poverty, and urbanicity and its impact on food store availability in the United States. Prev Med 2014;58:33–9.
58. Powell LM, Slater S, Mirtcheva D, et al. Food store availability and neighborhood characteristics in the United States. Prev Med 2007;44(3):189–95.

59. National Kidney Diseased Education Program. Chronic kidney disease (CKD) and diet: assessment, management, and treatment. Bethesda (MD): National Institutes of Health; 2015.

60. Moser M, White K, Henry B, et al. Phosphorus content of popular beverages. Am J Kidney Dis 2015;65(6):969–71.

61. Palmer SC, Hayen A, Macaskill P, et al. Serum levels of phosphorus, parathyroid hormone, and calcium and risks of death and cardiovascular disease in individuals with chronic kidney disease: a systematic review and meta-analysis. JAMA 2011;305(11):1119–27.

62. Banerjee T, Crews DC, Wesson DE, et al. Dietary acid load and chronic kidney disease among adults in the United States. BMC Nephrol 2014;15:137.

63. General Accounting Office. Siting of hazardous waste landfills and their correlation with racial and economic status of surrounding communities. Washington, DC: GAO; 1983.

64. Bell ML, Ebisu K. Environmental inequality in exposures to airborne particulate matter components in the United States. Environ Health Perspect 2012;120(12): 1699–704.

65. Clark LP, Millet DB, Marshall JD. National patterns in environmental injustice and inequality: outdoor NO2 air pollution in the United States. PLoS One 2014;9(4): e94431.

66. Blake KS, Kellerson RL, Simic A. Measuring overcrowding in housing. Bethesda, MD: US Department of Housing and Urban Development; 2007.

67. Agency for Toxic Substances & Diseases Registry. Lead toxicity: who is at risk of lead exposure? Atlanta, GA: Center for Disease Control and Prevention; 2007. Available at: http://www.atsdr.cdc.gov/csem/csem.asp?csem=7&po=7. Accessed June 30, 2015.

68. Ekong EB, Jaar BG, Weaver VM. Lead-related nephrotoxicity: a review of the epidemiologic evidence. Kidney Int 2006;70(12):2074–84.

69. Powell LM, Slater S, Chaloupka FJ, et al. Availability of physical activity-related facilities and neighborhood demographic and socioeconomic characteristics: a national study. Am J Public Health 2006;96(9):1676–80.

70. Moore LV, Diez Roux AV, Evenson KR, et al. Availability of recreational resources in minority and low socioeconomic status areas. Am J Prev Med 2008;34(1): 16–22.

71. Escarce JJ. Racial and ethnic disparities in access to and quality of health care. Princeton (NJ): Robert Wood Johnson Foundation; 2007.

72. Agency for Healthcare Research and Quality. 2014 national healthcare quality and disparities report. Rockville (MD): US Department of Health and Human Services; 2015.

73. Richardson LD, Norris M. Access to health and health care: how race and ethnicity matter. Mt Sinai J Med 2010;77(2):166–77.

74. Call KT, McAlpine DD, Garcia CM, et al. Barriers to care in an ethnically diverse publicly insured population: is health care reform enough? Med Care 2014; 52(8):720–7.

75. Perneger TV, Whelton PK, Klag MJ. Race and end-stage renal disease. Socioeconomic status and access to health care as mediating factors. Arch Intern Med 1995;155(11):1201–8.

76. Jurkovitz CT, Li S, Norris KC, et al. Association between lack of health insurance and risk of death and ESRD: results from the Kidney Early Evaluation Program (KEEP). Am J Kidney Dis 2013;61(4 Suppl 2):S24–32.

77. Obrador GT, Arora P, Kausz AT, et al. Level of renal function at the initiation of dialysis in the US end-stage renal disease population. Kidney Int 1999;56(6): 2227–35.
78. Office of Disease Prevention and Health Promotion. America's health literacy: why we need accessible health information. Washington, DC: US Department of Health and Human Services; 2008.
79. Wright JA, Wallston KA, Elasy TA, et al. Development and results of a kidney disease knowledge survey given to patients with CKD. Am J Kidney Dis 2011; 57(3):387–95.
80. Devraj R, Borrego M, Vilay AM, et al. Relationship between health literacy and kidney function. Nephrology (Carlton) 2015;20(5):360–7.
81. Ricardo AC, Yang W, Lora CM, et al. Limited health literacy is associated with low glomerular filtration in the Chronic Renal Insufficiency Cohort (CRIC) study. Clin Nephrol 2014;81(1):30–7.
82. Kazley AS, Hund JJ, Simpson KN, et al. Health literacy and kidney transplant outcomes. Prog Transplant 2015;25(1):85–90.
83. Abdel-Kader K, Dew MA, Bhatnagar M, et al. Numeracy skills in CKD: correlates and outcomes. Clin J Am Soc Nephrol 2010;5(9):1566–73.
84. Adeseun GA, Bonney CC, Rosas SE. Health literacy associated with blood pressure but not other cardiovascular disease risk factors among dialysis patients. Am J Hypertens 2012;25(3):348–53.
85. Cavanaugh KL, Wingard RL, Hakim RM, et al. Low health literacy associates with increased mortality in ESRD. J Am Soc Nephrol 2010;21(11):1979–85.
86. Lai AY, Ishikawa H, Kiuchi T, et al. Communicative and critical health literacy, and self-management behaviors in end-stage renal disease patients with diabetes on hemodialysis. Patient Educ Couns 2013;91(2):221–7.
87. Green JA, Mor MK, Shields AM, et al. Associations of health literacy with dialysis adherence and health resource utilization in patients receiving maintenance hemodialysis. Am J Kidney Dis 2013;62(1):73–80.
88. Barnes LL, Mendes de Leon CF, Bienias JL, et al. A longitudinal study of black-white differences in social resources. J Gerontol B Psychol Sci Soc Sci 2004; 59(3):S146–53.
89. Sloan MM, Newhouse RJE, Thompson AB. Counting on coworkers race, social support, and emotional experiences on the job. Soc Psychol Q 2013;76(4): 343–72.
90. Rees CA, Karter AJ, Young BA. Race/ethnicity, social support, and associations with diabetes self-care and clinical outcomes in NHANES. Diabetes Educ 2010; 36(3):435–45.
91. Almeida J, Molnar BE, Kawachi I, et al. Ethnicity and nativity status as determinants of perceived social support: testing the concept of familism. Soc Sci Med 2009;68(10):1852–8.
92. Uchino BN. Social support and health: a review of physiological processes potentially underlying links to disease outcomes. J Behav Med 2006;29(4):377–87.
93. Finch BK, Vega WA. Acculturation stress, social support, and self-rated health among Latinos in California. J Immigr Health 2003;5(3):109–17.
94. Pascoe EA, Smart Richman L. Perceived discrimination and health: a meta-analytic review. Psychol Bull 2009;135(4):531–54.
95. Porter A, Fischer MJ, Brooks D, et al. Quality of life and psychosocial factors in African Americans with hypertensive chronic kidney disease. Transl Res 2012; 159(1):4–11.

96. Kimmel PL, Peterson RA, Weihs KL, et al. Psychosocial factors, behavioral compliance and survival in urban hemodialysis patients. Kidney Int 1998; 54(1):245–54.
97. Thong MS, Kaptein AA, Krediet RT, et al. Social support predicts survival in dialysis patients. Nephrol Dial Transplant 2007;22(3):845–50.
98. Clark S, Farrington K, Chilcot J. Nonadherence in dialysis patients: prevalence, measurement, outcome, and psychological determinants. Semin Dial 2014; 27(1):42–9.
99. Greene ML, Way N, Pahl K. Trajectories of perceived adult and peer discrimination among Black, Latino, and Asian American adolescents: patterns and psychological correlates. Dev Psychol 2006;42(2):218–36.
100. Barnes LL, Mendes De Leon CF, Wilson RS, et al. Racial differences in perceived discrimination in a community population of older blacks and whites. J Aging Health 2004;16(3):315–37.
101. Lopez MH, Morin R, Taylor P. Illegal immigration backlash worries, divides Latinos. Washington, DC: Pew Hispanic Center; 2010.
102. Dolezsar CM, McGrath JJ, Herzig AJ, et al. Perceived racial discrimination and hypertension: a comprehensive systematic review. Health Psychol 2014;33(1): 20–34.
103. Ryan AM, Gee GC, Griffith D. The effects of perceived discrimination on diabetes management. J Health Care Poor Underserved 2008;19(1):149–63.
104. Wagner J, Abbott G. Depression and depression care in diabetes: relationship to perceived discrimination in African Americans. Diabetes Care 2007;30(2): 364–6.
105. Lillie-Blanton M, Brodie M, Rowland D, et al. Race, ethnicity, and the health care system: public perceptions and experiences. Med Care Res Rev 2000;57(Suppl 1):218–35.
106. Wachterman MW, McCarthy EP, Marcantonio ER, et al. Mistrust, misperceptions, and miscommunication: a qualitative study of preferences about kidney transplantation among African Americans. Transplant Proc 2015;47(2):240–6.
107. Federal Bureau of Prisons. Inmate statistics. United States Department of Justice 2015. Available from: http://www.bop.gov/about/statistics/statistics_inmate_ethnicity.jsp. Accessed June 30, 2015.
108. Gates ML, Bradford RK. The impact of incarceration on obesity: are prisoners with chronic diseases becoming overweight and obese during their confinement? J Obes 2015;2015:532468.
109. Wang EA, Pletcher M, Lin F, et al. Incarceration, incident hypertension, and access to health care: findings from the coronary artery risk development in young adults (CARDIA) study. Arch Intern Med 2009;169(7):687–93.
110. Olubodun J. Prison life and the blood pressure of the inmates of a developing community prison. J Hum Hypertens 1996;10(4):235–8.
111. Defina R, Hannon L. The impact of mass incarceration on poverty. Crime Delinquen 2013;59(4):562–86.
112. Green JA, Cavanaugh KL. Understanding the influence of educational attainment on kidney health and opportunities for improved care. Adv Chronic Kidney Dis 2015;22(1):24–30.
113. Aratani Y, Wight VR, Cooper JL. Racial gaps in early childhood: socio-emotional health, developmental, and educational outcomes among African-American boys. New York: National Center for Children in Poverty; 2011.
114. Education Week Research Center. Early-childhood education in the US: an analysis. Education Week 2015.

115. Magnuson KA, Waldfogel J. Early childhood care and education: effects on ethnic and racial gaps in school readiness. Future Child 2005;15(1):169–96.

116. Grant LD, Davis JM, Sors AI. Lead exposure and child development. Dordrecht, Netherlands: Springer Netherlands; 1989.

117. National Center for Education Statistics. Public high school graduation rates. Washington, DC: US Department of Education; 2015.

118. US Census Bureau. Statistical abstract of the United States: 2012. Washington, DC: US Department of Commerce; 2015.

119. Harris MI. Racial and ethnic differences in health care access and health outcomes for adults with type 2 diabetes. Diabetes Care 2001;24(3):454–9.

120. Plantinga LC, Johansen KL, Schillinger D, et al. Lower socioeconomic status and disability among US adults with chronic kidney disease, 1999-2008. Prev Chronic Dis 2012;9:E12.

121. Choi AI, Weekley CC, Chen SC, et al. Association of educational attainment with chronic disease and mortality: the Kidney Early Evaluation Program (KEEP). Am J Kidney Dis 2011;58(2):228–34.

122. Lash JP, Go AS, Appel LJ, et al. Chronic Renal Insufficiency Cohort (CRIC) study: baseline characteristics and associations with kidney function. Clin J Am Soc Nephrol 2009;4(8):1302–11.

123. Ryan C. Language use in the United States: 2011. Washington, DC: US Census Bureau; 2013.

124. Schenker Y, Karter AJ, Schillinger D, et al. The impact of limited English proficiency and physician language concordance on reports of clinical interactions among patients with diabetes: the DISTANCE study. Patient Educ Couns 2010; 81(2):222–8.

125. Fernandez A, Schillinger D, Warton EM, et al. Language barriers, physician-patient language concordance, and glycemic control among insured Latinos with diabetes: the Diabetes Study of Northern California (DISTANCE). J Gen Intern Med 2011;26(2):170–6.

126. National Center for Education Statistics. National assessment of adult literacy. Washington, DC: US Department of Education; 2003.

127. Navaneethan SD, Aloudat S, Singh S. A systematic review of patient and health system characteristics associated with late referral in chronic kidney disease. BMC Nephrol 2008;9:3.

128. Navaneethan SD, Kandula P, Jeevanantham V, et al. Referral patterns of primary care physicians for chronic kidney disease in general population and geriatric patients. Clin Nephrol 2010;73(4):260–7.

129. Hall EC, James NT, Garonzik Wang JM, et al. Center-level factors and racial disparities in living donor kidney transplantation. Am J Kidney Dis 2012;59(6): 849–57.

130. Young CJ, Gaston RS. Renal transplantation in black Americans. N Engl J Med 2000;343(21):1545–52.

131. Boulware LE, Meoni LA, Fink NE, et al. Preferences, knowledge, communication and patient-physician discussion of living kidney transplantation in African American families. Am J Transplant 2005;5(6):1503–12.

132. Gao SW, Oliver DK, Das N, et al. Assessment of racial disparities in chronic kidney disease stage 3 and 4 care in the Department of Defense health system. Clin J Am Soc Nephrol 2008;3(2):442–9.

133. Chapman EN, Kaatz A, Carnes M. Physicians and implicit bias: how doctors may unwittingly perpetuate health care disparities. J Gen Intern Med 2013; 28(11):1504–10.

134. Haider AH, Schneider EB, Sriram N, et al. Unconscious race and class biases among registered nurses: vignette-based study using implicit association testing. J Am Coll Surg 2015;220(6):1077–86.e3.
135. Oliver MN, Wells KM, Joy-Gaba JA, et al. Do physicians' implicit views of African Americans affect clinical decision making? J Am Board Fam Med 2014;27(2): 177–88.
136. van Ryn M, Fu SS. Paved with good intentions: do public health and human service providers contribute to racial/ethnic disparities in health? Am J Public Health 2003;93(2):248–55.
137. Ayanian JZ, Cleary PD, Keogh JH, et al. Physicians' beliefs about racial differences in referral for renal transplantation. Am J Kidney Dis 2004;43(2):350–7.
138. Bostrom MA, Freedman BI. The spectrum of MYH9-associated nephropathy. Clin J Am Soc Nephrol 2010;5(6):1107–13.
139. Gutiérrez OM. Contextual poverty, nutrition, and chronic kidney disease. Adv Chronic Kidney Dis 2015;22(1):31–8.
140. Narva AS, Sequist TD. Reducing health disparities in American Indians with chronic kidney disease. Semin Nephrol 2010;30(1):19–25.
141. Green AR, Carney DR, Pallin DJ, et al. Implicit bias among physicians and its prediction of thrombolysis decisions for black and white patients. J Gen Intern Med 2007;22(9):1231–8.
142. Murray-García JL, Harrell S, García JA, et al. Dialogue as skill: training a health professions workforce that can talk about race and racism. Am J Orthop 2014; 84(5):590–6.
143. Byrne A, Tanesini A. Instilling new habits: addressing implicit bias in healthcare professionals. Adv Health Sci Educ Theory Pract 2015. [Epub ahead of print].

Kidney Transplant for the Twenty-First Century

Mandy Trolinger, MS, RD, PA-C

KEYWORDS

- Kidney transplant • Kidney allocation system • Domino transplants • Immunizations
- Immunosuppressant medications

KEY POINTS

- Kidney transplantation is vital in improving the length and quality of life in patients with chronic kidney disease.
- Transplant medications can have serious side effects and require a team approach to decrease complications among transplant patients.
- Shortage of donated kidneys remains a problem in transplantation; however, a new allocation system is in place to improve outcomes.
- Cardiovascular disease is the main cause of mortality in transplant patients; therefore, it is vital to monitor, manage, and prevent cardiovascular events. Preventative medicine including certain immunizations can decrease complications and increase the life of the transplanted kidney.

HISTORY OF KIDNEY TRANSPLANTATION

Kidney transplantation is an amazing medical advancement that has allowed those with kidney failure to live fairly normal lives. In the realm of treatment options for kidney failure, transplantation is one of the new kids on the block. Although the ancient Greeks first recognized kidney disease and various treatments have been tried over the centuries, transplanting a viable organ into a patient with a failed kidney seemed to be a pipe dream.[1]

In the early days of the twentieth century, European scientists successfully transplanted organs between animals. However, survival was an issue. In 1906, two French vascular surgeons, Mathieu Jaboulay and Alexis Carrel, attempted two kidney transplants using a goat kidney into one patient and a pig kidney into the other. Neither patient survived.

In 1909, slices of a rabbit kidney transplanted into a 2 year-old child were successful, but the child died 2 weeks later. In 1933 there was a successful human-to-human

No disclosures.
Denver Nephrology, 9695 South Yosemite Street, Suite 285, Lone Tree, CO 80124, USA
E-mail address: mtrolinger@denverneph.net

Physician Assist Clin 1 (2016) 205–220
http://dx.doi.org/10.1016/j.cpha.2015.09.012
2405-7991/16/$ – see front matter © 2016 Elsevier Inc. All rights reserved.

transplant but again, the recipient died. It was not until 1936 that Yu Yu Voronoy completed six renal transplants between humans. However, these failed postoperatively related to what is now thought to be the ischemic time of the kidney. The concept of transplant had to wait until the postoperative care could catch up to the surgical expertise.

The breakthrough came in 1954 with a successful kidney transplant between identical twins done at what is now Brigham and Women's Hospital in Boston; this landmark surgery was performed by Nobel prize–winning surgeon Dr Joseph Moore.[2] As the 1950s progressed, live kidney donors were used and the donor kidney was placed extraperitoneally in the iliac fossa. This led to improved outcomes. As the years went on, the true appreciation for the role the immune system played in kidney transplant outcomes became more apparent and continues to be redefined to this day. Major advances in tissue typing, immunosuppression, and techniques have developed.[1,3] Today, kidney transplantation is considered not only a treatment option for kidney failure but is the preferred option with better patient outcomes for mortality and morbidity.[4,5]

Kidney transplants have a lifespan: deceased donor average is survival of 12 years and living donor average survival is 15 years.[6] Thus patients may require more than one transplant in their lifetime, especially if transplanted at a young age. This means management of the graft is vital and all disciplines of medicine must assist in managing and preventing complications in transplant recipients. Prolonging the life of the transplant helps to improve the quality of life for thousands of patients and the entire management team plays a role. All transplant patients, no matter what the organ, are defined as patients with chronic kidney disease (CKD) and all precautions regarding treating the CKD patient extend to the transplant patient.[7]

PRETRANSPLANT EVALUATION

Patients qualify to be listed on the kidney transplant waiting list once they have a glomerular filtration rate less than or equal to 20 mL/min/1.73 m^2, dialysis dependent or not.[4] Initial evaluation involves a thorough laboratory work including multiple tests:

- Complete blood count
- Comprehensive metabolic panel
- Complete urine analysis
- Screening for hepatitis
- Screening for cytomegalovirus (CMV)
- Screening for HIV

In addition tests that determine the appropriateness of the donor kidney include blood ABO typing, human leukocyte antigen (HLA) typing, and panel reactive antibody assay (PRA). Diagnostic testing includes

- Chest radiograph and/or purified protein derivative testing
- Electrocardiogram
- Cardiac stress test or angiogram
- Colonoscopy
- Abdominal and pelvic ultrasounds
- For women, a PAP smear and mammogram
- For men, a prostate-specific antigen and testicular examination[8]

It should be noted that although there are some general commonalities among transplant centers, each center sets its own inclusion and exclusion criteria and requirements. For that reason, it behooves the PA to become familiar with local centers and their criteria.

Contraindications to kidney transplant are classified as absolute or relative. Each transplant center has its own relative contraindications. Absolute contraindications are

- Active cancer
- Active infections
- Active psychiatric disease
- A medical condition that makes perioperative survival unlikely[8]

Relative contraindications for kidney transplant include

- Drug or alcohol abuse (although states with legal marijuana laws are modifying this)[9]
- Medical nonadherence
- Malnutrition
- Dementia (this is center specific)
- Urologic abnormalities
- Hypercoagulable states
- Bleeding disorders
- Obesity (again, center specific)[10–12]

Recent studies have shown that graft and patient survival is not significantly different with obese patients and thus many transplant centers have relaxed their body mass index requirements. However, the surgical technical challenges and the increased intraoperative time for the obese patient (donor or recipient) still remains a challenge.[12] Note that HIV status and hepatitis status are not included as either a relative or absolute contraindication for listing for kidney transplant. Patients with HIV and/or hepatitis accepted on the transplant list, but again this is center specific.[13] With the new Hepatitis C medications now available, some centers treat preoperatively while other centers treat post operatively. This is center specific. Age alone is not an absolute contraindication to kidney transplant and the new kidney allocation system introduced in late 2014 attempts to match the expected survival of the patient with the expected survival of the donated kidney.[14,15]

When a patient who is active on the list develops a serious medical illness he or she is placed on "hold," or Status 7 until the issue is believed to be resolved.[16] The patient will not lose the time accrued on the list and may still accrue time but would not be contacted for a transplant until taken off Status 7 and reactivated.[8] Early referral for kidney transplant is associated with better outcomes. It has been found that minorities, those with lower education levels, those treated by practitioners who do not refer to nephrology, and those without insurance are less likely to be referred and listed for transplant.[17,18] A new kidney allocation system, introduced in late 2014, seeks to promote fairness in allocation.

On December 4, 2014, this new allocation system was activated with the goal of improving allocation of organs, increasing the number of transplants and reducing the number of discarded organs. Although not perfect, this system represents an improvement over the former system, which often resulted in discarded kidneys, decreased transplants, and organs that were not well age-matched between donor and recipient. These changes should improve the process, create a more equitable system, and decrease the need for retransplant. The new allocation system includes scoring for the patient: the expected posttransplant survival score. The expected posttransplant survival score includes age, time on dialysis, diabetes status, and prior organ transplant. Over many years, these factors have been shown to be predictive of future survival of the kidney patient.[15] The deceased donor is assigned a kidney donor profile index score that includes age, body mass index, ethnicity, hepatitis C status, history of hypertension or diabetes, cause of death, serum creatinine, and donation after circulatory death. The expected posttransplant survival score and kidney donor profile index scores are correlated to better match the donor kidney and the patient thus increasing survival rates and decreasing retransplant rates.

The point system for the wait list is very specific: 1 year on the transplant list = 1 point, prior donor = 4 points, and a good match (DR genotype matching) = 1 to 2 points. Pediatric patients and those who have previously donated are also given extra points and thus priority. However, patients with high PRA levels who are much, much harder to match are given highest priority. A patient with a 99% or 100% PRA (meaning 99% or 100% of all kidneys would be rejected by this patient's immune system) is given 50 or 202 points, respectively, taking them to the top of the transplant list.[19] This has made a huge difference in these very hard to match patients with an increase from 2.4% of these patients transplanted in December 2014 to 17.7% in January 2015 (Fig. 1).

The ideal donor is an identical twin. However, the donor may be a blood relative, unrelated, or even a total stranger. What is essential is the compatibility of the donor and the patient.

A living kidney donation has better survival for the graft and the recipient. However, this puts a donor at risk medically and surgically, with the only upside being beneficence on the part of the donor. Recently two large studies looked into complications after donation from the point of view of the donor. For the female who delivers a child after kidney donation, the rate of hypertension and preeclampsia is twice that of nondonor female.[20] There is no difference in fetal or maternal death or in low birth weight for either cohort. For all other kidney donors, the risks seem to be minimal and related to age-appropriate CKD changes in the donor over the years.[21,22]

A kidney patient may have a living donor but the donor may not be compatible either by ABO typing or in antigen/antibody matching. To increase the number of living transplants and decrease rejection rates, a process known as domino or paired kidney

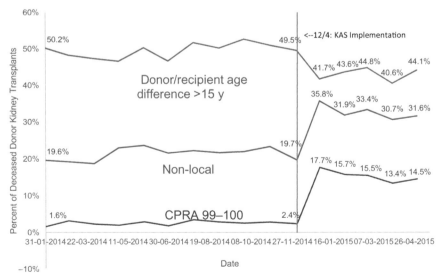

Fig. 1. Patient characteristics before and after implementation of the new kidney allocation system. (*From* USDA Organ Procurement and Transplantation Network. OPTN Kidney Allocation System (KAS) out-of-the-gate monitoring report. Available at: http://optn.transplant. hrsa.gov/learn/professional-education/kidney-allocation-system/.)

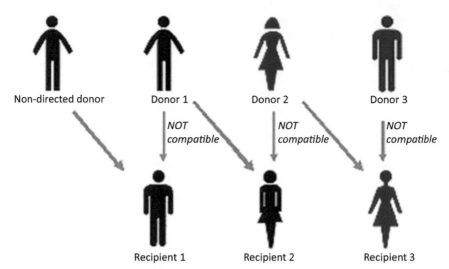

Fig. 2. Domino kidney swap. (*From* Available at: https://www.kidney.org/transplantation/livingdonors/incompatiblebloodtype/; with permission.)

transplants was developed at Johns Hopkins.[23] The living donor donates to a third party and the third party donor swaps or donates a kidney to the original pair (**Fig. 2**).

This requires matching via computer of kidneys from either a local transplant center or a nationwide group. This can be as simple as a two-person swap or as complicated as a 32-person swap. In the last 10 years, the domino kidney transplants have allowed patients who had incompatible donors to have a living transplant.

Another innovation is the kidney chain. This is initiated by a Good Samaritan donor who offers a "nondirected" donation or a willing donor who is not a match. This follows the rules of the domino kidneys or swaps but is started by the Good Samaritan donor and the final donor in the chain donates to the top of the wait list. Typically, a potential donor and a potential recipient are not a compatible match. A third patient, who is compatible with the first potential donor and also has a incompatible donor, receives the first kidney. The second potential donor then agrees to donate to the first match in the registry (see **Fig. 2**). The chain has made transplants possible all across the country beginning with one willing donor.[24]

KIDNEY TRANSPLANT PROCEDURE

Transplanted kidneys are usually placed in the right iliac fossa because the iliac vein is easier to access. If the need arises for a second kidney transplant, it is placed in the opposite iliac fossa of the first transplant. Third and fourth kidney transplants have been performed with differing surgical techniques.[25] Some centers remove a previous transplant if there are signs infection and/or rejection but that is center and patient specific.[26,27]

The donor renal vein and artery are connected to the recipient's external iliac vein and artery. If multiple renal veins are present on the donor kidney, they are usually ligated. There are several approaches to connect the ureter to the bladder including using the donor ureter to the recipient bladder or recipient ureter to the transplanted kidney. In most transplants an indwelling ureteral stent is placed and usually removed about 3 to 4 weeks after transplant surgery.[8,25] Often this is the procedure that causes the most postoperative complaints from patients.

Dual kidneys may be used if the donor is very young and the kidneys are small. For example, if the donor is less than 2 year-old then both kidneys may be placed into a larger donor, because one kidney would not be enough to sustain the recipient. Centers are able to achieve good outcomes with this technique.[8]

Previously, before the new kidney allocation system, for the younger patient (a 20–40 year-old) who was given an older, borderline kidney (>60 year-old donor), previously referred to as an extended donor criteria kidney, often the center would transplant both kidneys. With the new allocation system matching survival of kidney and recipient, it is expected that this will rarely or never occur.[28]

Native kidneys are not usually removed unless there are issues with significant proteinuria, chronic infection, uncontrolled hypertension, unmanageable pain caused by polycystic kidney disease, or recurrent nephrolithiasis.[8,29] The most common group who have pre-emptive nephrectomies are the patients with autosomal-dominant polycystic kidney disease where the size of the kidneys can be prohibitive to the surgeon's ability to place another transplanted kidney into the abdominal area (**Fig. 3**). Unless there is an issue with pain, bleeding, or chronic infection, the autosomal-dominant polycystic kidney disease kidneys can be removed at the time of transplant rather than before surgery. However, this again is surgeon and center specific.[30]

IMMUNOSUPPRESSION

One of the most comprehensive sets of guidelines for transplant patients is the Kidney Disease Improving Global Outcomes (KDIGO) series.[7] KDIGO is an international organization of experts that compiled evidence-based guidelines for managing the transplant patient. The guidelines include immunosuppression and management of immediate and long-term complications. Lifelong immunosuppression of the transplant is required to prevent rejection unless the donor is an identical twin. There are two main groups of immunosuppression: induction and maintenance therapies. Induction therapies include biologic antibodies, calcineurin inhibitors (CNI),

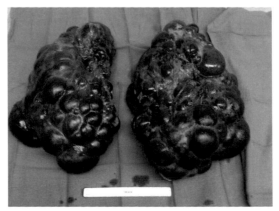

Fig. 3. Autosomal-dominant polycystic kidney disease kidneys. (*Courtesy of* Gilbert A. Transplant Nephrologist, Kidney and Pancreas Transplant Program. Medstar Georgetown Transplant Institute; with permission.)

antimetabolites/antiproliferative medications, and glucocorticoids.[7] These therapies are started preoperatively, perioperatively, or immediately postoperatively with a goal of preventing acute rejection. Induction therapies are used in most cases except for some living donor and well-matched grafts; however, this is very center and surgeon specific.

Maintenance immunosuppression is required for the life of the transplant. Maintenance medications include CNIs, antiproliferative/antimetabolites, and steroids. Commonly used are prednisone, mycophenolate mofetil, cyclosporine, tacrolimus, sirolimus, and/or azathioprine. More transplant centers are trying to go steroid free to eliminate long-term side effects of prednisone. A common successful regimen has been found to be tacrolimus and mycophenolate mofetil with or without steroids.[31]

Immunosuppressants are potent medications with a very high risk profile and should only be prescribed by someone who manages or is experienced with immunosuppressants. CNIs, such as cyclosporine and tacrolimus, must also be monitored by measuring trough levels.

Most transplant centers use a trough level 12 hours after the dose of Tacrolimus or Cyclosporine is taken; however, recent research has noted that a level 2 hours after the dose is more accurate for Cyclosporine. This is vital because low CNI levels increase the risk of rejection; whereas high CNI levels can lead to nephrotoxicity[32] (**Table 1**). However, these ranges are just a starting point and some goals might be lower depending on the type of induction therapy or if the patient is also on an antiproliferative medication.[33]

Immunosuppressant medications have very high side effect profiles (**Table 2**). Immunosuppressants also have significant interactions with many common medications (**Table 3**) and any medication that interacts with cytochrome P-450 can alter CNI levels.[8] This makes managing the transplant patient very difficult and many practitioners defer to the transplant center for most questions from a rash to pneumonia to vaccinations. A newer immunosuppressant showing promise is belatacept, which may allow patients to lower or stop CNIs, therefore decreasing side effects and rejection.[34] Because management of immunosuppressants is difficult and causes graft loss if mismanaged, a call to the transplant center is prudent if a question arises.

LONG-TERM MANAGEMENT OF THE KIDNEY TRANSPLANT PATIENT

Most transplant centers prefer to follow their patients long-term greater than 1 year posttransplant. Yet many patients return to their original nephrologist and visit the transplant center yearly.[7,32] Quarterly follow-up is important for all transplant recipients but because of distance or difficulty in travel, many community nephrology practices are the point of care for the long-term transplant recipient. Electronic communication between the community nephrology practice and the transplant centers has helped decrease errors in management and give needed follow-up feedback to the transplant centers.[35]

| Table 1
CNI therapeutic levels		
	0–3 mo Posttransplant	**3 or More Months Posttransplant**
Cyclosporine	2 h postdose: 800–1000 ng/mL 12 h postdose: 200–300 ng/mL	2 h postdose: 400–600 ng/mL 12 h postdose: 50–150 ng/mL
Tacrolimus (12 h trough)	8–10 ng/mL	3–7 ng/mL

Table 2 Side effects of common immunosuppressants	
Immunosuppressant	**Side Effects**
Cyclosporine	*Severe*: infection risk, BK virus nephropathy, nephrotoxicity, hepatotoxicity, hyperkalemia, leukopenia, thrombocytopenia, malignancy *Common*: increased BUN and creatinine, hypertension, hirsutism, gingival hyperplasia, acne, hypomagnesemia, hyperglycemia, hyperkalemia, hyperuricemia, hypertriglyceridemia
Tacrolimus	*Severe*: lymphoma, severe infection, BK virus nephropathy, cytomegalovirus, nephrotoxicity, neurotoxicity, severe hyperkalemia, myelosuppression *Common*: tremor, hypertension, increased serum creatinine, infection, nausea, vomiting, hypomagnesemia, elevated liver function tests, diabetes, hypokalemia, leukopenia, photosensitivity
Azathioprine	*Severe*: leukopenia, thrombocytopenia, infection, pancreatitis, hepatotoxicity, lymphoma, malignancy *Common*: leukopenia, thrombocytopenia, infection, nausea, vomiting, elevated AST/ALT, malignancy
Mycophenolate	*Severe*: thrombocytopenia, leukopenia, neutropenia, severe infection, viral reactivation, malignancy, polyomavirus-associated nephropathy, GI bleeding, pregnancy loss, congenital malformations *Common*: hypertension, infection, diarrhea, anemia, abdominal pain, leukopenia, hypercholesterolemia, hypokalemia, tremor, acne, insomnia
Sirolimus	*Severe*: malignancy, lymphoma, severe infection, BK virus–associated nephropathy, myelosuppression, impaired wound healing, hepatotoxicity, hypokalemia, osteonecrosis *Common*: hyperlipidemia, hypertension, increased creatinine, infection, thrombocytopenia, acne, proteinuria, leukopenia, hypokalemia, ovarian cysts
Corticosteroids	*Severe*: adrenal insufficiency, Cushing syndrome, infection, hypertension, diabetes, steroid psychosis, gastrointestinal ulcer, glaucoma, osteoporosis, cataracts, growth suppression, withdrawal symptoms if stopped abruptly *Common*: sodium and fluid retention, insomnia, mood swings, edema, muscle weakness, glucose intolerance, Cushing syndrome, hypertension, menstrual irregularities, hypokalemia, hirsutism
Belatacept	*Severe*: posttransplant lymphoproliferative disorder, malignancy, severe infection, neutropenia, polyomavirus-associated nephropathy, diabetes *Common*: infection, anemia, hypertension, peripheral edema, nausea, vomiting, leukopenia, dyslipidemia, proteinuria, hyperglycemia, hypotension, hematuria, increased creatinine, dysuria

Abbreviations: ALT, alanine aminotransferase; AST, aspartate aminotransferase; BUN, blood, urea, nitrogen; GI, gastrointestinal.

Laboratory values are serially followed on all transplant recipients. These include not only a complete blood count, urinalysis, and comprehensive metabolic panel but often the usual CKD laboratory studies: hemoglobin A_{1C}, lipid panel, phosphorus, albumin, intact parathyroid hormone, and vitamin D levels.[7] Immunosuppression levels are also monitored quarterly. Even though nephrology follows the patient quarterly, the primary care practice has an essential role in the management of the transplanted patient.

Table 3	
Medication and herbal remedies that affect CNI levels	
Increases CNI levels	Clarithromycin, clotrimazole, diltiazem, erythromycin, fluconazole, itraconazole, ketoconazole, nicardipine, nifedipine, troleandomyin, verapamil, voriconazole
Decreases CNI levels	Carbamazepine, caspofungin, phenobarbital, phenytoin, rifabutin, rifampin, sirolimus, St. John's wort

INFECTION RISK

Infection is the second leading cause of death in transplant recipients.[7] The first 6 months posttransplant are higher risk for infections because of higher doses of immunosuppression. Many of the infections encountered in primary care include upper respiratory and gastrointestinal organisms. Infections particular to the transplant patient are usually viral with the most common being CMV. Several other viral infections that must be considered in the transplant population besides CMV are Epstein-Barr virus, hepatitis B or C, BK virus, and papillomavirus.[36] Urinary tract infections are also common in transplant patients. Urine analysis and cultures should be done on all transplant patients and treated appropriately; however, pyelonephritis requires hospital admission because these patients may lose their graft due to infection.[37] Overall, infection rates have improved over the years because of better prophylactic antibiotic use during the immediate posttransplant period along with improved prevention methods.

CARDIOVASCULAR DISEASE

Cardiovascular disease (CVD) is the leading cause of mortality in kidney transplant patients, causing 23% of all-cause mortality at 15-year posttransplant. CVD risk factors must be addressed and corrected, if possible.

The usual risk factors for everyone including the kidney patient include family history, hypertension, dyslipidemia, obesity and inactivity, smoking, diabetes, and age. Transplant-specific risk factors are use of CNI, proteinuria, anemia, hyperparathyoidism and inflammation.[7,36]

The Framingham Heart Score underestimates the CVD risk in kidney transplant recipients.[7] All symptomatic patients should undergo appropriate cardiovascular testing, even if invasive. The usual precautions to prevent contrast-induced nephropathy in the CKD patient should be followed: intravenous hydration, N-acetylcysteine, and same day holding of high-risk medications (CNI, angiotensin-converting enzyme inhibitors, and angiotensin receptor blockers).[7,36]

Kidney transplantation does decrease CVD incidence by about 5% when compared with dialysis patients; however, kidney transplant recipients are still at greater risk for CVD when compared with the general population.[37] It is recommended that transplant recipients with a history of atherosclerotic CVD take aspirin, 100 to 650 mg daily, unless contraindicated.[7]

DIABETES

Posttransplant patients may develop new-onset diabetes after transplantation. This has been linked to multiple factors: CNIs, corticosteroids, and viral infections (CMV and hepatitis C).[38,39] The kidneys are gluconeogenic and metabolize several hormones including insulin.[40] This means that the patient with previously nonfunctioning kidney, who needed no diabetic management while on dialysis, suddenly needs medications again. KDIGO recommends a fasting plasma glucose, hemoglobin A_{1c}, or oral glucose tolerance test annually after 1 year posttransplant.[7] Because diabetes is a risk factor for CVD, and CVD is the leading cause of death in transplant recipients, strict management of diabetes is vital.[38]

HYPERTENSION

Hypertension is common in transplant recipients because it is often the precipitating diagnosis that caused the kidneys to fail in the first place. It is vital to have tight blood pressure control to prevent damage to the transplanted kidney. Hypertension can result from transplant rejection, steroids, CNIs, renal artery stenosis, and essential hypertension.[37] Hypertension goals are not defined because the leading experts disagree; KDIGO recommends a goal blood pressure of less than 130/80 mm Hg, but the Joint National Committee on Hypertension-8 guidelines recommend less than 140/90 mm Hg.[7,41] That said, the Joint National Committee on Hypertension-8 guidelines are for CKD patients and do not differentiate between the transplanted CKD patient and the nontransplanted patient.[42] Treatment includes weight loss, exercise, limited alcohol intake, discontinuation of smoking, and a low-salt diet. If albuminuria greater than 1 g/day is present, then angiotensin-converting enzyme inhibitors or angiotensin receptor blockers should be considered first because they decrease albuminuria in addition to controlling blood pressure. It is important to remember that nondihydropyridine calcium channel blockers can increase CNI levels, so close monitoring is required if these are prescribed.[37]

DYSLIPIDEMIA

CNIs, sirolimus, and steroids can have unfavorable effects on lipid and thus serial lipid monitoring is warranted every 2 to 3 months posttransplant for 1 year and then after a change in treatment and/or annually.[7] Lipid goals in transplant patients are low-density lipoprotein less than 100 mg/dL, non-high-density lipoprotein less than 130, and triglycerides less than 150 mg/dL. Lifestyle interventions, weight loss, exercise, and low-fat diet are tried first but often medication is needed in this patient population. Statins are the usual medication for the CKD patients and transplant recipients are considered CKD patients. Patients with elevated triglycerides and on CNIs must be monitored closely because there is a higher risk of myopathy if fibric acid derivatives are prescribed. Hypertriglyceridemia can be successfully treated using gemfibrozil, niacin, or fish oil. Another option is to consider decreasing the causative factors (immunosuppressant) but this must be done with input from the transplant team.[37]

IMMUNIZATIONS

Immunizations play a key role in preventing transplant complications but close attention must be paid to which vaccines should be administered to a transplant recipient. There was some concern in the past about the possibility of vaccines triggering a rejection episode, but this has been disproved.[43] Transplant patients should avoid all live vaccines, unless the benefit outweighs the risk and the transplant team approves.[44] It is recommended that required live vaccines be given before transplantation (this is more common in the pediatric population) and under the guidance of the transplant team. Family and household members of transplant recipients should also avoid receiving the live flu vaccine (**Table 4**).[36]

Table 4	
Inactive and active immunizations	
Inactive Immunizations	**Active Immunizations – AVOID**
Cholera	Bacille Calmette-Guérin
Haemophilus influenza B	Intranasal influenza
Hepatitis A	Japanese encephalitis (active)
Hepatitis B	Measles
Human papilloma virus	Mumps
Influenza (type A and B)	Polio (oral)
Japanese encephalitis (inactive)	Rotavirus
Meningococcal	Rubella
Pneumococcal	Smallpox
Polio (inactivated)	Typhoid (oral)
Tetanus, diphtheria, pertussis	Varicella
Typhoid Vi (intramuscular)	Varicella zoster
	Yellow fever

Data from Avery RK, Michaels M. Update on immunizations in solid organ transplant recipients: what clinicians need to know. Am J Transplant 2008;8(1):9–14.

OBESITY

Obesity is also prominent in the transplant population and it is recommended that patients lose weight with diet and exercise. Improved appetite, kidney function, and/or use of corticosteroids are thought to be major contributors to weight gain posttransplant. Obese patients have a higher risk of delayed transplant function and loss of the transplant.[10] Some weight loss medications, for example orlistat and cyclosporine A, should be avoided in transplant patients because they can interfere with the CNIs.[11] Bariatric surgery may also be an option; however, there are limited data on bariatric surgery in the transplant population. The overall bariatric mortality rate ranges from 2% to 5% and seems similar between transplant and nontransplant populations.[45] Because obesity can increase the risk of kidney failure and graft loss, the benefit of surgery must outweigh the risks.

CANCER

Kidney transplant recipients are at greater risk for developing cancer, any type, because of the immunosuppression regimen. The most common posttransplant cancers are melanoma, oral cancer, skin cancer, Kaposi sarcoma and non-Hodgkin lymphoma are 20 times more common than the general population.

Compared with the general population, these cancers are two times as likely in transplant recipients: colon, lung, prostate, stomach, esophagus, pancreas, ovarian, and breast cancer.[46] Although minimum age-appropriate cancer screening is recommended, there should be a low threshold to screen more frequently in this patient population.[47]

BONE AND MINERAL DISEASE

Transplant recipients are at greater risk for bone and mineral disease because most have a history of secondary hyperparathyroidism before transplant. Steroid use, calcium and vitamin D deficiencies, and CNIs also increase incidence of secondary hyperparathyroidism. Corticosteroids use can increase fracture risk four times that of the general population.[36,37] The first 3 to 6 months posttransplant are when the greatest bone loss occurs. Bone density examinations are not routinely performed but are recommended for those at high risk. They may also be included in study protocols at the transplant centers. Treatment methods include calcium, vitamin D supplementation, management of acidosis, weight-bearing exercises, and phosphorus control. Bisphosphonates may also be prescribed, but should be used with caution because of the risk of adynamic bone disease.[36,37] That said, there are some transplant centers that routinely place most posttransplant patients on bisphosphonates. Again, this is center and surgeon specific (M. Brazie, MD, personal communication, 2014).

FERTILITY

Kidney transplantation often restores regular menstrual cycles in women allowing pregnancy to be possible.[48] Before conception it is recommended that the recipient's serum creatinine be less than 1.5 mg/dL with albuminuria less than 500 mg per 24 hours. Reports have noted increased rates of graft loss with a serum creatinine greater than 1.3 mg/dL, thus there is a gray zone between 1.3 mg/dL and 1.5 mg/dL.[49] Medication discontinuations, most commonly for mycophenolate or angiotensin-converting enzyme inhibitors, are important and are done in consultation with the transplant and obstetric teams. Pregnancy is considered high risk and immunosuppressant drug levels must be monitored frequently during and right after the pregnancy. There are limited data on the use of birth control pills in the transplant population. However, studies up to this point have shown higher risks with pregnancy than with the use of any method of birth control.[50]

There is not a recommended waiting time for males to father a child and transplantation usually returns sperm motility to normal but does not change sperm count or morphology. If a transplant recipient, male or female, is on a teratogenic immunosuppressant it is recommended that birth control be used.[49] Careful planning and preconception counseling is necessary to improve pregnancy outcomes. Data continue to be limited on pregnancy and offspring outcomes in kidney transplant recipients but transplant pregnancy registries throughout the world, including the US-specific National Transplant Pregnancy Registry (http://www.ntpr.giftoflifeinstitute.org/), collect data and allow clinicians to offer knowledge and improved outcomes for pregnancy after kidney transplant.[48]

THE FUTURE OF TRANSPLANTATION

The field has come a long way since 1954 when the first kidney transplant between identical twins was performed. Improved surgical techniques and immunosuppression regimens have contributed largely to increasing the quality of life for transplant recipients. However, the biggest or main barrier to completing more transplants is the organ shortage. Even though transplant rates have grown each year, the need has out-stripped the available organs (**Fig. 4**).

Currently, there are more than 100,000 people in the United States waiting for a kidney. Most of those will die before a match is found. Research continues into creating a means to decrease the organ shortage: xenotransplantation, creating artificial organs. and cloning kidneys.[51,52] For now promotion of organ donation, advancements in immunosuppressant medications and increasing the graft life are the best options to try to decrease the organ shortage.

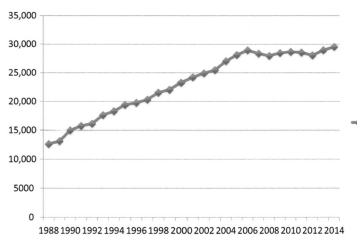

Fig. 4. Transplantation growth between 1998 and 2014.

REFERENCES

1. Watson CJ, Dark JH. Organ transplantation: historical perspective and current practice. Br J Anaesth 2012;108(Suppl 1):i29–42.
2. Schatzki S. The first kidney transplantation. AJR Am J Roentgenol 2003;181(1):190.
3. Vella J, Cohen D. Syllabus transplant. Nephrol Self-Assessment Program 2013;(12):314–21.
4. Abecassis M, Bartlett ST, Collins AJ, et al. Kidney transplantation as primary therapy for end-stage renal disease: National Kidney Foundation/Kidney Disease Outcomes Quality Initiative (NKF/KDOQITM) conference. Clin J Am Soc Nephrol 2008;3(2):471–80.
5. Knoll GA. Is kidney transplantation for everyone? The example of the older dialysis patient. Clin J Am Soc Nephrol 2009;4(12):2040–4.
6. 2014 Organ Procurement and Transplant Data. 2014 Annual Report of the U.S. Organ Procurement and Transplantation Network and the Scientific Registry of Transplant Recipients: Transplant Data 1994-2014. Department of Health and Human Services, Health Resources and Services Administration, Healthcare Systems Bureau, Division of Transplantation, Rockville, MD; United Network for Organ Sharing, Richmond, VA; University Renal Research and Education Association, Ann Arbor, MI. This work was supported in part by Health Resources and Services Administration contract 234-2005-37011C. The content is the responsibility of the authors alone and does not necessarily reflect the views or policies of the Department of Health and Human Services, nor does mention of trade names, commercial products, or organizations imply endorsement by the U.S. Government. Available at: http://optn.transplant.hrsa.gov/converge/latestData/rptData.asp. Accessed June 27, 2015.
7. Kidney Disease: Improving Global Outcomes (KDIGO) Transplant Work Group. KDIGO clinical practice guideline for the care of kidney transplant recipients. Am J Transplant 2009;9(Suppl 3):S1–157.
8. Danovitch GM. Handbook of kidney transplantation. 5th edition. Philadelphia: Lippincott Williams and Wilkins; 2010.
9. Weis B. Kidney disease education update, NKF Spring clinical meetings. Dallas, TX, 2015.

10. Gore JL, Pham PT, Danovitch GM, et al. Obesity and outcome following renal transplantation. Am J Transplant 2006;6(2):357–63.

11. Barbaro D, Orsini P, Pallini S, et al. Obesity in transplant patients: case report showing interference of orlistat with absorption of cyclosporine and review of literature. Endocr Pract 2002;8(2):124–6.

12. Krishnan N, Higgins R, Short A, et al. Kidney transplantation significantly improves patient and graft survival irrespective of BMI: a cohort study. Am J Transplant 2015;15(9):2378–86.

13. Sibulesky L, Javed I, Reyes JD, et al. Changing the paradigm of organ utilization from PHS increased-risk donors: an opportunity whose time has come? Clin Transplant 2015;29(9):724–7.

14. Pondrom S. What you need to know about the new Kidney Allocation System. Am J Transplant 2014;14(7):1470.

15. The New Kidney Allocation System (KAS) Frequently Asked Questions. 2015 Annual Report of the U.S. Organ Procurement and Transplantation Network and the Scientific Registry of Transplant Recipients: Transplant Data 1994-2015. Department of Health and Human Services, Health Resources and Services Administration, Healthcare Systems Bureau, Division of Transplantation, Rockville, MD; United Network for Organ Sharing, Richmond, VA; University Renal Research and Education Association, Ann Arbor, MI. This work was supported in part by Health Resources and Services Administration contract 234-2005-37011C. The content is the responsibility of the authors alone and does not necessarily reflect the views or policies of the Department of Health and Human Services, nor does mention of trade names, commercial products, or organizations imply endorsement by the U.S. Government. Available at: http://optn.transplant.hrsa.gov/converge/ContentDocuments/KAS_FAQs.pdf Accessed January 2015.

16. Huang E, Shye M, Elashoff D, et al. Incidence of conversion to active waitlist status among temporarily inactive obese renal transplant candidates. Transplantation 2014;98(2):177–86.

17. Bratton C, Chavin K, Baliga P. Racial disparities in organ donation and why. Curr Opin Organ Transplant 2011;16(2):243–9.

18. Navaneethan SD, Aloudat S, Singh S. A systematic review of patient and health system characteristics associated with late referral in chronic kidney disease. BMC Nephrol 2008;9:3.

19. Gilbert A. Kidney allocation: a new system to correct old disparities. Presented at the RPA AP meeting. Annapolis, MD, July 2015.

20. Garg AX, Nevis IF, McArthur E, et al, for the DONOR Network. Gestational hypertension and preeclampsia in living kidney donors. N Engl J Med 2015;372(2):124–33.

21. Glotzer OS, Singh TP, Gallichio MH, et al. Long-term quality of life after living kidney donation. Transplant Proc 2013;45(9):3225–8.

22. Rossi AP, Vella JP. Hypertension, living kidney donors, and transplantation: where are we today? Adv Chronic Kidney Dis 2015;22(2):154–64.

23. Segev DL, Gentry SE, Warren DS, et al. Kidney paired donation and optimizing the use of live donor organs. JAMA 2005;293(15):1883–90.

24. Flechner SM, Leeser D, Pelletier R, et al. The Incorporation of an advanced donation program into kidney paired exchange: initial experience of the National Kidney Registry. Am J Transplant 2015;15:2712–7.

25. Halawa A. The third and fourth renal transplant; technically challenging, but still a valid option. Ann Transplant 2012;17(4):125–32.

26. Pham PT, Everly M, Faravardeh A, et al. Management of patients with a failed kidney transplant: dialysis reinitiation, immunosuppression weaning, and transplantectomy. World J Nephrol 2015;4(2):148–59.

27. Dinis P, Nunes P, Marconi L, et al. Kidney retransplantation: removal or persistence of the previous failed allograft? Transplant Proc 2014;46(6):1730–4.

28. Denecke C, Biebl M, Pratschke J. Optimizing clinical utilization and allocation of older kidneys. Curr Opin Organ Transplant 2015;20(4):431–7.

29. Patel P, Horsfield C, Compton F, et al. Native nephrectomy in transplant patients with autosomal dominant polycystic kidney disease. Ann R Coll Surg Engl 2011; 93(5):391–5.

30. Dengu F, Azhar B, Patel S, et al. Bilateral nephrectomy for autosomal dominant polycystic kidney disease and timing of kidney transplant: a review of the technical advances in surgical management of autosomal dominant polycystic disease. Exp Clin Transplant 2015;13(3):209–13.

31. Guerra G, Ciancio G, Gaynor JJ, et al. Randomized trial of immunosuppressive regimens in renal transplantation. J Am Soc Nephrol 2011;22(9):1758–68.

32. Schiff J, Cole E, Cantarovich M. Therapeutic monitoring of calcineurin inhibitors for the nephrologist. Clin J Am Soc Nephrol 2007;2(2):374–84.

33. Kalluri HV, Hardinger KL. Current state of renal transplant immunosuppression: present and future. World J Transplant 2012;2(4):51–68.

34. Vincenti F, Larsen CP, Alberu J, et al. Three-year outcomes from BENEFIT, a randomized, active-controlled, parallel-group study in adult kidney transplant recipients. Am J Transplant 2012;12(1):210–7.

35. Shih FJ, Fan YW, Chiu CM, et al. The dilemma of "to be or not to be": developing electronically e-health & cloud computing documents for overseas transplant patients from Taiwan organ transplant health professionals' perspective. Transplant Proc 2012;44(4):835–8.

36. Djamali A, Samaniego M, Muth B, et al. Medical care of kidney transplant recipients after the first post transplant year. Clin J Am Soc Nephrol 2006;1(4):623–40.

37. Gupta G, Unruh ML, Nolin TD, et al. Primary care of the renal transplant patient. J Gen Intern Med 2010;25(7):731–40.

38. Sarno G, Muscogiuri G, De Rosa P. New-onset diabetes after kidney transplantation: prevalence, risk factors, and management. Transplantation 2012;93(12): 1189–95.

39. Woodward RS, Schnitzler MA, Baty J, et al. Incidence and cost of new onset diabetes mellitus among U.S. wait-listed and transplanted renal allograft recipients. Am J Transplant 2003;3(5):590–8.

40. Triplitt CL. Understanding the kidneys' role in blood glucose regulation. Am J Manag Care 2012;18(1 Suppl):S11–6.

41. James PA, Oparil S, Carter BL, et al. 2014 evidence-based guideline for the management of high blood pressure in adults; report from the panel members appointed to the Eighth Joint National Committee (JNC 8). JAMA 2014;311(5):507–20.

42. Mahvan TD, Mlodinow SG. JNC 8: what's covered, what's not, and what else to consider. J Fam Pract 2014;63(10):574–84.

43. Fischer AS, Møller BK, Krag S, et al. Influenza virus vaccination and kidney graft rejection: causality or coincidence. Clin Kidney J 2015;8(3):325–8.

44. Avery RK, Michaels M. Update on immunizations in solid organ transplant recipients: what clinicians need to know. Am J Transplant 2008;8(1):9–14.

45. Modanlou KA, Muthyala U, Xiao H, et al. Bariatric surgery among kidney transplant candidates and recipients: analysis of the United States renal data system and literature review. Transplantation 2009;87(8):1167–73.

46. Kasiske BL, Snyder JJ, Gilbertson DT, et al. Cancer after kidney transplantation in the United States. Am J Transplant 2004;4(6):905–13.
47. Wong G, Chapman JR, Craig JC. Cancer screening in renal transplant recipients: what is the evidence? Clin J Am Soc Nephrol 2008;3(Suppl 2):S87–100.
48. Coscia LA, Constantinescu S, Moritz MJ, et al. Report from the National Transplantation Pregnancy Registry (NTPR): outcomes of pregnancy after transplantation. Clin Transplant 2010;65–85.
49. Josephson MA, McKay DB. Women and transplantation: fertility, sexuality, pregnancy, contraception. Adv Chronic Kidney Dis 2013;20(5):433–40.
50. Paulen ME, Folger SG, Curtis KM, et al. Contraceptive use among solid organ transplant patients: a systematic review. Contraception 2010;82(1):102–12.
51. Zuber K, Howard T, Davis J. Transplant in the 21st century. JAAPA 2014;27(11): 26–34.
52. Sayegh MH. Looking into the crystal ball: kidney transplantation in 2025. Nat Clin Pract Nephrol 2009;5(3):117.

ELSEVIER

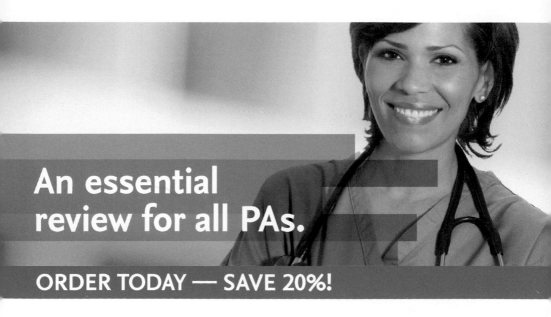

An essential review for all PAs.

ORDER TODAY — SAVE 20%!

Physician Assistant Board Review, 3rd Edition

Whether preparing for the **PANCE** or **PANRE**, PAs of all experience levels will appreciate the **concise** format and **comprehensive** coverage of important topics.

By James Van Rhee, MS, PA-C
2015 | eBook and Online Access
ISBN: 978-0-323-35611-4

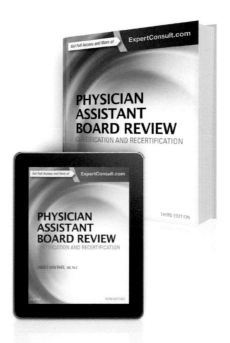

ORDER TODAY!

us.elsevierhealth.com/VanRhee · Free Worldwide Shipping!

Moving?

Make sure your subscription moves with you!

To notify us of your new address, find your **Clinics Account Number** (located on your mailing label above your name), and contact customer service at:

Email: journalscustomerservice-usa@elsevier.com

800-654-2452 (subscribers in the U.S. & Canada)
314-447-8871 (subscribers outside of the U.S. & Canada)

Fax number: 314-447-8029

Elsevier Health Sciences Division
Subscription Customer Service
3251 Riverport Lane
Maryland Heights, MO 63043

*To ensure uninterrupted delivery of your subscription, please notify us at least 4 weeks in advance of move.

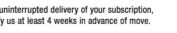